Adolescent Development, Psychopathology, and Treatment

Adolescent Development, Psychopathology, and Treatment

H. Spencer Bloch, M.D.

INTERNATIONAL UNIVERSITIES PRESS, INC.
Madison   Connecticut

Library of Congress Cataloging-in-Publication Data

Bloch, H. Spencer
    Adolescent development, psychopathology, and treatment / H.
Spencer Bloch.
        p.   cm.
    Includes bibliographical references and indexes.
    ISBN 0-8236-0065-3
    1. Adolescent psychopathology. 2. Adolescent psychology.
3. Adolescent psychotherapy. I. Title.
    [DNLM: 1. Mental Disorders—in adolescence. 2. Psychotherapy—in
adolescence. 3. Adolescent Psychology. 4. Human Development—in
adolescence . WS 463 B651a 1995]
RJ503.B55 1995
616.89'022—dc20
DNLM/DLC
for Library of Congress   95-4490
                                                                           CIP

Grateful acknowledgment is made to the following:
Centuries of Childhood by Philippe Aires, translated by R. Baldick. Copyright (©) 1962 by Jonathan Cape Ltd. Acknowledgment is made to the Estate of the author. Reprinted by permission of Alfred A. Knopf Inc.
Confessions by Saint Augustine, translated by R. S. Pine-Coffin. Copyright (©) 1961 by R. S. Pine-Coffin. Reprinted by permission of Penguin Books Ltd.
The Wild Boy of Aveyron by Jean-Marc-Gaspard Itard, translated by George and Muriel Humphrey. Reprinted by permission of the publisher.
The Sorrows of Young Werther and Other Writings by Johann Wolfgang van Goethe, translated by Catherine Hutter, translation copyright (©) 1962 by Catherine Hutter. Used by permission of Dutton Signet, a division of Penguin Books USA Inc.
"I WANT TO HOLD YOUR HAND" Words and Music by John Lennon and Paul McCartney. © 1963 Northern Songs. All rights controlled and administered in the U.S. and Canada by Duchess Music Corporation. Duchess Music Corporation is an MCA company. Copyright Renewed. All Rights Reserved International Copyright Secured. Used by Permission.
"Identity and the Creative Surge in Adolescents" by Sidney Werkman in *Adolescence, Dreams and Training, Science and Psychoanalysis, Vol. IX*, edited by J. Masserman. Published by Grune and Stratton, Inc., 1966. Reprinted with permission.
My Life by Havelock Ellis. Reprinted by permission of Constable Publishers.
Memoirs of Childhood and Youth by Albert Schweitzer. Copyright (©) 1949 by Macmillan. Used by permission of Rhena Schweitzer Miller.
"Discovery of a Father" in *Memoirs* by Sherwood Anderson. Copyright 1939 by *The Reader's Digest*. Copyright renewed 1966 by Eleanor Copenhaver Anderson. Reprinted by permission of Harold Ober Associates Incorporated.

Manufactured in the United States of America

Contents

PART IV:
FURTHER CONSIDERATION OF INTENSIVE THERAPY FOR
SEVERE PSYCHOPATHOLOGY

Acknowledgments

My late, younger sister was a theatrical press agent in New York. Much of her livelihood depended on disseminating the printed word. Once, during a moment of frustration in that high-pressure business, she decried the "scourge of Johann Gutenberg." Were she alive today, I suppose the inventor of laser printers might have been the object of her pique. I share that moment to acknowledge that despite having so much yet to learn, we currently may be in as much danger of being choked as further enlightened by the volume of information bearing down on us along mental hygiene's own superhighway. Harboring such a sentiment inclines me to explain what sets this book apart from others on the topic.

I began writing it in 1979 to provide a resource I was unable to find as I prepared to teach psychoanalytic candidates. That was an easy-reading, clinically oriented text that enunciated the long-standing view of adolescent development, discussed the challenges to that theory, summarized relevant contributions from other fields, and included references for those who wished to explore the latter areas in depth. Additional teaching of therapists from all the mental health disciplines prompted me to broaden the book's scope to include findings from more recent research that seemed relevant to adolescent development and treatment. And ultimately I attempted to reconcile those of the older and newer findings that I have found serviceable into a view of the developmental process—a view which provides understanding of how psychopathology develops during adolescence and thus how therapeutic interventions can be oriented. The finished product, some fifteen years in the making, is thus an original view of adolescent development but presented with sufficient background that it retains features of a clinical textbook.

In the background of this endeavor the appropriate recipients of the author's appreciation are many. I had the good fortune to learn about adolescents from exceptional mentors during my psychiatric and psychoanalytic training—at the Massachusetts Mental Health Center, the Judge Baker Guidance Center, and the Children's Hospital Medical Center in Boston during the 1960s and at the San Francisco Psychoanalytic Institute during the 1970s. By this time, however, their collective influence has been on my intellectual heritage in the field rather than bearing directly on this work. For that reason I will forgo naming them in favor of acknowledging with utmost gratitude the specific contributions of a few: Calvin Settlage, M.D., meticulously critiqued and Philip Speilman, M.D., trenchantly reviewed the chapter on development prior to adolescence. Steven Frankel, M.D., gave unstintingly of his time and energy in critically appraising each draft of the manuscript. Joseph Weiss, M.D., helped me immeasurably both to clarify and articulate many points and concepts. The generosity of Drs. Weiss and Frankel throughout this project certainly tested the reasonable bounds of collegiality and friendship. And Dr. Margaret Emery, Editor-in-Chief of International Universities Press, and her staff maintained uncompromising attention to the details of the manuscript, while still managing to make the publishing part of this process more painless than I would have anticipated.

Part I

Background for the Study of Adolescent Psychological Development

CHAPTER 1

Prologue

This book describes a distinctive, practical way of understanding and treating adolescents. It is centered on the premise that development during adolescence involves three basic issues: (1) adolescents' internal strivings to complete their development; (2) their need for parental sponsorship of those strivings; and thus, (3) a wish to retain a positive relationship with their parents. Successful emancipation to an adult level of psychological independence can only occur when adolescents' strivings are supported and sponsored by their parents. Conversely, when adolescents conclude that what is required to please their parents runs counter to their strivings to move ahead, then the developmental process becomes problematic or abortive, often in characteristic, predictable ways. Typically adolescents will sacrifice their forward movement in favor of gratifying their parents.

I realize that the latter conclusion is contrary to traditional thinking and the common wisdom that self-centeredness and rebelliousness are the norm in adolescents. Behavior which appears very rebellious against parental dictates, however, often reflects adolescents' efforts to comply with what they have accurately or inaccurately perceived to be their parent's or parents' underlying wishes. In fact, in contrast to the common view, it is hard to overemphasize the importance of such compliance in the lives of individuals who are having difficulty negotiating the years of adolescence. This dynamic has been portrayed poignantly with ironic humor. For example, in the following illustration, an adolescent compromised his forward movement after concluding that his father did not want him to succeed.

3

The 1979 movie *Breaking Away* (now available on video) chronicles the experiences of four best friends during the summer following their graduation from high school. In one scene, while talking about their future plans and their parents, Dave asks Cyril why he gave up playing basketball, his great passion:

> Cyril: Ah, I don't know . . . Agh! I was sure I was going to get that scholarship. My dad, of course, was sure that I wouldn't. When I didn't, he was really understanding, you know. He loves to do that. He loves to be understanding when I fail. [Imitating his father's tone]: "That's okay, Cyril, I understand. . . ." He even bought me that guitar 'cause he was sure I'd never learn to play it.
> Dave: Well, I'm supposed to take this college entrance exam.
> Cyril: [Disbelieving] Are you going to college?
> Dave: Hell no . . . I just want to see if I can pass.
> Cyril: Uh . . . maybe I'll take it too and flunk it. My dad's birthday is coming up.

Cyril apparently did not feel supported by his father in his wish to go to college and complied with that parent's unstated preference. More subtle variations of the dynamics dramatized in this example, with equally profound results to the adolescents, are more common than have been considered in the psychiatric literature. Conflicts like this one, which Cyril resolved by failing, are internal (intrapsychic); but they are not instinctual in the manner described in psychoanalytic theory, that is, between drives and ego/superego. Rather, such conflicts involve the internal reconciliation of ego-oriented motives which have become mutually incompatible. Conflict develops because the child is motivated to secure all three of the goals of adolescence noted above.

Studies of campus activists during the 1960s and 1970s illustrate the same phenomenon of compliance. Researchers found that the activists were not rebelling against their parents' political views but were acting out what they were taught in the home. That is, radical youth followed the intellectual, expressive, humanitarian, and political views of their parents. Moreover, amongst young people who held similar political beliefs, those who acted upon them came from more harmonious family backgrounds with social support for their views compared to those who did not act on their similar beliefs. The latter, who did not act, more often risked moving considerably further from their parents' beliefs and values were they to have done so (Braungart, 1980).

THE THREE BASIC ISSUES IN ADOLESCENT PSYCHOLOGICAL DEVELOPMENT

Manifestations of "strivings to complete development" are so pervasive from early in life as to be taken for granted (Jones, 1922; Bibring, 1937; Deutsch, 1944; A. Freud, 1965, 1968). They are part of the individual's constitution. Commonplace manifestations include the infant, toddler, and young child's drive to master walking and talking through repetition; the blatant efforts of younger sibs during the school-age years to accomplish what their older brothers and sisters have already achieved; and the urgency with which most adolescents attempt to arrogate adult prerogatives, such as self-regulation regarding curfews and driving, and freedom of choice regarding everything from personal appearance to association with peers.

With respect to the goal of maintaining the relationship with one's parents, growing children's sense of security is so dependent upon their parents that they are motivated to please them above all else (Freud, 1930; Bowlby, 1969, 1973, 1980). Adolescents retain this need while also striving to complete their development; the latter urge becomes intensified by puberty and by societal expectations. For this reason adolescence becomes the period during development when conflict is most likely to occur normally between these streams of development.

The conclusions of some academic research on adolescents are compatible with this view of the importance of a positive relationship with parents. Analyses of communication patterns show that independent-type behaviors in adolescents correlate most closely with families in which both individuality and connectedness are expressed when family members are performing a formal research task together (Cooper, Grotevant, and Condon, 1983; Grotevant and Cooper, 1985, 1986). Based on their own study of adolescents and their families plus studies of several other researchers, Hauser, Powers, and Noam (1991) find that ego development during adolescence correlates with parents expressing acceptance of their adolescents.

The last feature of my model of adolescent development, parental sponsorship (Erikson, 1950; Blos, 1985), is necessary because of the tendency for conflict to arise between the other two motives of wishing to maintain a positive relationship with parents and strivings to complete development. When adolescents feel in conflict between pleasing their parents and striving to complete their development, then a clear message of support for their forward movement helps reduce any ambiguity adolescents may experience about their parents' wishes.

The importance of parents sponsoring and demonstrating confidence in the ability of their adolescent children to progress developmentally is little more than great common sense. Yet it is remarkable how often this feature of the child–parent relationship becomes anywhere from subtly undermined to blatantly disregarded during the child's adolescence. Nonetheless, the importance of this clinical concept of sponsorship can be inferred from research in areas ranging from infancy through young adulthood.

Studies of children during the first two years of life illustrate the importance of the emotional availability of the parent, of sharing positive feelings, and of social referencing in advancing the child's development (Emde, 1991). (Social referencing refers to the tendency of people of any age, when faced with a condition of uncertainty, to look toward a significant other person for an emotional signal to help the uncertain one resolve and respond to the situation.)

Research has identified the importance of supportive, personal teacher-student relations, and familiarity and comfort with the school environment in promoting motivation and academic progress. Sixth and seventh graders who remain in kindergarten–grade 8 schools were compared with students who change to junior high schools. Those development-promoting conditions are more typically experienced by students in K–8 schools. The inference I draw from this finding is that the teachers in the K–8 schools are fulfilling a more sponsoring role than those in junior high schools are able to do (Eccles, Midgley, Wigfield, Buchanan, Reuman, Flanagan, and MacIver, 1993).

A study which compared highly functioning adolescents from black American working-class families with those from white American middle- and upper-middle-class families found that the families of both groups were intact and provided their adolescents with a strong sense of emotional support and human connectedness (Looney and Lewis, 1985). This work both implies the existence of sponsorship and illustrates that it cuts across racial and socioeconomic lines.

Adolescents who prove resilient to stress have been found to receive more parental support; they also often have extensive contacts outside the family with other adults or peers compared to nonresilient adolescents (Hauser and Bowlds, 1990).

From a study in which adolescents and their parents together attempted to resolve difficult, hypothetical moral dilemmas, Hauser, Powers, and Noam (1991) identified "enabling" interactions which promote ego development and "constricting" interactions which restrict ego development in adolescents. The "enabling" interactions include explaining things to the adolescent, taking a problem-solving approach toward the research task, and expressing curiosity about the adolescent's views. "Enabling" interactions also encompass helping the adolescent focus in the discussion, and demonstrating acceptance of the adolescent which implies a warm, nurturing, and supportive relationship. Those "enabling" parental behaviors reflect a sponsoring attitude toward their adolescents' efforts to move forward developmentally.

Studies have suggested that adolescents' general level of self-esteem correlates directly with their perception of the regard in which they are held by parents and others who are important to them. Conversely, low self-esteem is correlated with a perceived lack of support and regard from parents and significant others (Harter, 1990). I presume that positive self-esteem correlates with or promotes developmental advance.

The research of a sports psychologist to the U.S. Olympic team led to his conclusion that "support and encouragement of parents is the No. 1 thing Olympic athletes say got them to this level of competition" (Murphy, 1994).

Thus, research on infants, middle school children, competent black adolescents from working-class homes and white adolescents from middle-class homes, and Olympic athletes is consistent with the idea that parental sponsorship is important for adolescents' development to progress.

CONTRAST BETWEEN THE THESIS I AM ADVANCING AND STAGE THEORY

This view that adolescent psychological development evolves gradually through the continuing interaction of these three issues has implications for theory; for each of the three issues is dealt with throughout the course of development. Thus, development is not presented here as a process which occurs in stages. Most clinicians would probably agree in principle with the view that development is continuous. For example, Esman observes that "Development is a continuous process; the seams of its web are imposed by the observer seeking to order his data into conceptual segments" (1980, p. 421). Most existing developmental theories are stage theories, however. In contrast to what I have described, stage theories maintain that psychological development progresses by the stepwise enhancement of capacities which enable the individual to master stage-specific developmental tasks. Stage progression models may have retained their popularity because the most widely promulgated developmental theories, those of Freud, Piaget, Erikson, and Mahler, are stage theories.[1]

Each of the existing stage theories of adolescent development posits a specific, fixed relationship between either puberty (psychoanalysis) or cognitive changes (Piagetian-oriented psychology) or deidealization of parents (self psychology) on the one hand, and the onset of adolescents' efforts to emancipate on the other hand. I will illustrate, however, that no invariable relationship exists between those phenomena and the onset of adolescence.

The problem of defining the end of adolescence has been frequently described and addressed (Adatto, 1980; Staples and

---

[1]Freud himself demonstrated the compelling tendency to think in such terms. For he retained his stage theory model after he had discovered strong evidence against it. Specifically, he found that all the critical elements for symptom formation observed in the phallic–oedipal stage were also present in the antecedent, preoedipal stage (1931) (see chapter 3).

Smarr, 1980; Brockman, 1984; Scharfman, in Panel, 1987). I will discuss the difficulty in identifying a group of either external behaviors or internal changes which invariably occur close enough together in time to justify concluding that the advent of adulthood occurs in a discrete, stage-specific manner. That is, there is so much variation (both amongst adolescents in general and within any individual adolescent) in the time when they achieve goals which stage theories use to mark the transition to adulthood,[2] that stage theory conceptualizations confuse rather than clarify our understanding of the developmental process.

Moreover, research on adult development raises questions about the validity of some criteria which have traditionally been used to demarcate adolescence from adulthood. For example, Vaillant (1977) and Levinson, Darrow, Klein, Levinson, and McKee (1978) report that men seek mentor relationships until young middle age. Those findings call into question whether psychological independence, the hallmark of emancipation, is achieved by the end of adolescence. At the very least, their observations suggest that psychological independence is a multifaceted phenomenon, all features of which are not achieved simultaneously during development. Also, Vaillant (1987) observed from his longitudinal study that men progressively reduce their use of immature defense mechanisms at least until midlife. This implies that individuals eventually mature out of several adolescent behavior patterns that they were still exhibiting at the threshold of adulthood. Empirical research on both men and women from the Institute of Human Development[3] supports the idea that development occurs via a continually evolving, dynamic configuration of personality characteristics rather than in discrete stages (Block with the collaboration of Haan, 1971; Eichorn, Clausen, Haan, Honzik, and Mussen, 1981). Thus, character traits appear to be more dynamic and less immutable than they

---

[2] Those goals have typically included being emotionally ready for a permanent love relationship; conscience functioning which is independent of parental values and proscriptions (implying psychological autonomy); and readiness to make a realistic career commitment.

[3] The Institute of Human Development comprises the combined populations of the Berkeley Guidance Study and the Oakland Growth Study, perhaps the largest and longest running longitudinal study in this country.

have previously been considered. That finding makes it more difficult to accept as an indication of the difference between adolescent and adult psychological organization certain "structural" criteria which have been suggested, like resolution of residual traumata from earlier life into fixed character traits (Blos, 1977).

DEVELOPMENT IN WOMEN COMPARED TO THAT IN MEN

Comparable studies bearing on the issue of mentorship in women have not been published and the issue of sponsorship in the development of women is considered in chapter 7. Much research during the past quarter century has been oriented toward emphasizing gender differences, often on the basis of laboratory studies of behavioral and communicative styles. An implication of such findings is that development differs significantly in women and men. I suspect that these differences have been overdrawn, in part because research studies in the behavioral sciences are not immune from political influences, in this case the liberation movements; and researchers like people in general have a remarkable capacity to find what they are looking for, especially when the cause is just. I suspect that the pendulum of understanding development will move back toward a realization that the similarities are greater than the differences. In fact that has already begun to happen. For example, recently popular ideas that women's conception of morality is, or more often is, based on caring and connectedness while that of men is more devoid of humanity and based on principles of justice (Gilligan, 1982, 1986) have not stood the test of further formal research. Rather, it seems that both sexes tend to use a "caring orientation" when solving personal dilemmas and a "rights orientation" when resolving impersonal dilemmas (Torney-Purta, 1990).

After reviewing more than 300 studies on gender differences, Aries (Wilson, 1994) has recently concluded that many studies did not consider alternative plausible explanations other than gender for the different responses of men and women. She concluded that sex differences are small. This stands to reason because at base men and women share the same developmental needs and range of adaptive responses, and thus the developmental psychology of men and women is likely to be more similar than different. Thus, sponsorship in adolescence and its derivative in adult life, mentoring, is as important in the development of women as it is in men.

If sponsorship continues into adult life, for example, in the form of mentor relationships, then what is the ultimate developmental importance of sponsorship? It promotes the progression from dependence to independence to interdependence (Emery, 1994, personal communication). Psychological interdependence, mutuality in important relationships, would seem to be the desired endpoint of the development of autonomy. As the most "reasonable" way to live vis-à-vis other people, interdependence represents a necessary and continuing strength throughout adult life, a matter of truly shared responsibility with another or others, and the stance which best prepares one for the anticipated infirmity of old age.

COMPARISON WITH OTHER THEORIES OF ADOLESCENT DEVELOPMENT

The view of the adolescent developmental process I am presenting is consonant with later Freudian theory (1930, 1940), and with Erikson's ideas about the influence of the larger community on ego development in the child (1950, 1956). My view is also compatible with recent empirical research on adolescence (Offer and Offer, 1975), on infant development (Stern, 1985; Emde, 1988a, 1991) and on the therapeutic process in adult patients in psychoanalysis and psychotherapy (Langs, 1985; Weiss, Sampson, and the Mount Zion Psychotherapy Research Group, 1986).

The existing theories of adolescence do not completely explain the developmental process in any individual adolescent nor the developmental process and developmental psychopathology in all adolescents. I believe that the model I am presenting comes closer to doing so by integrating more accurately the role of real experience and ego maturation in the developmental process than have other theories. My focus on adolescents' ongoing adaptation to their real experiences renders this view particularly suitable for providing a theoretical, clinical explanation for the findings of recent empirical and academic research on adolescence; that is because the latter have a similar emphasis on adaptation (Offer and Offer, 1975; Feldman and Elliott, 1990; Hauser, Powers, and Noam, 1991).

PSYCHOANALYTIC THEORY

Psychoanalysis stresses that the hormonal changes of puberty create an upsurge of genital drive which causes a resurgence of oedipal yearnings. The adolescent's efforts to avoid guilt engendered by these regressive, incestuous, and parricidal urges and fantasies motivate the emancipatory process to psychological independence (Freud, 1905b). The "emancipatory process" refers to the ways in which the adolescent distances him- or herself from parents, their influence, control, and values. Thus, the common psychoanalytic definition of adolescence as adaptation to pubescence (Blos, 1962) means adaptation to the psychological reactions to the pubertal hormonal changes.

Emancipatory behaviors in some individuals do occur around the time of puberty. That temporal coincidence does not necessarily mean, however, that the motive for striving to become more independent is to ward off resurgent oedipal conflicts. In fact, that psychoanalytic definition is usually incomplete in my experience. More often I find that what appears to be an oedipal conflict involves more reality-based issues along with emancipatory guilt; emancipatory guilt is more like separation and survivor guilt than oedipal guilt.

OEDIPAL GUILT, SEPARATION GUILT, SURVIVOR GUILT, AND EMANCIPATORY GUILT

The operative "agent" in the Oedipus complex and in driving oedipal guilt is castration anxiety, the punishment that the oedipal child and the adolescent fears for harboring incestuous and parricidal urges. I have found that castration anxiety and the castration complex are a separate and distinct entity from oedipal urges and fantasies. Castration anxiety (and penis envy) are common features of child and adolescent development; they arise from observations of the differences between male and female genitals. By contrast, I find that the Oedipus complex, when it is discernible in childhood or adolescence, arises normally only in weak, muted form when it is based on inner drives. When it is a prominent feature of development in a child or adolescent, it has become so by virtue of certain parental attitudes and child–parent interactions; that is, because the child's real experiences have caused this construction to develop and burgeon. (The bases for making this distinction between the castration and Oedipus complexes are outlined in chapter 3 [pp. 68–71] and summarized in footnote 3, chapter 8, pp. 228–229.)

An implication of finding the Oedipus complex less significant in normal development than the position it has been accorded in traditional Freudian theory involves the ongoing nature of the child–parent relationship (object relationship). For without the intrusion of two periods of preordained, internally generated hostility toward parents (during the oedipal stage and adolescence), the quality of the child/adolescent–parent relationship is more consistent throughout developmental time. That more continuous relationship is characterized by the child seeking both age-appropriate protection and nurture from his parents; for it is those qualities that provide the major source of his sense of security.[4] The emancipatory process becomes one in which the adolescent moves toward greater autonomy while concomitantly needing to retain parental support.

Thus, emancipating adolescents are concerned about the impact of their gathering autonomy on their relationship with their parents. If they sense that their growing independence somehow threatens their parents' equanimity, then they feel conflict and experience guilt—not because they harbor hostile and incestuous wishes toward the parents, but because they fear losing the historical source of their own sense of security if their parents become alienated by their behaviors or attitudes. The following prosaic example illustrates this underlying concern in normal daily life:

---

[4] The adolescent's underlying strivings to complete development provide an inherent source of security, or at least confidence, as well; however, that source can be influenced strongly by parental attitudes and behaviors.

> A college freshman was home for her first vacation since entering a distant college. While chatting with her high-school aged sister and their mother she casually mentioned something she wanted to do "before going home" (to college). Immediately upon uttering those words both girls simultaneously looked intently at their mother's face to see whether the coed's reference to her dorm (rather than the life-long family house) as "home" was distressing or hurtful to their mother.

This type of compunction resembles separation and survivor guilt rather than oedipal guilt, but those conditions do not quite convey this developmental phenomenon. Separation guilt (Modell, 1965) is experienced by people who feel that their wishes to have more than their fair share will destroy others who are important to them (basically their mothers); and because of that greed they do not deserve to or cannot have an independent life of their own. The guilt I am describing also involves the wish to separate from childhood ties to parents, but it does not relate to wanting more than one's fair share. To the contrary, it is associated with a wish to have one's fair share, namely the freedom to emancipate to an autonomous existence.

Survivor guilt (Modell, 1971) is at the other end of a continuum from separation guilt. It arises when people fear that their success or advantage has occurred at the expense of others (usually a close relative), toward whom the survivor harbors no ill wishes; for example, a normal child who has a defective older sibling. (This phenomenon is illustrated in footnote 4, chapter 6, pp. 163–164). Survivor guilt resembles the guilt I am describing in that adolescents wish no harm to befall their parents. The definition of survivor guilt does not, however, emphasize a crucial developmental aspect of the phenomenon I am describing, namely the importance to the survivor of preserving the other person. For adolescents ultimately feel that their own sense of security depends upon maintaining the relationship with their parents. In addition, survivor guilt usually refers to faits accomplis. Also, the classical example of survivor guilt, the syndrome of concentration camp survivors (Niederland, 1981), is so dramatically different from normal adolescent development, that use of the term *survivor guilt* might confuse rather than elucidate the phenomenon I am detailing. So, although separation and survivor guilt together encompass in pathological proportions most elements of what I am presenting, I will refer to guilt associated with efforts to become more autonomous as *emancipatory guilt.* I have found these distinctions crucial in understanding adolescents' conflicts. Emancipatory guilt, separation guilt, and survivor guilt are common in human psychology; oedipal guilt is relatively uncommon. This stands to reason, since the oedipal relationship includes love as well as parricidal wishes toward the same-sexed parent.[5] And, for example, it is common for adolescents to wish to surpass their parents' achievements, but they do not want this to occur at their parents' expense.

The following example illustrates the distinction I am making between oedipal, emancipatory, separation, and survivor guilt. I frequently find that adolescents who appear to be stumbling on incestuous conflicts prove on closer examination to be primarily struggling with emancipatory guilt. The adolescent's real experiences are a critical contributant to this phenomenon. (While the following is an extreme example of brevity, many of the clinical cases in this book are presented in abbreviated form to illustrate rather than "prove" my points.)

> A late adolescent seemed unable to date girls because of his close relationship with his chronically ill mother. Exploration revealed that he was being held back by fear that she would die without his constant presence and ministrations and by guilty feelings that her fate was in his hands. These attitudes had become instilled in him by his mother's possessive manner toward him. Her attitudes were communicated in unhappy expressions, withdrawal, and complaints of greater pain when he talked to her about girls who were interested in him or whenever he left to spend time with friends.
>
> Intensive psychoanalytic therapy failed to reveal evidence that incestuous yearnings played a significant role in his distress or in his social inhibitions.

---

[5]Oedipal guilt arises from the desire to supersede a parent toward whom one feels competitive. As such, I consider it a subspecies of the separation–survivor guilt continuum. For survivor and separation guilt encompass the special case of an individual who feels competitive toward the other person. Oedipal guilt does not account, however, for the experience of an individual who feels guilty about surpassing another person toward whom he or she does not feel rivalrous.

The thesis I am presenting offers understanding of this youth's development. His urge to move ahead into dating engendered emancipatory guilt, because he felt that his involvement with girls would compromise his mother's well-being. The latter idea had been communicated to him by her possessive attitudes and expressions of medical setbacks whenever he left her. In fact, his motives were opposite from those of someone experiencing an oedipal conflict; for he wanted to leave his mother. But I find that many therapists would interpret such emancipatory guilt as oedipal guilt.

THE SIGNIFICANCE OF SEXUAL MATURATION IN ADOLESCENCE

The integration of adult sexual capacity is important in adolescence, but not because threatening, incestuous urges are invariably aroused. Rather, the importance of puberty lies in it being the last biological function to mature, which, in concert with cognitive and physical maturation, gives adolescents full adult potential; that is, puberty consolidates a physiological adult, though not a psychological one.

My thesis assumes the same forward orientation exhibited by adolescents' burgeoning physical, physiological, and intellectual growth. To further clarify its difference from a feature of psychoanalytic theory which has remained very influential, in my view the wish to progress is primary; regression can occur to accommodate perceived parental wishes (compulsive dependency). By contrast, in the traditional psychoanalytic theory of adolescence, the regression (to oedipal urges) is primary; progression arises secondarily to defend against castration anxiety.

OTHER THEORIES OF ADOLESCENCE

Unlike psychoanalysis, the other psychological theories have not yet offered a comprehensive view of adolescence, though self psychology and Piagetian-oriented cognitive psychology have each offered a perspective on adolescent development. My consideration of these theories will be limited in this book to their perspectives on adolescent development. The contributions from both assume, as does my model, a positive thrust in adolescent development. Self psychologists Wolf, Gedo, and Terman (1972), for example, posit that the process of psychological emancipation commences when adolescents become disillusioned with their idealized view of their parents. This disillusionment occurs under the influence of peer relationships.

Piagetian-based cognitive psychology, which is not clinically oriented, considers that the acquisition of a newly acquired capacity for abstract thinking enables adolescent development to occur. This incremental advance in cognitive ability motivates and allows adolescents to establish values independent from those of their parents (Kagan, 1971; Kohlberg and Gilligan, 1971).

One occasionally observes individuals whose course through adolescence demonstrates features described by both of these theories; however, both describe only part of the adolescent developmental process, and neither explains the developmental process in all adolescents. For example, the following adolescent became progressively more independent while retaining ideals, values, and moral standards similar to those of her parents. She did not demonstrate striking evidence of a capacity for sophisticated abstract thinking until late in the adolescent emancipatory process:

> A girl, who had always looked forward to growing up, treated her menarche as she subsequently did the acquisition of her driver's license, namely as one more milestone in the process of developing to maturity. She remained affectionate toward her father and close to her mother as she embarked on dating. She functioned with increasing independence from parental influence in attitude and action. Her parents relinquished control over her comings and goings with relative ease because of her dependability and because her basic values remained consonant with their own. Furthermore, it was not until relatively late in her adolescence, at age $17^1/2$, and with the help of a rigorous teacher, that she developed a level of intellectual sophistication in her capacity to analyze problems which she had not previously exhibited.

This girl's adolescent development does not conform, in the overview or specifics, to the self psychology or cognitive psychology models. It is better explained by the view I am advancing.

Her strivings to complete development were not in conflict with her need to maintain a relationship with her parents. Her parents in turn were readily able to support her progress, in part because her values remained congruous with their own. Her intellectual development emerged gradually, through hard work and practice, as she matured in other respects.

ADOLESCENT TURMOIL

Although it is common, adolescent turmoil, a hallmark of the psychoanalytic theory, is not invariably exhibited by normal adolescents (Offer and Offer, 1975) as the last example illustrates. When it does arise it can have several sources, including problems integrating adult sexuality (which is the explanation of psychoanalytic theory), or aggression or enhanced cognitive abilities. Amongst the most frequent sources of turmoil are adaptive efforts to try on new identities for fit with established patterns and talents; to experiment with newly emerged capacities and potentials, to practice as it were; and to attempt to resolve problems in relatedness to parents, that is, reconcile earlier traumata of all degrees of severity that often involve the issue of autonomy, as demonstrated in the following example:

A high-school freshman exhibited all of the latter three motives. He had some talent for surf boarding to which he began to devote more time while also adopting the hairstyle, hair coloring, clothes, and language of admired upper-class surfers. At the same time that this formerly intense lad was attempting to affect the "laid back" manner of surfers, he developed a particularly scathing tone in denouncing his parents. They had looked upon this as the rebelliousness they had half-anticipated during their son's adolescence; then one day his mother heard herself in her son's tone and words. This reminded her that on occasion during the boy's childhood (perhaps more times than she would like to acknowledge), when intensely frustrated by his obdurate, headstrong ways, she had addressed her son in just such a belittling manner. She recalled that on those occasions he had exhibited a consistent reaction: he would struggle not to cry and would develop a hang-dog expression and withdraw to his room for awhile. Now, older, bolder, and bigger, he was reversing the trauma he had experienced passively as a child into active experiences as an adolescent. The lad's motive was to master residual, internal effects of those traumatic moments which, while not overwhelming, had nevertheless been telling upon his developing sensibility and the freedom he had felt to assert himself as he wanted.

DEVELOPMENTAL PSYCHOPATHOLOGY

The model I am presenting explains psychopathology arising during the adolescent developmental process in a way that provides direction for effective psychotherapeutic and psychoanalytic intervention.

When conflict arises between the three motives in development, adolescents frequently experience, consciously or unconsciously, several attitudes, feelings, and ideas which strongly influence the form of their resulting behaviors or symptoms: (1) They blame themselves when the relationship with parents goes awry (Freud, 1930, 1940; Beres, 1958); however, this self-blame is often defended against by reversal (i.e., acting blame-less), and by externalization (i.e., blaming parents). (2) Adolescents feel responsible for maintaining that relationship. (3) They often feel that they have great influence over parents in that relationship (Weiss, Sampson, and Mt. Zion Psychotherapy Research Group, 1986).

Symptoms arising from conflicts which have been influenced by these attitudes often are either: (1) behaviors which represent a compliance with parental wishes (Weiss, Sampson, et al., 1986), as Cyril demonstrated (p. 4) by failing in order to please his father; or (2) behaviors equivalent to those of the adolescent's parents (defensive identifications) (Weiss, Sampson, et al., 1986). An example of the latter is the adolescent boy who starts to fail in school after his father loses his job.

CONCLUSION

Stated oversimply and schematically, the developmental conflict I am elaborating is between psychological dependency and psychological autonomy; and adolescents must feel support for this shift away from their parents. Clearly both dependence and autonomy are relative conditions. Or, as Spielman (personal communication, 1991) puts it, the conflict of life is not dependency versus independence; rather, it is how to live together with people and apart from people. Nevertheless, the balance between these conditions evolves during the course of development. And the level of autonomy we anticipate that youth will achieve by the end of adolescence is one which will enable them to pursue a life as close to their own design as their abilities and opportunities can afford them.

CHAPTER 2

Historical and Interdisciplinary Overview of Adolescence

Our civilization is doomed if the unheard-of actions of our younger generations are allowed to continue [inscription on a tablet found at the site of the Sumerian and Babylonian city of Ur which flourished during the 3rd millenium B.C. and was abandoned in the 4th century B.C. (Lauer, 1973)].

In the eighth century B.C., the Greek poet Hesiod complained, "I see no hope for the future of our people if they are dependent on the frivolous youth of today, for certainly all youth are reckless beyond words. . . . When I was a boy, we were taught to be discreet and respectful of elders, but the present youth are exceedingly wise and impatient of restraint" (quoted in Group for the Advancement of Psychiatry (GAP), 1968, p. 751). When that view of adolescents as willful, importunate, callow, and cavalier disrupters of the social order is compared with the idealization of youth presented in Plato's *Dialogues* four centuries later, we are left with the impression that parents in antiquity probably shared much the same spectrum of attitudes toward adolescents as do contemporary adults.

21

Moreover, from the standpoint of the behavior of youth, the examples which follow provide ample reason to temper any conceit we may harbor that phenomena like "liberated" behaviors in adolescent girls and radical student activism originated in the 1960s. The following observations were attributed to Martin Luther while teaching at the University of Wittenberg in 1544: "We have a great horde of young men here from all countries. The girls are getting very bold. They run after the fellows into their rooms and chambers and wherever they can, offering them free love. I hear that many parents have ordered their sons home" (quoted in *Marin Independent Journal,* 1991).

The next quotations are from the work of the French cultural historian Ariès (1960):

[I]n 1649 at Die the logicians barricaded themselves inside the college, prevented the masters and the pupils of the other classes from entering, fired pistol shots, fouled the rostra in the first and third classrooms, threw the benches in the second classroom out of the window, tore up the books, and finally climbed out of the windows of the fourth classroom, scandalizing the public. Sometimes indeed they would attack passers-by with their swords when they did not make do with the traditional fireworks [p. 318].

At Winchester, in the late 18th century, the boys occupied the school for two days and hoisted the red flag. In 1818 two companies of troops with fixed bayonets had to be called to suppress a rising of the pupils. At Rugby the pupils set fire to their books, their desks, and withdrew to an island which had to be taken by assault by the army. There were similar incidents at Eton. In 1768 . . . —the good pupils—of the Sixth Form seceded and left the school. In 1783 there was a revolt against the headmaster, with rooms pillaged and windows broken. In 1818 the school authorities brought forward the time when the gate was locked, to prevent the boys from going hunting: the latter, after pelting their master with rotten eggs, knocked down part of the wall, and the troublemakers had to be taken by force. Mutiny had become one of the typical and picturesque aspects of the idea contemporaries had of school life. . . . In England, the last important mutiny occurred at Marlborough as late as 1851. At Eton there was none after 1832, when the last one ended with the flogging of eighty boys: order was then restored [pp. 318–319].

COMPARATIVE LITERATURE/PSYCHOLOGY

Studies of diaries and autobiographies also demonstrate certain universal and timeless attitudes and behaviors on the part of adolescents themselves which the parental generation reacts to or perpetrates (Kiell, 1964). For example, in the year 1009, a 12-year-old Japanese girl wrote in her diary that "Mother was a person of extremely antiquated mind." This differs only in the delicacy of her expression from a current-day agemate who declares her mother "behind the times." In 1012, the 13-year-old daughter of a Japanese provincial governor recorded a daydream about a "shining prince" who in every respect was like the later-day "knight in shining armor" (Kiell, 1964).

Similarities across centuries and culture have also been identified in language, ambivalences and contradictions, delinquency, gambling, lying, conformity and peer culture, intellectualism, rejection of parents, use of teachers, and preoccupation with religious and suicidal thoughts (Kiell, 1964). A further example, from the autobiography of Saint Augustine, *Confessions*, written in 360 A.D., describes his delinquency at age 16:

> Yet I was willing to steal, and steal I did, although I was not compelled by any lack, unless it were the lack of a sense of justice or a distaste for what was right and a greedy love of doing wrong. For of what I stole I already had plenty, and much better at that, and I had no wish to enjoy the things I coveted by stealing, but only to enjoy the theft itself and the sin. There was a pear-tree near our vineyard, loaded with fruit that was attractive neither to look at nor to taste. Late one night a band of ruffians, myself included, went off to shake down the fruit and carry it away, for we had continued our games out of doors until well after dark, as was our pernicious habit. We took away an enormous quantity of pears, not to eat them ourselves, but simply to throw them to the pigs. Perhaps we ate some of them, but our real pleasure consisted in doing something that was forbidden [Saint Augustine, p. 47],

SOCIOLOGY

In addition to this first point that certain behaviors of adolescents and certain attitudes of adults about them have persisted throughout civilized time, there are certain consistent ways in which adults and adolescents in primitive and civilized cultures deal with each other. For example, sociologists Herbert A. Bloch and Alfred Niederhoffer demonstrate striking similarities between puberty rites in primitive societies and the practices of contemporary lower and middle-class gangs. Some features which were compared include self-decoration (tattooing, scarification, dress); rituals; customs and ceremonies (hazing); exploitation of initiates by elders for their own gain; acquisition of a new name and language; sexual ambivalence and homosexuality; seclusion from women, bachelor huts, and age grading; education for new roles and incorporation into adult men's groups. These authors conclude that adolescence contains certain universal imperatives which are unrelated to culture. The most basic is the wish to attain adulthood, and puberty rites basically serve to induct children into adulthood; that is, they celebrate social or sociological puberty, not biological puberty. They further conclude that when societies refuse to impose satisfactory standards for admission to adulthood and ordeals for acceptance, the young aspirant frequently demands to be put to the test. Gangs have arisen in certain cultural settings as a spontaneous attempt on the part of adolescents to accomplish this imperative on their own. They emerge in those primitive societies where the elders are overwhelmingly hostile to the youths as competitors or where there are insufficiently formalized pubertal rites for admission to adulthood. And they are formed in cultures like our own, where prolonged adolescence predisposes to ambiguity in these regards (Bloch and Niederhoffer, 1958).

CULTURAL ANTHROPOLOGY

A clinical report by a psychoanalytically oriented anthropologist, Muensterberger (1961), sheds further light on the relationship between the individual adolescent, his or her family, and society:

The patient was the elder child of a middle class, second generation Jewish couple. Muensterberger characterized the boy's father as a "little Napoleon." For years the boy suffered in being physically the smallest in his class. His father rubbed salt into those wounds by reproaching his son about his height, and with sentiments like, "You'll never amount to anything"; "You are a nobody"; and "You have no character, no backbone." As the boy approached puberty and lacked pubic hair, his father, considering the lad deficient, took him to doctors to see if the hair could be made to grow. Thus, Muensterberger observed that the boy's father stressed repeatedly that his adolescent son would never grow up and become a rival.

The lad was prepared for bar mitzvah. He anticipated the event with great anxiety as though he were to pass through an inexplicable ordeal. The author reported that the boy felt very alone on the day he was to become a man. On the morning of his bar mitzvah, he awoke with a backache which became increasingly more painful until he finally lay on the floor, unable to move. A doctor found no physical cause for this. Nevertheless, he was unable to stand erect and did not become bar mitzvah. Symbolically stated, he proved his father correct—he had no backbone.

At 15 he left high school against his father's wishes and ran away to earn his own living. He searched for security in groups which certain jobs might afford. He eventually joined the Army, and subsequently achieved some success in a career.

Muensterberger concluded that the father's hostility predisposed this lad to a neurotic solution. By contrast, fathers in primitive tribes institutionalize their aggression, and in doing so, normalize it. That is, if the harshness of the adult generation toward the initiates is institutionalized, youngsters who are social misfits will not emerge in the way that they might in response to individualized expressions of an instinctual drive within the family. From the standpoint of my own thesis, I would like to call attention to three features of Muensterberger's account. The first is the aloneness (the lack of parental sponsorship) that this lad felt on the day he was symbolically to become a man. The second is his compliance with his father's apparent wish that he not grow up, exemplified in the bar mitzvah experience. The third is this adolescent's efforts to find an environment in which he could surmount the interpersonal and ensuing intrapsychic impediments to his development encountered in his home. That is, he demonstrated internally motivated efforts to complete his development.

HISTORICAL APPROACH

The word *adolescence* derives from the Latin verb meaning "to grow up to." According to the Oxford English Dictionary, the term was first recorded in the late fourteenth century. Some dictionaries define it as the period between ages 14 and 25 years in boys and 12 and 21 in girls.

Ariès (1960) traced the origins of family life from the Middle Ages (400–1400 A.D.) by analyzing changes in such things as written records of schooling, artworks, biographical material, evolving patterns of speech and language (idioms) and the evolution of games and pastimes. For example, he concluded that it was probably common practice in western European countries during medieval times to send boys and girls away from home at age 7 or 9 years. They were raised in the households of other families where they were treated as adults. This custom was gradually forsaken in favor of sending 7- to 9-year-olds away to school where they would often be grouped in classes which included 18- to 20-year-olds. This practice was then supplanted by having children live at home and attend age-graded day schools.

Ariès concludes that the concept of the family was unknown in the Middle Ages, when loyalty was to the clan. During the fifteenth century children began to be viewed as different from adults and accordingly in need of different treatment. As this concept gained wider acceptance, the importance of the child and the family to each other grew, evolving to its full expression in the seventeenth century. Ariès concluded that the concept of adolescence was merged with that of childhood until the latter part of the eighteenth century. Then, under the influence of conscription and the Cartesian philosophy of keeping things separate, the concept of adolescence emerged from that of childhood. This conclusion has been more recently disputed by at least one other historian of French culture (Davis, 1975).

Davis (1975) reports that both youth groups and youth rituals were common in sixteenth century France. Also, medical, religious, and popular printed material all distinguished adolescence as a period of sexual maturation (cited in Elder [1980] and in Modell and Goodman [1990]).

Other historians maintain that although the term *adolescence* existed, it was not commonly used before the nineteenth century. The term *youth* was more typically used and the time frame it encompassed overlapped that designated by the term *childhood.* The explanation given for this ambiguity is that during the agrarian period of the sixteenth and seventeenth centuries there was no transition between childhood and adulthood. Individuals simply emerged from the period of childhood dependency as soon as they were able to perform adult tasks. The overriding consideration in "classifying" a person was not the individual's age but rather what he or she was capable of doing (Modell and Goodman, 1990). The term *youth* seemed to refer to individuals who were in a transitional period between a relationship of full dependency on one's parents and complete economic and social independence from them. These authors report that in western Europe and colonial America girls and boys from all classes were "fostered out" at ages 12 to 15 to be raised and work in the homes of other families. Whether motive for or effect of this practice, Modell and Goodman conclude that apprenticing out children of the adolescent age range served a rite of passage function; it also facilitated a smoother transition to adulthood than would have occurred if the adolescents had remained with their own families.

SOCIOPOLITICAL INSTITUTIONS APPROACH

Other social scientists have reached different conclusions about what adolescence is and how it arose. For example, Bakan (1971) distinguishes between adolescence as a romantic idea and adolescence as a social fact. The idea of adolescence may have been around since the fifteenth century; and it was particularly consolidated and popularized by Rousseau's ideas in the 1760s of adolescence as a second childhood (one is born first a human being and then reborn later as an adult). At least in America, this concept was adopted, and adolescence was invented as a specifically definable period, to accommodate economic and social conditions which arose after the Civil War. Prior to the Post-Civil War period of urban industrialization, there had existed a chronic shortage of laborers, dating from the first settling of America. This problem had previously been mitigated by slavery, by encouraging immigration, and by industrializing. The incompatibility between slavery and industrialization was resolved by the Civil War in favor of the latter. The rapid urban industrialization which followed that war resulted in a large number of young people who, to that point, had been mature in the sense that they were part of the work force. They now became immature in the eyes of society. In response to this new social class, three major sociopolitical movements arose in the late nineteenth and early twentieth centuries. While ostensibly humanitarian, they were in fact motivated by the need to deal with the potential and perhaps actual increase in crimes to property which typically characterize delinquent behaviors. These movements were compulsory education, child labor legislation, and special legal procedures for juveniles. With the implementation of these laws, a specific time frame supplanted the previous vagueness of the time when adolescence ended. Thus, adolescence as a social fact became that period from the onset of biological puberty to the time when compulsory education and those special legal procedures which presumably protected children/adolescents ended, and eligibility for employment as an adult began.

These views of adolescence as, respectively, the evolved product of secular trends in civilization or a societally imposed institution to maintain social order (i.e., adolescence as an institution imposed on youth by its society) contrast sharply with clinical views which focus on the importance of changes within the individual as defining features of this developmental period. I am not presenting this distinction to pose an either/or versus a both/and dilemma. Rather, I want to point out, for example, the very different ways in which proponents of these views would understand such adolescent phenomena as rebellious behavior. From Bakan's perspective, youth who rebel against school attendance prove to be those who quite appropriately perceive that attending school will not, as society promises, result in successful employment (1971). Those students do not rebel who can pass through school with at least reasonable assurance that doing so will lead to a successful life. On the other hand, theorists who

perceive adolescence as a response to internal psychological restructuring and an imperative to emancipate from childhood attachments would anticipate some manner of rebelliousness
regardless of the confidence young people have in their society's
institutions. And viewed from the extended time-frame studied
by Ariès, one can understand that far from representing an institution which is in decline, family life has been accorded an increasingly paramount position in modern society. (See
Furstenberg [1990] for a consideration of the latter idea in relation to more recent trends in family life.)

DEMOGRAPHIC STUDY

In addition to the historical and social institutions approaches,
demographic analysis has also become popular amongst academic students of adolescence during the past quarter century.
Demographic analysis attempts to integrate historical and social
phenomena with individual lives in a general way. Demographers
have studied the influence of birth cohort status on individual
lives and the way this correlates with developmental time and
family experience. For example, an individual born in 1937 be-
longed to a cohort whose parents had been adolescents during
the Depression. Furthermore, there was a good chance that this
person lived in a fatherless household during that part of his or
her preteen years that coincided with World War II. By contrast,
a child born in 1947 was a member of a cohort distinguished by
its very large size. This factor influenced the individual's opportunities for college and job placement as teenagers.

One study which compared demographic trends over three
centuries reported that social and revolutionary changes have occurred during those periods when the youth cohort (ages 15–29
in this study) was of ascending size (Moller, 1968). This does not
say how the cohort effect influences change, just that it does.
Moller concludes that "Social change is not engineered by
youth, but is most manifest in youth" (p. 260). The direction of
such change is determined by the total situation in which the
youth find themselves; this includes the types of leaders with
whom they interact and the traditions and institutions they have

inherited. Moller supports a supposition that most youth in Western countries, even if they are in a state of unrest, usually remain stabilized emotionally and socially within the established adult society. By contrast, in developing countries adults are also involved in the unstable social conditions. So, in those nations, adolescents may be more in touch with the tenor of the society as a whole and of the wishes of their elders. These youth are more politically involved and play a dominant role in overthrowing their governments. Again, the implication is that, at least in some contexts, rebellious youth are acting in concert rather than in opposition to the sentiments of their elders.

ECONOMIC CONDITIONS AND THEORIES OF ADOLESCENCE

Articles on adolescence appearing in the *Journal of Genetic Psychology*, which is devoted to developmental psychology and has been published for more than a century, were studied during two periods of economic depression and two periods of rapid economic expansion (wartime). The authors found statistically significant stereotyping of adolescents depending upon the economic demands of society. Specifically, during periods of economic depression theories of adolescence depict youth as immature, psychologically unstable and in need of prolonged education. In periods of wartime when manpower is needed, the opposite view emerges in theories of adolescence; youth are then portrayed as mature, psychologically competent, and less needful of protracted education. One would not anticipate basic conceptions of development to alter on the basis of short periods of differing economic conditions (19th century depression, 1894–1895; period of American involvement in World War I, 1917–1918; Great Depression, 1933–1935; later period of American involvement in World War II, 1943–1945). From this conclusion that economic conditions are a significant independent variable in the theories advanced about youth in the direction described, an inference can be drawn similar to those raised in the sections on demographic influences and on sociopolitical influences. That is, youth are manipulated to serve the social order (Enright, Levy, Harris, and Lapsley, 1987).

LONGITUDINAL RESEARCH

Naturalistic studies present researchers with a tremendous challenge in sorting out patterns from voluminous and complicated data. Their results probably provide the clinician with more benefit to his or her appropriate professional humility and fund of general knowledge in the field than predictive value for any individual case. As with the other academic contributions to adolescence, I will outline representative findings rather than surveying the field exhaustively. Probably the best known longitudinal research relating to adolescence is that which describes the progression of physical changes associated with puberty. These invariant sequences in the maturation of boys and girls are reviewed in chapter 4.

Efforts have been made to correlate these biological sequences with the psychosocial attributes of the individual and to relate the psychosocial to the biological. An example of the former is the finding that the rate of structural maturation in adolescent boys predicts leadership capacity and success in work as an adult better than such psychosocial phenomena as demonstrated leadership qualities with peers during adolescence (Ames, 1957). Studies relating the psychosocial to the biological have found that early maturing adolescent boys became, in their thirties, more successful, self-controlled, reliable, and sociable, though also more inflexible, conforming, and moralistic than late maturing adolescent boys. The latter, while less self-contained and more self-assertive as adults, were more perspicacious and better able to adapt to the unfamiliar (Jones, 1965).

Early maturing adolescent girls were found to be less self-confident, popular, and active, and more submissive and withdrawn than their late maturing counterparts. The early maturers, however, ultimately became more confident and competent in adapting to life stress as adults (Peskin, 1973).

Many longitudinal studies were established to demonstrate continuities in phenomena throughout developmental stages. One is often impressed though by the discontinuities between pre- and postadolescent patterns in such studies, as well as by the degree of intrastage variability of behaviors amongst adolescents. For example, low levels of activity in boys between ages 3 and 6 years followed by high levels between ages 10 and 14 (pre- and early adolescence) predicted dependency on the love object in adulthood (Kagan and Moss, 1962).

Preadolescent girls who were independent and self-controlled, confident and rarely whiny, but who became whiny, dependent, explosive, and lacking in confidence as adolescents, ultimately adapted best as adults. On the other hand, psychological health for boys was predicated less on such switches into the opposite traits from preadolescence to adolescence, and more on strengthening of preadolescent traits. Specifically, while a shift from being emotionally self-contained and having a hearty appetite to being irritable and having a poor appetite in adolescence predicted psychological health in adulthood, generally, remaining socially at ease, expressive, and upbeat in mood from preadolescence through adolescence predicted psychological health at age 30 (Peskin, 1972).

These latter findings suggest that behavior patterns can change dramatically from childhood to adolescence and this overall pattern correlates with better adaptiveness in adulthood. Those studies also suggest that better adaptiveness is associated with continuity of some traits, at least in boys. So, the situation is not nearly as simple as whether continuity or change in prior behavior patterns during adolescence promotes psychological health in adulthood. The challenge remains to determine which kinds of traits can change, which serve the individual better by remaining stable and which by changing, and what factors in the environment or individual determine whether and how traits can change.

Block and Haan (1971), studying the personalities of the Institute of Human Development subjects from junior high school age to their mid-thirties, have factored out several, statistically distinct groupings of personality traits. The developmental courses of the different groups in their typology ranged through a spectrum: This comprised girls and boys in whom a core of adaptive personality traits remained basically constant from junior high to young adulthood; some whose personality characteristics changed from more to less adaptive and others for whom the opposite situation occurred. And, as noted above, regarding girls particularly, some exhibited more psychological stability in junior high than in senior high school but then recouped their adaptive advantage by the time they were young adults.

From the same study population, Eichorn, Clausen, Haan, Honzik, and Mussen (1981) have identified adolescent anteced- ents of adjustment during midlife (approximately age 50) with respect to personality development, IQ, psychological health, physical health, social maturity, marital adjustment, midlife drinking patterns, careers, resemblances amongst three genera- tions of family members, and political ideologies. Although tan- gential to the focus of this book, I will mention a few of their general findings that relate to the questions posed above. They reported, as had Block and Hann (1971), that sets of personality traits do not necessarily remain prominently continuous over time. Traits that were in greater evidence during early adoles- cence as opposed to late adolescence were better predictors of psychological health in midlife (ages 40–47) than in earlier adulthood (ages 30–37). Thus, it was posited that individuals can selectively draw upon traits from the past at different periods of adulthood. The appearance of specific personality traits during the different age periods of adult life studied seems to reflect both internal factors and environmental exigencies in the lives of the members of each cohort. Cognitive style, impulse control, and tendencies toward introversion or extroversion were the characteristics that most consistently distinguished amongst indi- viduals over long periods of time; and, in most general terms, interest and competence in intellectual activity and self-control over emotions in adolescence predicted psychological health in midlife—moreso for men than women.

STUDIES OF COGNITIVE DEVELOPMENT

Academic psychologists, expanding upon Piaget's work, have of- fered a different understanding of the adolescent developmental process. They conclude that adolescence is a discrete develop- mental stage because a capacity to think in new and different ways emerges in early adolescence. This notion of stage progres- sion to the capacity for formal operational thinking is perhaps the only idea developed outside psychoanalysis that has been incorporated by analysts into their theory of adolescence. Specifically, the 12-year-old becomes able to examine the logic and consistency of his existing beliefs. This acquisition may depend on biological changes in the nervous system; however, the environment must contribute catalytic experiences for this capacity to develop (Kagan, 1971).

The environment confronts adolescents with phenomena and attitudes that are not readily reconcilable with their existing ideology. Such intrusions into their existing belief systems predispose adolescents to reexamine their own knowledge and premises. This school of thought considers biological puberty to be a universal source of conflict-inducing information; yet, other issues serve a similar function of inducing cognitive conflict in youth (Kagan 1971). These latter issues may be unique to each generation, and might include school, drugs, sexual behavior, authority—each of which generates uncertainty which the child resolves by creating new beliefs.

To illustrate this shift in cognitive development, the political ideas of a large number of adolescents from ages 11 to 18, in the United States, West Germany, and Britain have been studied (Adelson, 1971). The ideas of 12-year-old German boys about politics proved to be closer to those of 12-year-old American boys than to those of their 15-year-old German brothers. Typical responses demonstrate the change in manner of thinking described above. In response to the question, "What is the purpose of laws?," typical responses of 12- and 13-year-olds included: "They do it, like in schools, so that people don't get hurt"; "If we had no laws, people could go around killing people"; "So people don't steal or kill." In contrast, adolescents two or three years older responded: "To ensure safety and enforce the government"; "To limit what people can do"; "They are basically guidelines for people. I mean, like this is wrong and this is right, and to help them understand." The younger adolescents responded concretely, and even in situations which embodied a general principle, the 12- and 13-year-olds generally had difficulty articulating it. By contrast the 15-year-olds could abstract from the concrete and use the latter for examples.

It does seem clear that the older a child gets the more inclined he or she is to use abstract thinking. The research data do not, however, convincingly support the concept that this enhanced cognitive capacity is acquired in a discrete, incremental way. Piagetian tests do demonstrate different performances. Yet preadolescent children can be demonstrated to use the same capacities, though in a less sophisticated manner. The younger child's poorer performance may reflect factors other than lack of the necessary cognitive "structures." For example, younger children may have more difficulty holding all the premises in mind simultaneously. Also, the reliability of Piagetian testing is not high and relatively modest numbers of subjects pass the tests at the highest level; this raises questions about whether universal features of cognitive functioning are being identified. In sum, while the validity of considering adolescence discrete by virtue of the stage-type acquisition of a new cognitive mode is questionable, there is agreement that adolescents tend to use cognition in a more sophisticated manner than do children; and this supports Piaget's conclusion that adolescence is a transitional period in the development of critical thinking (Keating, 1980, 1990). In addition to the capacity to retain and consider a greater number of options simultaneously, other cognitive achievements during this period include a greater base of knowledge, a wider range of strategies for gaining and applying knowledge, an improved capacity to work with these tools spontaneously and automatically, and greater appreciation of the relativity of knowledge. More recent research on cognitive development has concluded that the content and context in which this process occurs is a more critical factor in acquiring these capacities than had been previously considered. Furthermore, the use of these enhanced skills and capacities is not stable or static. That is, adolescents do not always utilize their most sophisticated capacities. Their strategic approach to any problem is very situation-specific, depending on such factors as their familiarity and comfort with the issue, and whether it is a hypothetical or real situation (Keating, 1990; Torney-Purta, 1990; Feldman and Elliott, 1990).

An alternative understanding for this changed mode of thinking and problem solving in adolescents posits a more gradual maturation of several cognitive functions which sum to this enhanced capacity. The great variation in cognitive abilities (and tendencies) exhibited by adolescents may reflect an overriding genetic contribution. In this model, environmental factors would have greater influence on the tendency of any individual to utilize and capitalize upon these capacities, rather than having a primary effect on their acquisition. This concept of the accretion of evolving abilities rather than stage acquisition is more compatible with concepts of development emerging from recent infant research (chapter 3).

PSYCHOANALYTIC CONCEPTS ABOUT ADOLESCENCE

Because it has been the most comprehensive theory of adolescent development and has had the most influence on clinical understanding of adolescent behaviors, the psychoanalytic theory of adolescent development and the history of its development and views from other clinical fields will be summarized here.

HISTORY

The development of psychoanalytic concepts about adolescence began with Freud's *Three Essays on the Theory of Sexuality* (1905b). In Part Three of that treatise, entitled "The Transformations of Puberty," Freud wrote that sexuality takes its final form with genital primacy. The pregenital drives continue to be expressed in forepleasure. Freud ascribes a biological basis to this transformation.

At the same time, G. Stanley Hall, the American psychologist, published his two-volume work, *Adolescence: Its Psychology, and Its Relations to Physiology, Anthropology, Sociology, Sex, Crime, Religion and Education* (1904), which catalogued the phenomenology of adolescence. It was Hall who characterized this period as one of "sturm und drang" (storm and stress).

Next, in 1922, Ernest Jones contributed his recapitulation theory. His idea is that each individual proceeds through the adolescent phase in a manner which precisely recapitulates the way he or she had worked through the phase of infantile sexuality. Thus, there is a reinstinctualization, remodeling, and a reintegration of psychic components.

Also during the 1920s, two Viennese analysts studied different aspects of adolescence. Bernfeld concentrated on its progressive aspects. He described two different ways in which individuals negotiate this period. One group appears, from the time of puberty, to be impatiently eager to achieve adulthood and adult prerogatives (Bernfeld, 1935). These individuals act as if they feel that the adult generation simply stands in their way. Bernfeld characterizes this as "simple adolescence"; he considers that individuals who take this route emerge with less complicated personality structures than the second group which exhibits "protracted adolescence" (Bernfeld, 1923). The latter individuals seem to avoid facing and dealing with their biological maturity. Bernfeld concludes that there is a relationship between this form of adolescence and creativity, and that these individuals emerge with richer personality structures. At the same time, Aichorn(1925) was studying the regressive aspects of adolescence in his work with juvenile delinquents, and developed a concept and technique for rendering such youth amenable to psychoanalytic therapy.

In 1936 Anna Freud devoted part of *The Ego and the Mechanisms of Defense* (1936) to adolescent defenses. She identified two defense mechanisms of the ego which gain ascendance during this developmental period, namely intellectualization and asceticism. Although both may be present earlier in development, either in rudimentary or full form, they are uniquely equipped mechanisms to deal with the problems presented by the upsurge of drive at puberty. For a while, this contribution and Jones' recapitulation theory were the major points of view about adolescent development.

During World War II, the opportunity to study adolescents who had been exposed to extreme stress brought forth a resurgence of interest in adolescence. Then, with the development of ego psychology in the 1950s, more attempts were made to analyze adolescents.

In 1951 Spiegel attempted to pull together features which would comprise a psychoanalytic theory of adolescence. In discussing adolescent phenomenology, Spiegel underscored Bernfeld's point that the great multiplicity of phenomena render classification of this phase difficult.

In 1958 Anna Freud elaborated the long-held "sturm und drang" idea that adolescent turmoil is an inevitable and universal feature of normal development; or at least the maintenance of a steady state is more abnormal during adolescence. Subsequently, in the 1960s, Masterson (1967) published his studies which challenge the normality of adolescent turmoil. And the Offers (Offer, 1969; Offer and Offer, 1975) presented research findings which question the universality of adolescent turmoil.

Two popular areas of clinical research during the past twenty-five years which have a developmental perspective are object relations theory and self psychology. The work of Peter Blos exemplifies how insights developed from these orientations have been applied to adolescent phenomena. For example, Blos detailed a second individuation process in adolescence (1967). He contrasted it with the first individuation process in which the outcome is the achievement of psychological separateness from objects. The second individuation during adolescence allows for the opposite condition to occur, namely, finding external love and hate objects. Blos has also written about the development of the ego ideal in males. He concludes that it is contributed to in equal measure by the idealizing pregenital relationship to the father and the competitive oedipal relationship to the father (1985). These strands should become consolidated at the end of adolescence. In this conclusion Blos follows the trend of object relations theorists in ascribing increasing importance to pregenital experiences in development. In also focusing on the importance of an idealizing relationship to the father, Blos is adapting an idea stressed by self psychology. Blos presents these views as clinical theoretical refinements to the traditional psychoanalytic view that are intended to complement rather than contradict or supplant it.

Wolf, Gedo, and Terman (1972), writing from the self psychology perspective, suggest that the crucial developmental step in adolescence involves disillusionment with the child's ego ideal which follows disillusionment with the parents. Peer group pressures catalyze this change by offering new values. The peer group serves a transitional function in maintaining the cohesion of the young adolescent's self prior to the integration of new guiding principles. Since this process can occur at any time during the span of adolescence, these authors do not consider sexual maturation to be the precipitant for adolescent development. Rather, the need to acquire new ideals and the transformation of the self fuel this process. Thus, these authors propose a process not unlike that of the cognitive psychologists and one more akin to an adolescent recapitulation of early childhood development than embodying the emergence of a new organizing principle for development during adolescence.

THE PSYCHOANALYTIC THEORY OF ADOLESCENCE

In the commonly accepted clinical view, the terms *prepuberty* and *preadolescence* refer to a period of generalized increase in drive activity that occurs before puberty. The original descriptions of these stages maintain that boys regress to pregenital messiness and orality because their greatest fear is castration. Girls, on the other hand, respond by ego strengthening, observed in greater self-control and self-discipline, because libidinal regression is more threatening to them than castration. These behavioral patterns represent efforts on the part of both boys and girls to prepare for the upsurge of genital drive at puberty.

   Puberty is ushered in by the hormonally induced changes in body build and genitals, by menstruation and ejaculation, and by the unsettling sensations which accompany these physiological changes. The upsurge of genital drive is the psychological correlate of these biological changes. It brings incestuous urges closer to consciousness. Young adolescents' need to escape awareness of these desires becomes the motive force for efforts to disengage from childhood attachments to their parents, the incestuous objects. In this process of disengagement, adolescents withdraw libido from mental representations of their parents into the self. Then libido is reinvested in mental representations of different people who represent new relationships. Typically the first new recipient of the adolescents' love is someone of the same sex, who usually turns out to be very much like the adolescent or like some ideal they harbor about the way they would like to be. Thus, this relationship is based more on love of self than on love of the other person, which is why it is considered a narcissistic rather than a bona fide homosexual object choice. The back and forth nature of this process—from parents to self to peers and groups—accounts for the mood swings, loneliness, self-centeredness, experimentation with new roles and styles (new identities), the unpredictability, and unmitigated activity or passivity (either pole of which can grow into pathology), which we observe in adolescents.

If this process renders the incestuous wishes less pressing, adolescents move toward consolidating their heterosexuality. The development of formal operational (abstract) thinking contributes by enabling the effective use of the defense mechanism of intellectualization which flowers in adolescence. The capacity for abstract thinking also probably contributes to the evanescent spurt of creativity in midadolescence that serves the process of internal restructuring. Masturbation helps integrate physical, emotional, and fantasy elements of sexuality, including empathy and feelings of romance. When masturbatory fantasies become stereotyped and boring, adolescents search for partners and sexual intercourse.

The initial sexual encounters between boys and girls have historically been fraught with devaluation of the self and partner following intercourse, by aggressive overtones (especially on the part of boys), and other features which reveal lingering incestuous and pregenital remnants, some of which endure for life. The latter (remnants) usually remain subordinated to nonincestuous genitality. The playing-at-love, almost caricatural quality of late adolescents' romances, bears witness to their ongoing efforts to become comfortable in the role of heterosexual partner.

The process of development is further consolidated by the reworking of conscience and ideals during later adolescence. By taking risks and testing the limits of their own endurance and their society's tolerance, late adolescents temper their omnipotence and enhance their sense of reality. Delinquent activities, in the face of eagerness to usurp adult prerogatives, even if not adult responsibilities, provide additional evidence of their efforts to establish ethical codes which are not simply carbon copies of their parents' standards. In their intense, albeit shifting devotion to causes, which are often embraced as intensely as a loved person, we witness a similar reworking of their ego ideal. These efforts toward more mature superego and ego ideal functioning afford adolescents greater internal freedom to turn toward career choices based on a realistic appraisal of their abilities and opportunities, rather than simply on possibilities or the wishes of parents. Erikson (1956) considers that the consolidation of what he has termed ego identity is a psychosocial feature of this process. Ego identity refers to the development of a felt sense of conviction that the adolescent's self-view is congruent with the way the community views him or her. Significant progress toward accomplishing these interrelated tasks places the adolescent at the threshold of adulthood.

For psychoanalysis, therefore, adolescence refers to the process of adapting to pubescence, which importantly involves defense against reactivated, regressive urges. From the structural metapsychological viewpoint, this period of psychological restructuring should consolidate the ascendance of ego over id and superego. This should occur in such a manner that the superego allows for adaptation to the social order without either too great prohibition of instinctual gratification or without a loss of productive energy.

SUMMARY

In developing an understanding of what adolescence is, I reviewed data from social scientists which point to universal features of adolescence that transcend history, culture and subculture, and familial relatedness. In addition data were touched upon that suggested both commonalities associated with later success and the uniqueness of any adolescent's experiences depending upon cohort status and the social institutions during his or her era, as well as the adolescent's reaction to biological and peer group changes. If anything, such inherently contradictory theses complicate rather than clarify the relative contribution from within the individual and from his or her environment in producing the particular behaviors and attitudes that are displayed. This book suggests that these disparate views can be reconciled by considering the interaction of three principles of development: the maturational force termed "strivings to complete development," the adolescent's need to do so in the context of a positive relationship with his parents, and a specific need from the latter for ongoing sponsorship of their adolescent's progress.

CHAPTER 3

A Review and Critique of Psychological Development Prior to Adolescence

PSYCHOANALYTICALLY ORIENTED VIEWS OF DEVELOPMENT

FREUD

Psychoanalysis has provided the most comprehensive, clinical developmental psychology to date. As such, it has been the most influential theory underlying the psychotherapeutic treatment of children. Freud's early clinical writings and his late theoretical writings contain most elements of the view I am presenting. But he never segregated and integrated these into a coherent model distinct from an alternative view he favored during much of his career which supported different basic premises about development. Specifically, Freud started with a traumatic theory of neurosis (the seduction theory, 1896) and never completely abandoned that idea. Yet he subsequently deemphasized the importance of real experiences compared to ontogenetic fantasies (the theory of infantile sexuality, 1905b). The crucial differences between Freud's most popular theories and newer findings are two-fold. They involve the degree to which development is motivated by sexual and aggressive drives as opposed to maturational features inherent in the ego apparatus, and the role of inner-derived fantasies as opposed to real experiences in advancing development and in creating psychopathology.

BASES/BACKGROUND OF FREUD'S THEORY

Freud's theory of normal development derived from his ideas about how psychopathology (specifically neurosis) develops in adults. While undergoing his early cathartic treatment, adult neurotics reported having been seduced during childhood by adults. Freud concluded that their illnesses stemmed from the specific psychological trauma of premature sexual stimulation. Having decided that the adult neurosis originated in childhood, it would seem a natural step for Freud to theorize about the difference between the childhoods of future neurotics and of normal adults. This historical perspective suggests not only how Freud may have become interested in childhood development, but also why sexuality played such a central role in his understanding of development.

FREUD'S THEORY OF NEUROTIC PSYCHOPATHOLOGY

This was based on two assumptions which reflected his efforts to align psychological illnesses with popular ideas from the natural sciences about how physiological systems functioned (Freud, 1920): (1) The nervous system of an organism could be stimulated from outside or inside itself; (2) organisms strove to deplete themselves of excitation so as to exist with at least a constant, if not the lowest possible, level of excitation (Fechner's principle of constancy [1873]; see also Breuer and Freud [1893–1895, p. 197]). This latter idea, described in Freud's writings as the pleasure principle, the nirvana principle, and later as the basis for the death instinct became a central tenet of development. According to Strachey (1955), it was "the most fundamental of Freud's theories" (p. xix). When carried to its logical conclusion in an abstract sense, living matter would strive to become dead matter (Freud, 1923, p. 47). At the clinical level, however, people strove for pleasurable gratification through discharge of (sexual) tension.

DEVELOPMENT OF NEUROSIS

This theory of psychopathology explained neurotic illness as follows: If the child was prematurely sexually stimulated, his or her nervous system would strive to discharge the resulting heightened sexual tension/energy (termed libido). Not only was the child's immature genital apparatus incapable of mature sexual functioning (orgasm), but also, parents and caretakers (the child's environment) opposed his or her involvement in sexual activities. Thus, the child's ego, which Freud at that time considered a conscious, repressing force, augmented by the environment's efforts to instill the repressing forces of shame, disgust, and morality, strove to push the sexual excitement out of consciousness. Sexual excitement/energy then became trapped within the individual's Unconscious by these efforts, creating anxiety. Thus, anxiety, in this topographic model of the systems Conscious, Unconscious, and Preconscious, was sexual energy (libido) which had no outlet. This predisposed the person to neurotic illness in later life. In fact, the symptoms of the later neurosis were simply expressions of the individual's sexual functioning, displaced from genitals to other organ systems, for example, to a limb in hysterical paralysis. Future neurotics repressed sexual trends excessively while future normals repressed them less completely and more selectively (Freud, 1906, p. 277).

INFANTILE SEXUALITY REPLACES THE SEDUCTION THEORY

Freud was persuaded by further clinical experience, and evidence from parapraxes, momentary forgetting, and dreams, that mental functioning was based on a different mechanism. Consequently, he altered his ideas about how neuroses develop. The crux of this change was his determination that some ego functioning was unconscious. This led to the concept of defense mechanisms of the ego and an opposite view of the genesis and function of anxiety. He concluded that anxiety and symptoms arose when children could not retain in their unconscious those sexual (and aggressive) wishes which were unacceptable to themselves and their parents. In the new formulation, anxiety, rather than being a direct expression of undischarged libido, was conceived of as a signal, originating from the unconscious part of the person's ego, that unacceptable libidinal wishes were in danger of erupting into consciousness (Freud, 1926). This was a warning to the individual that greater efforts were needed to maintain repression. Symptoms arose when these efforts were insufficient and represented a compromise between complete repression and full, conscious expression of the unacceptable wishes.

Additional clinical experience, his own self-analysis, plus observations and analyses of children, prompted Freud to retract his traumatic theory of neurosis in favor of what he termed infantile sexuality. He concluded that sexual drives were present from birth; and it was these and their associated wishes, desires, and fantasies, rather than real experiences of seduction, which caused neuroses. In this later theory, socially unacceptable sexual and (subsequently) aggressive[1] drive-based wishes were maintained in repression (i.e., unconscious). Repression was accomplished by the joint efforts of the ego, which interpreted the disparity between unconscious drive wishes for expression (pleasure principle) and environmental tolerance (reality principle), and the superego, a part of the ego which mediated conscience functions. The role of the environment shifted from being an essential feature for symptom formation to one of curtailing, reinforcing, or otherwise influencing fantasies, that is, oedipal yearnings; such fantasies arose from within the individual as the ideational component of drives rather than from real experiences.

Despite these radical changes in the way he understood the mind to function and form symptoms, Freud retained basic premises of his developmental theory, namely, the libido theory

---

[1]Freud developed conviction about an independent aggressive drive only gradually over a number of years. Originally, in the *Three Essays*, he observed it clinically in the form of sadism and considered it a pregenital component of the sexual instinct. At the same time he wrote that it originated with the self-preservative, as opposed to the species-preservative, sexual instincts. He seemed to go back and forth on the matter until 1920 (*Beyond the Pleasure Principle*), when he formulated the more abstract, self-destructive death instinct, of which the aggressive drive was a derivative. From that point on he retained the idea of coequal sexual and aggressive drives (Strachey, 1961, editor's note, pp. 61–62).

and the pleasure principle. Rather, he shifted his attention toward the role of the individual's endowment compared to that of his environment. Nevertheless, during and after making this change in his orientation, Freud continued to refer to the importance in development of the individual's adaptation to his real experiences. For example, in *The Interpretation of Dreams*, Freud wrote that "the bitter experience of life" turned the infant from seeking gratification of drive wishes in hallucinations (based on the pleasure principle) to pursuing actual gratification from his environment (based on the reality principle) (1900, p. 566). And regarding the origins of developmental psychopathology, he wrote that Little Hans' castration complex derived from his mother's threat to have him castrated (1909, pp. 7–8). Nevertheless, Freud primarily investigated the ways in which experiences influenced drive pressures rather than the ways in which experiences influenced adaptation in the process of development.

From 1923 on, references to the importance of trauma, real experiences, and adaptation to the environment reemerged in Freud's writings. These appear scattered throughout his works. For example, anxiety was now understood not only as an anticipatory signal of danger erupting from within the individual; it was also the ego's response of helplessness when overwhelmed from without (i.e., from the environment) or from within (1926). Also, Freud identified paradigmatic danger situations in development related to the real experience of separation. These encompass a developmental progression from fear of loss of the parent, to fear of loss of the parent's love, to fear of castration, to fear of the superego (1926). Another example is his revised view of the manner in which the Oedipus complex arises and is resolved in girls and boys (see pp. 64–68); he specifically invokes the importance of real experiences, namely, observations of the anatomical differences between male and female genitals (1924, 1925b). Then there is identification, which basically amounts to imitation of parental behaviors or style, and which assumed greater importance in his view of the resolution of the Oedipus complex in both girls and boys (1923, 1924).

Such ideas about the importance of adapting to real experiences were added onto rather than reconciled with Freud's other ideas about development (e.g., 1924, pp. 173–174). In fact, his most cogent reformulation of the relationship between the child and his environment (parents) appears in "An Outline of Psychoanalysis" (1940) which was published posthumously. Thus, it is not surprising that a perusal of clinical articles in the psychoanalytic literature today leads to the conclusion that many therapists still do not apply Freud's later ideas in their therapeutic work.[2]

THE COMPLEMENTAL OR ETIOLOGICAL SERIES

Freud's consideration of innate and experiential factors in development led to the other premise upon which his theory of neurosis was based, namely, the complemental or etiological series: He posited a spectrum of causal factors in the development of neuroses. One end of the spectrum is the innate, reflecting an individual's endowment, heredity, or constitution (i.e., his or her nature). At the other end of the spectrum are environmental factors (i.e., his or her nurture). The cause of any individual's neurosis falls somewhere along this spectrum, with varying contributions from the innate and experiential (see Freud, 1895, editor's note, pp. 121–122).

FREUD'S DEVELOPMENTAL THEORY

Freud incorporated both the principle of constancy and the complemental series into his theory of development.

The Stimulus Barrier and Origin of Thinking. Additional features of Freud's developmental model have had a far-reaching influence on subsequent theory and research. These appear to have arisen from his premises about the susceptibility of organisms to being stimulated and the imperative to discharge excitation. He considered the newborn very vulnerable to stimulation from its environment. For he postulated that the infant is protected from external stimuli during the early months of life by a

---

[2]Hartmann and Erikson have also stressed the importance of adaptation in development. Hartmann's consideration is more theoretical/abstract (1939). Erikson's psychosocial model of development is more theoretical/clinical (1950, 1956).

biologically based stimulus barrier. Thus, the infant's attention is primarily focused on stimuli arising from within rather than from outside his or her body (Freud, 1920, p. 29; Esman, 1983); that internal milieu consisted of the infant's physiological needs. Freud (1905b) linked these normal physiological needs to the sexual component of the infant's inherited endowment. Thus, the earliest manifestations of the sexual drive arise in conjunction with suckling in response to hunger. The lips and mouth become the locus of age-appropriate sexual gratification (erogenous zone) in the form of nonnutritive sucking. The mother's breast is the object of the infant's nutritive and sexual desire. By so linking sexuality to other bodily functions such as feeding and defecation, it becomes easy to see how Freud could conclude that nonsexual functions like eating and bowel functions can be affected in neurotic illness.

As noted, the stimulus barrier kept the infant more focused on stimuli arising from inside itself. When hungry the infant would experience increasing excitation, with frustration mounting when the excitation went unrelieved. Freud postulated that this tension caused the infant to hallucinate his mother's breast. Thus, a cognitive mode developed to reduce tension as a substitute for real gratification. This process of hallucinating gratification initiated the infant's capacity to think. Only when this mechanism was insufficient to reduce tension would the infant become aware of the outside world (i.e., his mother). Thus, cognitive activity and the ability to mediate with the outside world developed postpartum from frustration of drive gratification and its accompanying feelings.

MENTAL OBJECT REPRESENTATION (PART TO WHOLE)

Freud thought that the infant initially conceived of the external world, his or her mother, as those parts of her which afforded the infant gratification, rather than perceiving her as a whole person. Thus, the breast was the first part object representation of the outside world. It was only during the second and third years, after many experiences with these part object representations, that the young child coalesced a gestalt of the mother as

one whole person and the same person who frustrated and gratified him.

THE ROLE OF OBJECT RELATIONSHIPS

The foregoing paragraphs document that Freud did not neglect
the role of object relationships in his theory; they represented
the environmental end of the complemental series; but his interest turned to drive development. Thus, his focus on object relationships centered on their role in gratifying and frustrating
discharge of the infant's drives. This process (gratification/frus-
tration) became the source of what Freud later called the origin
and development of the ego—the psychic structure which attempts to control drives and mediate between drive demands
and the outside world. This frustration/gratification paradigm
also accounted for the development of the superego; that
"grade" within the ego is the psychic repository of parental/
societal standards and expectations that became integrated into
the child's developing personality a few years after birth.

Only late in his career did Freud reassess his view of the
interaction between the child and its parents and emphasize the
degree to which the child strives to gratify the wishes of the important objects rather than its own drives in an effort to insure
his or her safety and security. This was different from his earlier
frustrating-the-infant aspect of object relationships, in which the
reality principle was only tolerated as a necessary means to the
end of pleasure principle gratification. These later ideas, which
I find crucial to understanding development, have never enjoyed
the popularity of his drive-centered theory.

SUMMARY AND STAGE PROGRESSION

In Freud's paradigm of development, the infant is inner-
directed, driven by physiological needs, relying first on fantasy to
achieve gratification and only attentive to the environment as a
last resort to reduce internal excitation. The role of the environment, the child's mother, is certainly to insure the infant's survival by fulfilling basic needs, but that only insures its physical

survival. Her major function is otherwise to optimally frustrate the infant's drives. For such proper balancing of frustration and gratification of drive wishes forces the infant both to begin thinking (the origin of mental life), and to engage with and adapt to the outside world. The infant's adaptation is accomplished by developing a psychic agency to mediate between inner wishes/ needs and the environment's limits; and, as a corollary, the infant develops mechanisms by which that agency can accomplish this task. These are the ego and its adaptive and defense mechanisms. Those defense mechanisms, which develop during the first year or oral stage, include denial, projection, and incorporation (considered by some an oral precursor of identification).

If the mother optimally balances frustration and gratification of the primarily oral based drives (and normal biological maturation of his motor apparatus also occurs), the infant progresses in the second year to a greater interest in his or her anal zone. The expulsion (and later, the retention) of feces now becomes a greater source of libidinal (sexual) pleasure than oral activities (sucking and biting). The environment's role in socializing the now toddler has its paradigm in toilet training. This is one of many types of experience in which the toddler learns to substitute self-control for pleasurable, immediate discharge of excitement/tension. Another commonplace example is the process by which the toddler is helped to forsake grabbing delicate objects. The defense mechanisms of the ego which have their roots in this anal phase include isolation (keeping things separate as stool in the toilet, thoughts from actions, and later, feelings from thoughts); reaction formation (reversing wishes to mess or to break things or to control and be aggressive into desires to be clean, careful, tractable, and loving toward rivals); and undoing (after-the-fact reversal of or regret for barbaric behavior).

LIBIDINAL FIXATION, ARREST, REGRESSION

If the environment is either too gratifying or too frustrating during either of these stages, or if the infant or toddler's endowment is loaded with high levels of drive for gratification from either the oral or anal erogenous zones, then the child can develop a fixation or arrest upon oral or anal gratification. Though he or she will progress to later psychosexual stages, these remain areas of vulnerability to which the child can regress when experiencing stress later in life. Depending upon its severity, such a factor predisposes the adult toward a preference for oral or anal gratification; or it becomes subsumed under the dominance of genital sexuality and is expressed in preferences for oral or anal (dominance/submission) foreplay; or it can predispose the individual to later neurosis and influence the choice of neurosis;[3] or it might lead to perversions. To Freud, perverse sexuality was nothing more than the persistence into adult life of preferences for pregenital (oral, anal, phallic) sexual gratification.

Concepts described in these latter paragraphs have had a profound influence on subsequent theories and research paradigms. These include the concepts of stage, that is, a stepwise, progression in development in which the consolidation of each stage evolves into the next one, and the ideas of arrest (developmental perspective), fixation (economic perspective), and regression (structural perspective) in the genesis of psychopathology.

More recently Erikson popularized a concept, attributed to Harvey in the fifteenth century, termed epigenesis, which relates sequential stage experiences to each other: The nature of a person's passage through any stage influences his or her experience during subsequent stages. This helps to explain the unique features of an individual's psychology within the confining commonalities of developmental experiences.

Freud termed the oral and anal stages the pregenital phase, thus separating them from the next one, to which the toddler progresses during his or her third year, the phallic–oedipal or genital phase.

AMENDMENTS AND REVISIONS TO FREUD'S THEORY OF THE PREGENITAL PHASE

These investigations have involved both ends of the complemental series. The earlier work focused on the environment while

---

[3]These ideas have persisted even though later Freudian child analysts have found no consistent correlation between the form of childhood neurosis and the later adult neurosis (A. Freud, 1965, pp. 151–152).

the more recent studies elaborate primarily upon the infant's innate endowment.

MAHLER'S SEPARATION–INDIVIDUATION THEORY

This theory, the most popular since Freud's and presented as supplemental and complementary to his psychosexual stages, was a natural next step after his ground-breaking ideas about development. Mahlerian researchers accepted drive theory, the pleasure principle/reality principle progression, and the libido theory-based concept that relatedness to others develops from autoerotism through narcissism to true object relatedness. They focused their investigations, however, on the mother–infant/ child relationship during the pregenital stages.

Also, unlike Freud who focused primarily on the developing ego's defensive reactions to drive frustration, Mahler and her co-workers studied the impact of threats posed by separation from its primary caretaker on the infant's developing identity. Thus, their interest is in the development and adaptation of the infant's ego capacities, as they emerge through a combination of interactions with his or her caretakers and maturation. This focus led it to becoming known as an object relations theory.

Mahler traces the roots of her theory to her observations of the mother–infant dyad. This led her to study infantile psychosis and then turn back to normal development (Mahler, Pine, and Bergman, 1975, p. 8). Notwithstanding this, her theory seems to have been profoundly influenced by her ideas about the core problems of children with autistic and symbiotic psychoses (Stern, 1985). So, Mahler's theory of development, like that of Freud, was strongly influenced initially by her theory and terminology of psychopathology, specifically infantile psychosis. These ideas in turn seem to have been greatly influenced by Freud's premises about the neonate's sensibility (see below).

SEPARATION–INDIVIDUATION

The separation–individuation process describes the "psychological birth of the infant." Individuation refers to the integration within individuals of those ego capacities which allow them to experience themselves as psychologically separate from mother and as individuals in their own right. Separation in her theory refers to the psychic experience of separateness from others, not the physical experience of separation.

Mahler and her coworkers defined four stages in this process. Progression from one stage to the next was accomplished by a combination of maturation and the same mechanism posited by Freud to explain movement through the psychosexual stages. That is optimal frustration, in this case of the infant and toddler's attachment behaviors to the mother.

The first phase, termed normal autism, encompasses the first few weeks after birth. Mahler's presumptions about the newborn, while identical to those of Freud, also rested on electroencephalographic (EEG) evidence regarding the P wave. The P wave, which was thought to indicate central nervous system processing of sensory inputs, did not appear until 1 to 2 months of age (Settlage, 1991, personal communication). A biological barrier against stimuli impinging from outside renders the infant primarily responsive to stimuli emanating from inside. The infant possesses little capacity even to perceive the outside world, and the newborn is essentially undifferentiated with regard to regulatory psychic structures. However, Mahler also emphasizes both the importance of an innate drive to individuate (Mahler et al., 1975, p. 9) and of maturational factors, especially locomotion, in propelling the infant forward (Settlage, 1974a). She also maintained a strong focus on adaptation. The latter ideas point to a neonate who is less of a tabula rasa than described by Freud.

At about 1 month of age, the combination of repetitive experiences with mother and maturation enables the infant to become aware of mother's existence, which is experienced as indistinguishable from the infant's own existence. The infant has now entered the symbiotic phase of "dual unity," and feelings of omnipotence emerge at this stage. The infant, unable to differentiate those tension-reducing efforts which emanate from him- or herself from those which mother provides, basks in the delusion that the power to minister to his or her every need is shared with mother.

At about four to five months, the separation–individuation process begins, with the infant "hatching" from the nondifferentiated state to beginning awareness of self versus nonself. This is enabled, fostered, and facilitated (or hindered and derailed) by the nature and quality of mother's interactions with the infant during the next four to five months, and by maturation of the motor and sensory apparatus.

This period of rapid differentiation, with the infant's increasing awareness of his or her own capacities (particularly motor functions), and growing interest in the outside world, culminates in the practicing subphase; this takes place between approximately 10 and 15 months. Borrowing Greenacre's term from another context, Mahler characterized the toddler's behavior in this phase as a "love affair with the world." This refers to the air of exhilaration communicated by toddlers when using their new ambulatory abilities to explore that part of their environment to which they can perambulate. They return to their mothers frequently for "emotional refueling." In contrast to the close physical proximity they maintained to her during the prior period and the apprehension they will experience when feeling too long or far away from her during the next phase, practicing toddlers seem relatively self-contained and independent of their mothers' nurturance. A full flowering of their elated mood during this practicing phase has been considered important for future self-esteem regulation (Settlage, 1974a).

Then, between about 14 and 22 months, these independent toddlers again become more dependent upon their mothers' presence, albeit at a higher level of interaction, because they are now developing language. This rapprochement subphase is predicated on enhanced cognitive and emotional awareness of separateness from mother. The toddlers now realize that mother can leave them, and that the omnipotent state of dual unity does not exist. The sensitivity with which mothers help toddlers deal with the inevitable deflation of those feelings of omnipotence is considered by Mahlerian researchers to have profound effects on later development; the features affected encompass self-esteem regulation and characterological mood states, and later psychopathology, including depression.

If the environment (mothers) facilitates toddlers' adaptation to this awareness, and they do not have special, constitutional (inherited) problems which preclude being able to respond to an average expectable environment, then toddlers are "on the way to" object constancy; this is achieved at a first level around the age of 36 months. This culmination of the separation–individuation process is characterized by the achievement of a capacity to retain an inner sense of the mother's safety-providing qualities; this enables the individuated child to retain a sense of security during mother's protracted absence. This achievement, termed libidinal object constancy, constitutes the primary basis in Mahlerian theory for psychological separateness and independence from other people.

The term *autonomy* has referred to different developmental conflicts in different theories. In Freudian theory it has been associated with self-control of both voluntary activity and sphincters, developing during the anal, pregenital phase. In Erikson's psychosocial theory it is the healthier pole of his second stage. As currently used, it seems to refer to inner independence from a compulsive/pervasive influence of another, at base the parents. Given this definition, autonomy and libidinal object constancy might most accurately be considered as different phenomena. Libidinal object constancy may relate to an inner sense of security, stability of mood, and self-confidence. But it may have only partial relevance to the broader based concept of psychological autonomy. The interpersonal factors which are important in the achievement of libidinal object constancy are different from factors which determine autonomy. The point of reference for libidinal object constancy is what toddlers accrue to themselves from the quality of their mother's constancy, consistency, and dependability. This may be a necessary but not sufficient condition for autonomy. Other dimensions of the mother–infant/child experience are involved in autonomy, importantly including the toddlers' accrued perceptions of their mothers' needs of them.

Mahler's theory is appealing on several counts. It gives credence to the infant's drives, but also places more weight on the importance of the nuances and totality of the mother–child relationship. The latter had been given short shift by Freud's emphasis on an individual driven from birth by drives which are simply blunted by his object relationships, forcing the detour through the reality principle to drive satisfaction. Freud's theory seemed a flatter, more two-dimensional representation of development.

From a historical perspective, separation–individuation theory was also appealing because it continued Freud's tradition of offering a developmental perspective on psychological illnesses. Many efforts to force all diagnostic conditions into some relationship to the Oedipus complex had proven unsatisfactory, however, from the standpoints of both adequately explaining the behavioral, ideational, and emotional phenomena of some psychiatric conditions and of helping to cure them. Separation–individuation theory held out the promise of explicating some pathology better than that of Freud. And what seems to have eventuated in recent years is that separation–individuation, particularly the rapprochement subphase conflict (i.e., fears versus wishes) over re-merging to a symbiotic state of psychological fusion/organization with another person, has come to replace the Oedipus complex and sexuality as the linchpin of much psychopathology, including borderline conditions, perversions, character pathology, depression, and eating disorders.

Infant research beginning in the 1970s and 1980s, using cleverly devised experiments, calls into question some basic theoretical premises of separation–individuation theory (Stern, 1985). Even if this accumulating data prove replicable, it is important not to lose sight of the basic ways in which Mahler and Freud advanced developmental psychology. By emphasizing the importance of environmental as well as internal contributants, Freud offset the then prevailing view that vicissitudes of development reflected hereditary taints. Mahler stimulated thinking away from the drive model to features of ego development through interpersonal experiences. Like Kohut more recently, Mahlerians served a rejuvenating function for practitioners and researchers, broadening their thinking about clinical and developmental phenomena, and keeping the field of psychoanalytic developmental psychology from stagnation.

BOWLBY'S ATTACHMENT THEORY

A competing theory to that of Mahler, developed during the same period, is Bowlby's attachment theory (1969, 1973, 1980).

It did not become a significant competitor in the minds of clinicians until publication of the more recent research on the infant's endowment provided findings which more readily fit within the framework of Bowlby's theory than that of Mahler.

Both of the latter theories have been extended to the whole life span; however, the research on which they are based has been focused on the period from ages 6 months to 3 years. Separation experiences are the primary source of research data for both groups of investigators. Separation–individuation theory focuses on the achievement of psychological separateness as the aim of development, while attachment theory posits attachment, that is, close physical proximity, as the ongoing aim of the child during these years. Thus, attachment theory posits the capacity for relationship from earliest on, rather than the need to develop a sense of one's individuated self as a prerequisite for forming attachments. Separation in attachment theory refers to an interpersonal event; separation in separation–individuation theory refers to an intrapsychic experience (Lieberman, 1987).

Bowlby derived his theory from studies of the effects on children of separation from and loss of their parents. It has roots in both psychoanalysis and ethology: The former are seen in his premise that attachment is a drive-driven behavior in its own right, akin to and on a par with drives for food and the dual sexual and aggressive drives of Freud's system. The ethological root can be identified in Bowlby's understanding of this drive for attachment as necessary for species survival; object relationships, or as he calls them, affectional relationships, are necessary for survival of the individual in the species and for the survival of the species itself (Bloom-Feshbach and Bloom-Feshbach, 1987, p. 26; Lieberman, 1987, pp. 113–114). It is not just relatedness which is being sought, but a specific kind, one in which the offspring feels secure and safe when interacting with primary caretakers.

Bowlby finds a universal pattern of response in young children to physical separation from their attachment figures. It comprises a three-step progression, depending on the length of the separation. The child's initial reaction is one of protest (loud expression of anger and tears). This is followed by a phase of despair (sadness, misery, grieving-type behavior). Then, if the separation is protracted, the specific length depending on the age of the child and other factors, the child exhibits detachment (avoidance of feelings associated with the attachment figure, and an attitude of seeming uninterest in the mother). Bowlby attributes the detachment to a massive defense against anger felt toward the mother. This same sequence of overt behaviors might well be compatible with Mahlerians' observations, although they would attribute detachment to libidinal object constancy not having been achieved (i.e., a lack of psychic structure). Attachment theory posits an infant who, at least from age 6 months, is preadapted in the sense of sufficiently neurologically developed to make an emotional bond with his mother.

RECENT EMPIRICAL STUDIES ON INFANT DEVELOPMENT

This sophisticated research has presented the most compelling challenge to psychoanalytic developmental theory and to those object relations theories which arose from psychoanalytic premises. Stern (1985) has summarized much of this research in conjunction with presenting his own empirical findings. These experimental studies have essentially expanded our understanding of what are known in psychoanalysis as the autonomous functions of the ego. These are ego functions not bred from conflict, though able to be drawn into intrapsychic conflict, like vision in hysterical blindness and motor function in hysterical paralysis. By establishing with greater precision the scope of infants' inborn endowment, these researchers have documented capacities which are not compatible with the assumptions and presumptions of the other theories. They find that infants are born with many more capabilities for ordering their experience and that they also demonstrate greater interest in engaging their environment from the first days of extrauterine life than the psychoanalytic view attributes to them (Osofsky, 1987).

In addition to being more socially oriented and with a more sophisticated endowment, infants exhibit abilities to group, order, sort, identify gestalts, and thus to abstract from experiences in nonverbal ways. The latter conclusion, accounted for by neurological connections, also calls into question long-standing

Piagetian ideas about how cognitive development occurs, and specifically the manner and age of onset of the capacity to deal with things abstractly. Stern (1985) concludes that infants are "prewired" for social interaction; he characterizes the process of development as the "continuous unfolding of an intrinsically determined social nature" (p. 234).

Infants seem to seek stimulation from early in life, for they are observed to quickly lose interest in repetitious stimuli, as measured by changes in heart rate (habituation) and by gaze aversion. Furthermore, from very early they use other modalities as prominently as the mouth to relate to and engage the outside world. These include vision, which is highly developed at birth, and hearing. Such observations are not compatible with a concept of development based on the pleasure–constancy principle (Freud, 1915, p. 121; 1920, p. 9), in which the infant tries to reduce stimulation to the lowest level. Such findings also raise questions about the legitimacy of having defined developmental stage progression solely in terms of features of the concept of erogenous zones (oral, anal, etc.).

It has long been known that infants seem to seek contact but turn away when their visual overtures are not responded to by caretakers (Provence and Lipton, 1962). Consistent observations that the infant actively engages his or her environment and is seemingly preoccupied with and learning from these real experiences, however, call into question the relative importance of fantasy over reality in the infant's psychological development. It will be recalled that psychoanalytic theory posits that cognitive activity, in the form of wish-fulfilling hallucinations, arises as the early infant's response to frustration. In Stern's view (1985), "ego instincts" and the reality principle must at least coexist from birth with the pleasure principle and libidinal drives, rather than follow them in development. Even granting the possibility that drive pressures arise in conjunction with physiological needs, these findings present a serious challenge ultimately to the psychoanalytic theory of neurosis. It will be recalled that in the psychoanalytic view, children's fantasies and wishes rather than their experiences are ultimately considered the culprits in necessitating symptom formation. Developmental researchers' studies raise questions about whether the kind of fantasies that

Freudians maintain arise ontogenetically from drive pressures, like the Oedipus complex during later verbal (postsymbolic expression) periods of development, exist or at least arise in this manner. Nor do the findings of the recent developmental studies support the validity of Kleinian ideas, currently experiencing a resurgence of popularity, which carry Freud's ideas to the extreme by positing intense, object-directed aggressive wishes and fantasies in earliest infancy as the driving forces of development and symptom formation.

These more recent conclusions have been based on studies such as the following:

From birth, the natural states of infants' level of arousal include periods of "alert inactivity" (Wolff, 1966). These intervals are initially brief but progressively increase in length. During these intervals the infant seems to be actively studying and taking in the immediate environment visually (not orally). This well-accepted finding casts doubt on both the Freudian view of an exclusively inward directed, stimulus barrier-protected infant and the normal autistic newborn phase of Mahlerian theory (Stern, 1985).

Experiments to determine the infant's capabilities can be conducted during these periods of attentiveness to the environment. Measures of response used in these experiments include such behaviors as looking, sucking, and turning of the (supported) head, all of which the infant is capable of at birth. Thus, for example, selective head-turning of newborns to the side of their own mother's breast pad led researchers to conclude that newborns can distinguish their own mother's milk by smell.

Infants between 3 and 4 weeks of age exhibit amodal or cross-modal perception. This refers to being able to transfer information from one perceptual system to another. It implies functioning neural connections between different sensory systems. For example, 26- to 33-day-old infants were blindfolded and then given either a smooth or a nubbed pacifier to suck, and then shown both, after the blindfolds are removed. A statistically significant number of the infants concentrated their gaze on the pacifiers they had just sucked (Meltzoff and Borton, 1979). Constellations of such findings suggest that the infant can perceive and then conceive whole object representations (gestalts) from the outset or close to the outset of extrauterine life. This finding calls into question the validity of theories which consider that infants initially perceive and conceive part object representations which later coalesce into whole object representations. Such findings undermine the developmental rationale for currently popular explanations of psychopathology that is characterized as borderline. These patients are thought to split their object representations within their egos, based on problems in developing object constancy during the pregenital stage. So, if the concept of splitting is valid, it is either a later developing capacity rather than a developmental failure, or else that particular developmental premise about the basis of borderline psychopathology needs to be reexamined.

While one cannot legitimately criticize one theory simply by invoking another one, the developmental researchers' observations challenge psychoanalytic theory to prove that the infant is more inward than reality oriented/directed/interested, and motivated by genetically developing fantasies stemming from two drives rather than from his interpretation of real experiences which are influenced by multiple motivations. These issues must be addressed and reconciled in order for Freudian theory to remain credible, and efforts are underway to integrate these new findings about infancy into Freudian clinical theory (Lichtenberg, 1983, 1989; Cramer, 1987; Emde, 1988a,b, 1991; Lichtenberg and Kindler, 1994).

From empirical studies of infants and their caregivers, Emde (1988a,b) has identified a set of inborn motives which are brought to fruition by an emotionally responsive caregiver. These motives are described as activity, self-regulation, social fittedness, affective monitoring, and cognitive assimilation (Emde, 1991). The idea of cognitive assimilation refers to a "biological propensity to process information, to structuralize such information according to what is familiar, and, more broadly, to seek out novelty" (1991, p. 36). This concept is consonant with one of the two basic ways in which Piaget considered that experience is integrated, namely assimilating the perception of the new experience in terms of one's previous perceptions or models (Bowlby, 1973, p. 172; Emde, 1991, p. 36). Emde also makes a good case for the importance of positive emotions as a motivational system which propels development independently from the system involving negative emotions. This proposition about positive emotions contrasts with the classical Freudian view that pleasure, rather than serving an expansive motivating function, is basically the experience of relief from unpleasurable tension.

From the research literature and clinical experience, Lichtenberg (1989) has extrapolated an integrated set of independent motivational systems which continue to interact dynamically throughout life, albeit in more sophisticated ways than during infancy. These five motivational systems are, respectively, the need for psychic regulation of physiological requirements; for attachment-affiliation; for exploration and assertion; to react aversively through antagonism or withdrawal; and for sensual enjoyment and sexual excitement. Lichtenberg's motivational systems are basic needs of the individual derived from "lived experience" (p. 2). Motives in Emde's model are inborn functional abilities that are capitalized upon to greatest developmental advantage by responsive interaction on the part of the infant's caregivers. Thus, a positively responding environment is a crucial feature of the models of development posited by both Lichtenberg and Emde. Most significant for our purposes is that both these sets of motivations are primarily involved with adapting to the environment. That is, the motivations in development posited by both Lichtenberg and Emde are most readily reconciled with the adaptive metapsychological point of view of Freudian psychology. The adaptive point of view is the one that relates the intrapsychic to the interpersonal, the individual to his or her environment. Thus, the importance of the individual's real interactions as opposed to inner-derived wishes, is emphasized in the research that is attempting to find common ground between Freudian developmental theory and recent empirical infant research. And this common ground seems to be the adaptive or adaptational perspective. Also, both models of infant development, but particularly that of Emde, seem consonant with the existence of strivings to complete development.

The object relations theorists (such as Mahler, Winnicott, Guntrip, and Kernberg) maintain that the infant separates himself psychologically from an undifferentiated or fused mother–infant state. Based on the type of data I have outlined, Stern (1985) suggests that the infant does not separate a sense of his psychological self from the environment. Rather, he has the wired-in outlines of himself from the outset. If anything, he separates the environment from his inherent, emerging sense of himself. This implies that rather than being an achievement of development during the first three years of life, the core of autonomy, namely a sense of oneself as separate from others, is more or less a given and autonomy an issue of the whole life span. The influence of development on autonomy is to define its unique qualities in the individual.

Just as Mahler's work represented a logical next step after Freud, adding understanding to an area which he had not studied as thoroughly (ego and object relations), the recent developmental research seems a natural next step after Mahler; it focuses more on the areas not studied by her, and has been facilitated by the development of more sophisticated experimental apparatus. We might anticipate that although developmentalists are trying to keep each pole of the complemental series in focus, the next advances will be made from understanding more about the environmental side.

FREUD: THE PHALLIC–OEDIPAL STAGE

Rather than tracing the evolution of Freud's ideas about this stage, I will summarize his penultimate and ultimate conclusions, and their influence on development in boys and girls.

All previous autoerotic and object-related components of the sexual instinct (oral, anal, sadistic, scoptophilic–exhibitionistic) now become subordinated and organized under the dominance of genital interests with a specific object for the young child's love in mind, namely, the parent. This is the oedipal part of the term *phallic-oedipal.* This newly evolved psychological organization is precisely similar to that which will subsequently occur when sexual development culminates at puberty—with one important distinction. At puberty all prior expressions of sexuality become subordinated to the genitals in the service of reproducing the species; the pregenital components retain expression in forepleasure, and the anatomical distinctions between male and female genitals are recognized accurately by boys and girls. By contrast, during the phallic phase, both boys and girls believe that there is only one genital, the male one (phallus). This explains the phallic part of the term *phallic-oedipal.* The reaction of both boys and girls to this realization has the most profound effect on development; it is responsible for the formation (in girls) and the resolution (in boys) of the Oedipus complex.

INITIAL AND LATER CONCEPTIONS OF OEDIPUS COMPLEX RESOLUTION

Freud originally thought that both boys and girls resolve the Oedipus complex in the same manner. Boys wish to cohabit with their mothers and eliminate their fathers, and girls wish for the opposite experience. Disappointments in their efforts to realize these wishes motivate both sexes away from these goals. Additional clinical experience, however, led Freud to a much more complicated formulation of the way in which boys and girls resolve their Oedipus complexes (Freud, 1924, 1925b).

He decided that when boys and girls observe genital differences they conclude that some females have been castrated, rather than that females have different genitals. That is, there are two states—male (phallic) and castrated, rather than male and female. In boys this generates anxiety associated with the idea that they too can lose their genitals (castration anxiety). The response in girls to considering themselves castrated is to experience more penis envy than castration anxiety.

BIPHASIC NATURE OF THE OEDIPUS COMPLEX

Clinical experience persuaded Freud that the oedipal complex itself is a double-phased phenomenon. This was based on Fliess' idea that humans are inherently bisexual—capable of and tending to absorb or adopt the sexual characteristics of either sex. Thus, in moving from preoedipal, dyadic relationships to oedipal, triadic ones, the boy and girl experience both sides of the triangle—loving the same-sexed parent and hating the opposite-sexed one (the negative oedipal constellation), as well as the better-known positive complex. Freud's very last ideas on the subject, published posthumously by a collaborator, Ruth Mack

Brunswick (1940), suggested that he felt more attention should be paid to the active versus passive role of the child with respect to the love object in each constellation, rather than equating passivity with femininity and activity with masculinity. The conventions of positive and negative complexes and the sex-linked associations of passivity and activity have nonetheless persisted.[4]

VICISSITUDES IN THE RESOLUTION OF THE OEDIPUS COMPLEX

Freud had also come to realize that the first love object of both boys and girls is their mother. So, girls have to change the sex of the object of their love from female to male as well as the zone of their genital sexual excitement from the male, phallic, clitoral zone to the vagina in order to establish reproductive desire (mature genitality). Boys by contrast have to make neither of those shifts. Becoming aware that females have no penis, at a time when caretakers are threatening him with castration for masturbating, motivates the boy to relinquish his sexual desire for his mother in favor of self-preservation, thereby saving his penis. This occurs by a process in which he gives up sexual interest in his mother and substitutes an identification with his father and the father's proscriptions and values. This is the prototype of the defense mechanism termed identification with the aggressor, even though its basic underlying component of turning passive into active is observed prior to the oedipal stage. Also, because

---

[4]The persistence of this convention may reflect a holdover from the cultural values of Freud's society in which passivity was considered a desirable trait in women. The persistence may also reflect an element of the inertia which characterizes change in psychological ideas. It is as likely though that this convention has persisted because Freud was trying to understand the implications of a difference which may exist between women and men. But by characterizing as passivity the discomforts and limitation of activity which women uniquely endure during defloration, menstruation, pregnancy, and childbearing, Freud may have misrepresented the effect on girls' development of any psychological anticipation of these later experiences by using a term that implied a less desirable trait than activity, at least in our culture. Had he instead considered these uniquely female experiences to represent the active pursuit of passive aims, the outcome of which is the ability to bear pain and to develop superior stamina, then Freud would have anticipated the results of more recent psychological research on physical strength and endurance in women compared to men, which traits including stoicism are considered admirable in our culture.

of bisexuality, an identification with his mother (who has also threatened him with castration) becomes part of this new identification which Freud characterized as a grade in the ego, and termed the superego, the psychic agency which mediates conscience function. Furthermore, while oedipal yearnings are literally dissolved in this creation of the superego, "the heir to the Oedipus complex" (Freud, 1923, p. 48), because he still loves both parents as well, the boy retains affectionate feelings toward his mother (a desexualized and repressed sexual component), and he becomes passive toward his father (negative oedipal complex). The latter complex has been assigned to the whole of the oedipal stage because of the importance Freud attached to bisexuality (Freud, 1923); but it seems to me most logical from Freud's own formulation that it follow the positive Oedipus complex and merge into the ensuing latency phase as the narcissistic, admiring attachment of the boy to his father, epitomized by the "my dad can beat up your dad" attitude.

The situation in girls is much different. Awareness of genital differences, which has prompted boys to give up their positive oedipal complex, causes the development of the positive Oedipus complex in girls. Disappointment in their mothers, for not having given them the desired penis, motivates girls to turn from their intense love of mother to love for father, in hopes of acquiring a penis from him in the form of a baby; that is, in a compensatory manner, girls unconsciously equate baby with penis. Moreover, castration anxiety never has the same impact on girls as it does on boys, because girls are already "castrated." Thus, the boy's strong self-preservative motive for resolving his Oedipus complex does not exist for the girl. This explains why girls both linger in their oedipal relationships and exhibit oedipal feelings more openly than do boys, who resolve them quickly and move on to the latency phase. Ultimately, fear of losing her mother's love motivates the girl to resolve her Oedipus complex, through identification mechanisms similar to those adopted by boys.

DIFFERENCES IN SUPEREGO FORMATION

Lacking the castration anxiety motive, however, girls repress their incestuous feelings more than they dissolve them. That factor accounted for females developing superegos which were qualitatively different from those of males. Specifically, Freud concluded that women are less unswerving with respect to standing by principles and more readily swayed by emotion. As such, their superegos are less impersonal than those of men. Freud concluded from those observations that the conscience of women is less strong than that of men. While he seemed to be emphasizing the differences more than making value judgments, the fact that he never considered that a penchant for judgment tempered by a sense of humanity might be as or more desirable, suggests that he was devaluing women's conscience function. Although those conclusions have brought him to grief in some quarters, some recent research has supported Freud's idea of differences in superego functioning of men and women along the lines he identified (Gilligan, 1982, 1986). Other recent research has not confirmed the ideas of Freud and Gilligan that the consciences of men and women function consistently or predominantly in these different ways. Rather, the tendency of the individual, male or female, to utilize a principled as opposed to a humanitarian approach in facing any moral dilemma is very situation-specific rather than sex-specific; the individual's approach depends on features like his or her familiarity with the situation and whether it is a real or hypothetical problem (Torney-Purta, 1990; Keating, 1990). My own clinical experience favors the latter conclusions. In any event, even if Freud did accurately describe a difference between the conscience functioning of men and women, his own explanation for the phenomenon is not necessarily accurate.

AN ALTERNATE UNDERSTANDING OF THE RELATIONSHIP BETWEEN CASTRATION ANXIETY, PENIS ENVY, AND THE OEDIPUS COMPLEX/OEDIPAL STAGE

Presumptive evidence of castration anxiety (e.g., touching and holding one's crotch, heightened fear of injury) is much more frequently observed in oedipal-aged boys than either direct expressions of oedipal yearnings or defenses against them. In light of this, it is pertinent to realize that Freud first brought the Oedipus complex and the castration complex together into one complex many years after he first described each.[5] Thus, it is possible

[5]Briefly, they arose independently and took somewhat parallel courses. The Oedipus complex apparently originated from his own analysis and turned him

that they are independent phenomena, and that each has a source different from Freud's idea that they are amalgamated by the threat of castration associated with oedipal yearnings. Castration anxiety, the more prevalent phenomenon, probably arises normally, as does penis envy (see below), from children's reactions to observed anatomical differences rather than from oedipal strivings. Children are acute observers and are sensitive to differences between people. Also, having more than someone else seems inherently to be considered preferable to having less than others. So, girls observing genital differences wish for boys' genitals (without necessarily wanting to be boys) and boys observing girls' genitals worry about losing their own. Oedipal yearning, on the other hand, rather than being a prominent, preordained developmental phenomenon, is usually a response of certain children to experiences with their parents or to psychic trauma. Thus, castration anxiety is a more normal, developmentally precipitated phenomenon and oedipal anxiety a more environmentally precipitated phenomenon. That is, there is a larger developmental component to castration anxiety and a larger environment-induced component to oedipal anxiety.

Castration anxiety and penis envy are the more common phenomena in normal development. The way children come to grips with castration anxiety and penis envy involves many factors, in which their own experiences are important. By contrast, I have found that whenever evidence of oedipal conflicts are clinically apparent and sustained rather than mild and fleeting, then as noted, there has been either psychic trauma in the family or the child–parent relationships are problematic.[6]

---

from his traumatic theory to infantile sexuality beginning in 1897 (Letters 69, 71). It was mentioned in *The Interpretation of Dreams* (1900), elaborated in the Dora case and the *Three Essays* (1905a,b), named in 1910, but not linked to the castration complex until 1913 (*Totem and Taboo*) (Calogeras and Schupper, 1972). Ideas about castration anxiety developed around symbols in dreams (1900), where he talked about oedipal dreams and castration dreams in children on the same page without connecting them (Ghannam, 1985). He mentioned it only in passing in the *Three Essays*, elaborated it as the conscious aspect of the more hidden Oedipus complex in 1908 ("On the Sexual Theories of Children"), and related it to awareness that women have no penis in 1910.

[6]Kohut (1982) maintained that the Oedipus complex only appears as a parricidal and incestuous constellation when the parent's self is "flawed" (p. 404). Jung (1917) had earlier considered the Oedipus complex to be an effort to cure development which had gone awry, and Adler (1938) concluded that

This different slant on the Oedipus complex and oedipal stage in normal development has particular relevance to the child–parent relationship throughout development. To frame this in terms which adhere more strictly to Freud's paradigm, psychological development is promoted by the parent optimally balancing gratification and frustration of the infant's and child's drives. Because some tension, dissatisfaction, and frustration is inevitable on the part of the infant/child, ambivalence in the sense of harboring negative as well as positive feelings toward the parent develops. In normal development the positive feelings outweigh the negative feelings toward the parents. This is accomplished or promoted from the parents' side by presenting conditions in which the child is relatively willing to forsake gratification of his or her impulses in favor of gratifying their (parental) wishes. The parents' role is one of providing age-appropriate nurturance and protection from which the developing child gains a sense of security. And while I believe from clinical work and observation that children have an inherent sense of security built into their strivings to complete development, this inner-generated sense of security is susceptible to influence from parental attitudes and behaviors.

According to Freudian theory, this general tone of the child–parent interaction is interrupted during the oedipal stage (and again at puberty) by internally generated hostility toward parents; this is preordained (spontaneously generated) in boys and prompted by frustration in girls. Without those two wrinkles of parricidal and incestuous urges, the nature and quality of the child–parent relationship remains more continuous throughout the course of development. Thus, the basic developmental conflict is different from oedipal conflict; it more continuously and undistractedly involves achieving one's autonomy through the maintenance of a secure relationship with parents rather than by avoiding the anticipated consequences of incestuous conflicts.

Some young children do exhibit possessiveness toward one parent and make efforts to exclude the other. In such cases I

---

the Oedipus complex is an unnatural response to maternal overindulgence. Thus, each of those authors considered the Oedipus complex to be a pathological formation (see also Calogeras and Schupper [1972]).

find that these behaviors much more often reflect the child's effort to gain the security-providing attention of the desired parent rather than to realize incestuous and parricidal wishes. Freud (1912) himself identified the "affectionate current" of love as older than the "sensual current" and based on the "self-preservative instinct" which was "directed to the members of the family and those who look after the child" (p. 180). These observations are congruent with my conclusion that this most important feature of the child–parent relationship, the wish to retain a positive relationship with parents, is continuous throughout development and a prerequisite for achieving psychological independence.

AN EXAMPLE OF THE OEDIPUS COMPLEX

The Oedipus complex is unconscious and thus under normal circumstances difficult to detect. When clinically evident, I have inevitably found that it has formed in response to a seductive or possessive or foundering or otherwise traumatizing interaction with a parental figure rather than from sexual desire in the child. The arousal of incestuous wishes and their integration with castration anxiety into an Oedipus complex occurs when a child attempts to reconcile normative castration anxiety or penis envy with traumatic experiences with parents. Thus, the relationship between castration anxiety and oedipal anxiety is opposite from Freud's paradigm quoted above in which the child experiences oedipal desire and later castration anxiety. I find that children develop castration anxiety (and penis envy) first on the basis of observations of genitals and subsequently, in their efforts to adapt to real experiences, can elaborate a developmentally incapacitating Oedipus complex as the following example illustrates:

> A 7-year-old boy presented with depressive and phobic symptoms, a lack of peer relationships, poor school performance, and avoidance of his father. The depressive features included a loss of his "joie de vivre" and intense self-criticism. The phobic elements included an inability to remain home alone (for fear of a burglar) or to leave his house unaccompanied (for fear of being attacked by a knife-wielding man). Night fears of monsters kept him from

venturing from his bed to the bathroom. He had just begun second grade with the "fast" group, but became so anxious when the child at the next desk seemed to be getting ahead of him that he would bluff his answers and was failing to learn.

At the age of 4 years, 8 months, he had had a tonsillectomy for which he was prepared psychologically and after which he had exhibited no psychiatric symptoms. Then, three months later, his career naval officer father was almost killed in a recreational boating accident while he was on leave. The boy had been furious that his father had not taken him on that outing. In the immediate aftermath of the accident the boy became uncontrollably anxious, voicing certainty that his angry thoughts had magical power and had caused his father's accident. Then, dating from the time when it became clear that his father would recover completely, the symptoms of the boy's neurosis began to develop and progressed increasingly until he was referred for psychoanalysis.

Blatant oedipal themes dominated his play during treatment. For example, in one typical sequence he had gained possession of the "king's jewel"; however, he lamented, "I've got it—but if I keep it, the cops will come and get me; but if I get rid of it, I won't be the richest person in the world anymore." Fears of retaliation for his wishes to have what wasn't his became supplanted by self-punitive demands. He concluded that his tonsillectomy had been punishment for having caused his father's accident. (He had reversed the sequence of events in his mind. This suggests that he had been attempting to develop cognitive understanding of why bad things had happened to him. His motive for doing so was to reverse the psychologically traumatic effects of the tonsillectomy and his father's accident [Weiss, Sampson, and the Mt. Zion Psychotherapy Research Group, 1986].) He developed a comparable, intense oedipal transference characterized by anxious, intense rivalry and hostility toward the analyst as well as an intense desire to monopolize his mother. Complete resolution of his neurosis was accomplished by interpretation and working through in the transference of his oedipal conflicts in relation to his fears and guilts about having a destructive impact on others.

While oedipal conflicts were significantly curtailing this child's development, physical traumata to both son and father, which were psychologically traumatic for the boy, were critical elements in the development of his oedipal conflicts and his illness. Traditional psychoanalysis typically relates such phenomena in the following way: Real experiences which coincide with normal developmental conflicts have the effect of intensifying and making the developmental issue more difficult to resolve (Coren and Saldinger, 1967). In this case, his father's near death at a time when this boy was experiencing the psychological aftermath of his tonsillectomy and presumably a normative oedipal conflict, served to confirm that his hostile wishes could come true. This boy's explanation in treatment was that his father's accident had confirmed his own idea that he had magic power; and for weeks afterward the little boy had gone around trying to put spells on people to determine whether he in fact did have such influence. The power to have had such a devastating impact on others rather than a parricidal wish seemed to be the greatest source of this lad's anxiety.

Sexual and aggressive drives are important in normal development, but their importance arises in direct proportion to their biological strength in the individual. Thus, sexual and aggressive urges normally become important after puberty, not during the period designated in Freudian theory as the phallic–oedipal phase. The degree to which such urges are prominent in a child's sensibility before adolescence is primarily a result of that child's experiences rather than his or her sexual or aggressive drives.

PENIS ENVY

Turning to these developmental phenomena in girls, observations of penis envy are too frequent and widespread, even if not universal, to be disputed on political bases. For example:

> A class of 3- to 4-year-olds, exposed to coeducational bathroom facilities, was sent into a turmoil. The mothers reported their daughters were experimenting with the standing position. One little girl wailed that she wished she had a pony tail like the little boys. Another became depressed, openly expressed her wish for a penis, and grew increasingly abusive of her baby brother, calling him "Peter Penis." Many of the girls took to hanging ornaments around their waists that dangled in the manner of a penis; a few, even more insistent, took to hiding bulky articles in their underpants [Marasse and Hart, 1975, p. 115].

The motive for penis envy may be different from that posited by Freud, namely that girls want to be boys. It would appear that some do but probably most do not. A more frequent motive was revealed when a 4-year-old girl announced to her mother that she wanted a penis. Her mother, taken by surprise and a bit aback asked, "You mean you want to be a boy?" "No," replied her daughter, "I want to be a girl with a penis." A 10-year-old in analysis may also have offered a more accurate explanation for this phenomenon than did Freud. She was reflecting on a previously acknowledged wish to pull off the penis of her boyfriend and of her analyst, about which she no longer evinced interest. When asked why she thought she had had such wishes, she replied, "Little kids want everything." She was observing that children are very sensitive to differences, especially of more and less, and that penis envy has less to do with sexuality than it does with not having what others do.

EFFECT OF THE OEDIPUS COMPLEX ON OBJECT RELATEDNESS

The traditional view holds that the child moves from being able to be involved only in two-person relationships to becoming engaged in three-person relationships during the oedipal stage. Since boys resolve their oedipal attachments more quickly and definitively than do girls, boys move on to latency with greater toleration for a peer group than do girls. Girls, by contrast, remain more involved with jealousies and cliques, that is, competitive rivalries in which two girls exclude a third. The reverse situation occurs in adolescence: Adolescent girls resolve their resurgent Oedipus complexes relatively quickly and move on to interest in and dating older boys. Boys by contrast take a long time resolving their recrudescent oedipal conflicts at puberty and move toward girls more slowly. These distinct patterns are frequently observed, and only the earlier interest of girls in boys can be explained by the fact that the process of puberty begins at a younger age in girls.

DEFENSE MECHANISMS WHICH DEVELOP DURING THE PHALLIC–OEDIPAL STAGE

Repression occurs with resolution of the Oedipus complex (though Mahler, Pine, and Bergman state [1975, p. 211] and

Kernberg [1966, pp. 247–248] has implied that it is a factor in development during the second year of life). The outcome of repression is the ability to differentiate between inner and outer reality. This suggests that conflicts can now be intrapsychic, not just interpersonal, thus necessitating defense mechanisms. Displacement, which develops as a way of dealing with sexual interests and questions, such as where babies come from and sexual differences, becomes the basis of another defense mechanism, sublimation. Boys move toy cars in and through tunnels, or begin to build structures. Girls play with baby dolls and create domestic scenes, and some girls and boys become interested in drawing and painting. The third defense mechanism which becomes elaborated during this phase, identification with the aggressor, was mentioned earlier in relation to oedipal resolution.

In summary, Freud felt that the Oedipus complex arises in boys on an inherited, genetic basis, and under normal circumstances its dissolution occurs in a preordained manner. In girls, however, the Oedipus complex arises as a secondary, compensatory phenomenon, in response to penis envy, rather than on an inherited basis. In boys the Oedipus complex is destroyed by castration anxiety, while in girls it is initiated by the castration complex.

EXTENSION OF THE OEDIPAL STAGE INTO THE PREGENITAL PHASE

To complicate matters further, Freud concluded late in his career (1931) that the girl's preoedipal attachment to her mother included the features of her negative Oedipus complex, that is, strong love for mother and a wish to exclude father. Thus, for girls, the negative Oedipus complex is a preoedipal phenomenon. He subsequently realized that all conflicts which occur in the oedipal phase could be identified in the preoedipal stages, but this did not present a problem for him. He simply concluded that the oedipal stage could be extended back in time, to include all parts of the preoedipal stage. He did not consider the alternatives, namely that his stage progression theory might not be the most accurate description of the developmental process or that oedipal resolution itself did not have the importance he attached to it. To the end of his career, Freud retained his conviction that resolution of the Oedipus complex is the cornerstone of individual development (and of civilization for that matter), and the shibboleth which separates Freudians from non-Freudians (1905b, 1920 footnote, p. 226).

DOES THE OEDIPUS COMPLEX EXIST AND IF SO, IS IT UNIVERSAL?

THE SIGNIFICANCE OF FREUD'S METAPHOR

The Oedipus myth was adopted by Freud as a prototype and demonstration that these attitudes have existed since antiquity and are thus universal in man. More complete renderings of the Oedipus myth, however, including the histories of Oedipus' father and stepfather, and the full role of Jocasta, suggest that parental infanticide rather than incest and parricide are the more blatant themes of the myth (Levin, 1948; Devereux, 1953). While not disproving the existence or universality of the Oedipus complex, this does suggest that Freud was either interpreting the myth idiosyncratically or neglecting its major theme.

RESEARCH DOCUMENTING THE OEDIPUS COMPLEX[7]

Attempts to demonstrate the existence of the Oedipus complex, by demonstrating that oedipal-aged children prefer the opposite-sexed parent, have been inconclusive (Fisher and Greenberg, 1977). Since the Oedipus complex is an unconscious configuration, failure to demonstrate its existence by tests involving conscious choice situations does not necessarily disprove its existence. In an uncontrolled study, responses of boys and girls to projective stimuli, as well as spontaneous stories at age 5 compared with similar material collected a year later at age 6, revealed a marked reduction of tension associated with oedipal themes (Scheffler, 1971, cited in Fisher and Greenberg, 1977, p.

---

[7]Fisher and Greenberg (1977) have reviewed many studies relating to this question. This section draws heavily from their compilation. Researchers whose work is quoted from Fisher and Greenberg are referenced to that work.

184). This is consistent with Freud's ideas about the transition from the oedipal stage to latency. Were it not for such observations and for phenomenological observations of oedipal play themes in many 3- to 6-year-old children, one might conclude that the Oedipus complex is a phenomenon which arises in adolescence or young adulthood, where more presumptive evidence has been accumulated.

The later developmental evidence which supports the existence of the Oedipus complex in adolescence demonstrates castration anxiety rather than oedipal anxiety; and as I pointed out, these may basically be unrelated phenomena. Studies have demonstrated the existence of castration anxiety in boys more than in girls, and in women with traditionally masculine interests (career, unmarried, no children) compared to women with traditionally feminine interests (homemakers with children) (Levin, 1966, cited in Fisher and Greenberg, 1977, p. 200).

Men are more influenced than women by castration anxiety, if this is a valid inference from fear of bodily injury (Blum, 1949, cited in Fisher and Greenberg, 1977, p. 194). College men are more likely to see their fathers as castrators and college women their mothers as castrators in responses to the "Blacky Test," a projective test in which pictures depict a dog with a knife poised over its tail (Schill, 1966, cited in Fisher and Greenberg, 1977, p. 180). In college men, castration anxiety, inferred from fear of death (which may not be a valid inference), was shown to heighten following exposure to heterosexually stimulating material (Sarnoff and Corwin, 1959, cited in Fisher and Greenberg, 1977, pp. 195, 220).

Women by contrast seem more influenced than men by fear of loss of love, as reflected in fears of being rejected (Manosevitz and Lanyon, 1965, cited in Fisher and Greenberg, 1977, p. 198), rendered anxious by a film with a loss-of-love theme (Lewis, 1969, cited in Fisher and Greenberg, 1977, p. 198), and associations to the meaning of death (Lowery, 1965, cited in Fisher and Greenberg, 1977, p. 198). This is consistent with Freud's view that males and females have different motives for forsaking their oedipal attachments. But, as Freud noted, this could reflect females experiencing less castration anxiety on a developmental basis when they realize that they do not risk losing something they never possessed. Data from preoedipal children demonstrate that they do not perceive the penis as the only genital. There is evidence that women perceive and accept their bodies with greater comfort than do men (Fisher, 1970, 1973), and that oedipal-aged girls are if anything more settled, stable, and confident in their developing femininity than their male age-mates are confidently masculine (Frankel and Sherick, 1979).

Data of the sort outlined in this section are convincing neither of the existence of the Oedipus complex as a universal phenomenon nor its inevitable relationship to the castration anxiety/penis envy issues, which as I suggested above, may be more universal developmental phenomena.

THE ROLE OF THE RESOLUTION OF THE OEDIPUS COMPLEX IN THE DEVELOPMENT OF SEXUAL IDENTITY

If we grant the existence of the Oedipus complex, do girls consider themselves boys until the oedipal stage, and is oedipal resolution in girls prompted by disappointment after learning that they have no penis?

Observations of biologically intersexed infants and children, and those born with ambiguous-appearing genitals have persuasively illustrated that gender identity, the knowledge and sense of oneself as a boy or girl, is established by parental attitudes at the time of the infant's birth, and this environmental factor can override biology (Kleeman, 1976; Stoller, 1976).[8] This sense of one's gender is expressed with confidence and conviction before 2 years of age. Penis envy and presumptive evidence of castration anxiety are observed in 18- to 24-month-old girls (Galenson and Roiphe, 1976). These might not be universal phenomena; however, as the earlier example from the nursery school suggests, it is observable in normal girls (p. 73).

---

[8]An experiment in nature illustrates that this is not invariably the case. Due to an autosomal recessive trait, some males found in three isolated, inbred groups from different parts of the world, are born with female-appearing genitalia. They are raised as girls but at puberty they develop masculine sex characteristics and feelings. Most then change their sexual identity and live the rest of their lives as males (West, 1994).

DO GIRLS ENTER THE OEDIPAL STAGE BY WAY OF THE CASTRATION
COMPLEX, THAT IS, AS A SECONDARY COMPENSATION, AFTER DISCOVERING
THAT THEY LACK A PENIS?

A very small sample, observational study reported that one girl
demonstrated a wish for a baby before she seemed aware of genital differences. In another girl the wish for a baby preceded evidence of castration anxiety (Parens, Pollock, Stern, and Kramer,
1976). The implication of this study is that the development of
the Oedipus complex in girls is not necessarily related to discovery of "castration"; thus, girls can enter the oedipal stage on the
same preordained basis as do boys.

DOES CONSCIENCE (SUPEREGO) FUNCTION DEVELOP DURING THIS PHASE
AND DOES IT OCCUR AS A PRECIPITANT FROM RESOLUTION OF THE
OEDIPUS COMPLEX?

Children have been described, from the Hampstead Clinic's in-
dexed analytic material, who exhibit autonomous, integrated de-
personalized (i.e., stage-mature) superego formation and
functioning, but who show no evidence of oedipal resolution
(Holder, 1982). Freud's theory cannot account for superego formation in such individuals.

A semantic distinction is often raised when the type of cri-
tique represented by the latter findings is considered: Some psychoanalysts characterize the superego as a psychic structure
which mediates conscience function. The term *conscience* describes the pertinent area of mental functions while superego is
the name for the "organ" which performs these functions. Thus,
the terms should not be used interchangeably as I have done—as
if the structure can be formed without any contents. The problems in making that distinction include the facts that the only
way we have of assessing the existence of the superego is through
evidence of conscience functioning; and the best conceptualization we currently have of psychic structures is that they are constellations of similarly related functions. So, it is difficult to
separate superego and conscience at the current state of our
knowledge. And thus, it is difficult to conclude anything other
than that conscience formation in the children described in the

last paragraph cannot be explained by Freud's theory of the superego as heir to the Oedipus complex.

In his later writings (1930, 1940), Freud himself laid the groundwork for a different and I believe more accurate understanding of the development of conscience. He emphasized the integration of parental standards which are more broadly gleaned from experiences with both parents, based on the overriding importance of maintaining parental favor because of the helpless dependency of the child on them. This implies a gradual adoption of conscience functions, developing from early in life through real experiences with parents and society; that is, via teachings, preachings, and examples. These are integrated by accruing identifications on bases which include fear of punishment as well as wishes to retain the love and acceptance of parents. Thus, conscience is not acquired in a stage-specific manner. Furthermore, it is likely that one's sense of values and conscience are always in flux in such a way that renders doubtful the value of distinguishing between superego as a structure and superego contents (conscience functions). Freud's later theory of conscience formation has never gained the acceptance or renown of his oedipal theory.

Freud's later theory, however, is consistent with research which has been interpreted as contradicting a major tenet of his oedipal resolution theory. Although Freud mentioned that the boy's love and good feelings for his father contribute to the resolution of his Oedipus complex, he posited that it is primarily fear of the father's harshness which motivates the boy to forsake his incestuous, oedipal strivings, form the superego, and move into latency. The strength of the boy's conscience/superego is directly proportional to the harshness of his father (Freud, 1928). Formal research, however, has consistently found the opposite (Fisher and Greenberg, 1977). Boys who have had a positive and nurturing relationship with their fathers form stronger, in the sense of more law-abiding, superegos than those with harsh, punitive fathers. Children of the latter are more likely to exhibit delinquent behavior, as expressed by a disregard for societal rules. Some of these delinquents may conform to Freud's model, especially since in one place he said that the child's superego is modeled after the parental superego not after the parents

(Freud, 1933, p. 67). For these delinquents may not be suffering, as they appear to be, from a lack of superego. Rather, they have developed such overwhelmingly harsh, punitive, untempered, and thus strong superegos that they defend against their super-egos' overweening dictates by flagrant disregard for conventional morality and laws. I have found, however, that the delinquent behavior exhibited by such individuals usually is not based on an overwhelming conscience. Rather, their delinquency involves efforts to please the harsh parent's perceived wishes to punish or reject.

LATENCY

The combined dissolution and repression of incestuous and parricidal urges, accomplished by oedipal resolution, ushers in the next developmental stage. Freud termed this the "latency" phase because of the notable absence of those sexual interests and manifestations which had been so prominent during the oedipal phase and which would again resurge at puberty. It occurs between ages 5 to 6 and 10 to 11 years. As was true for much of his developmental theory, Freud's clinical ideas about the genesis of this phase were entwined with or influenced by phylogenetic and anthropological ideas about the evolution of the human race.[9] For although he emphasized the importance of the environment (family, education) in instilling reaction formation defenses of disgust, shame, and morality in order to keep sexual interests unconscious, he nevertheless ascribed an inherited, physiological basis to the latency period. Thus, drive strength will diminish on a biological basis, without external influences (Freud, 1905b, pp. 177–178). He ultimately concluded, however, that latency can only accomplish complete interruption of sexuality in cultures which strive to suppress infantile sexuality

---

[9]Freud's conclusion about the diphasic character of sexual development in humans, with a peak at about 5 years and a second peak at puberty, led him to surmise that man's ancestor had reached sexual maturity at 5 years of age. He further speculated that a latency phase would figure importantly in the adoption of erect posture, and the importance of the sense of vision would supplant that of smell. This latter change would figure in the disconnection of sexual arousal from the esdrus cycle, characteristic of lower mammals, for which smell is the predominant stimulant for arousal (1930, p. 99n; 1940, p. 153).

(1925a, p. 37). Thus, a spectrum of sexual manifestations can be anticipated amongst latency children, ranging from those who experience occasional breakthroughs from sublimation of sexual urges to others in whom sexual activity persists throughout the latency phase (1905b, p. 179).

Freud considers the major task of the latency period to be fending off the temptation to masturbate, which would keep alive those very sexual interests which must be repressed in order that the child be educated. These efforts can give rise to obsessional symptoms (ritualistic behavior); for children typically regress from oedipal conflicts to anal sadistic ones which, when defended against, predispose to obsessional symptoms (1926, p. 116). Thus, Freud sees the early latency child still struggling to effect the massive wave of repression associated with oedipal resolution which gives rise to the amnesia people retain for their infantile sexuality. This continuing effort is most readily seen in the child's efforts to integrate the newly formed superego into his or her psychic structure; for superego formation is the vehicle by which these changes are effected. Many child analysts, following Bornstein (1951), consider this the most important structural change to occur in latency, and they divide the phase into early ($5^1/2$ to 8 years) and late (8 to 10 years) subphases on the basis of successful integration of the superego.

The early latency child experiences the superego as unfamiliar, a foreign body. Thus, auxiliary ego support is required from the environment to enable the child to do the "right thing." This fact, that the child's superego has not yet been comfortably integrated into his or her psyche, accounts for many typical behaviors of these children. They are sensitive to criticism and inclined to externalize and project the source of responsibility for their misbehaviors onto others. This is explained by their intolerance for the new, harsh superego, whose dictates they ward off by acting blameless. The severity of the newly formed superego's strictures is felt to be directly proportional to the strength of the latency child's lingering incestuous urges and wishes to follow his or her own dictates rather than those of society.

Another frequently noted behavior involves children's approach to playing competitive games. Early latency children spend as much, if not more, time debating the rules and accusing each other of cheating than concentrating on the competition. The child has not yet fully accepted a sense of conscience relatively independent from those around him. So, in accusing opponents, children externalize and project onto them their own readiness to cheat in order to achieve their aim of winning the game.

By contrast, late latency children play with a tacitly acknowledged acceptance of the rules and thus concentrate on developing their strategy to win. Children have now comfortably integrated the dictates of their own conscience, at least as it reflects their parents' and society's strictures about rules of games and fair play; thus, the child's ego can be turned more toward dealing with the outside world rather than controlling inner drives. Generally, at least when compared to adolescent children, latency children are "law and order" oriented, subscribing to conventional ideas about right and wrong, rather than challenging authority. This of course is too broad-based a conclusion about conscience function and insufficient to explain, for example, why children (and adults, too, for that matter), can be law abiding about certain issues and not about others. Freudians look for specific dynamic conflicts within individuals to explain such variations. It is likely, however, that the differences reflect the fact that conscience develops through a combination of identifications with parents or reactions against parental behaviors which have been gradually accruing since early childhood, rather than by the integration of a "structure" termed superego.

REVISIONS AND AMENDMENTS TO FREUD'S THEORY OF LATENCY

Working from orthodox Freudian premises about latency, Sarnoff (1976), focusing particularly on psychodynamics, observes from his clinical experience that far from being diminished, drives remain as strong as ever during the latency years. In fact, he concludes that the latency phase is a defense against infantile sexuality, which society must superimpose on the child's development in order to acculturate the child. The environment must render the child tractable to being educated about the mores, morals, standards, and lore of a complicated culture.

The specific defenses adopted by the child against oedipal impulses are unique to the phase. Foremost amongst these is the development of conscious fantasies as an alternate mode of drive discharge instead of direct instinctual repression. The fact that aggression is often the more prominent drive being defended against by latency children stems from the tendency of children to regress to anal sadism as a first-line defense against the oedipal conflicts. The sadism/aggression is then defended against by obsessional mechanisms, particularly reaction formation and undoing but also isolation, all of which become better developed during latency.

Sarnoff relies on Piaget's observations of maturational advances in cognitive functioning at this time to explain the enhanced capacity to array fantasy. Piaget also provided Sarnoff with an explanation for how drives can be discharged by fantasies whose content has no seeming relation to the drive. For Piaget had described early reflex activities, like sucking and grasping, which occur independently during the first months of life, but then become linked together in circular reactions which persist in organized patterns of activity. For example, hair stroking can be linked in this way with sucking. Later, the sexually based wish to suck can be repressed, but the linked activity, the hair twisting, can remain as a mode for discharging the libidinal urge. In a similar manner, consequent to the acquisition of symbol formation (words and ideas) during the second and third years of life, ideas which form the basis of fantasies can be linked with sexual or aggressive actions. It becomes possible to repress the linkage in the third year of life, and the more innocuous fantasy content remains to express the whole experience. Furthermore, such single fantasies typically become fragmented, and small pieces of different ones reassembled into a fantasy which ultimately bears little if any resemblance to the original wish, but serves to discharge the drive.

Sarnoff bolsters his conclusions about the high level of sexual drive in latency by noting that sexual intercourse has been reported amongst latency-aged children. He also cites anthropological studies of at least one primitive society, the Trobriand Islanders, in which no efforts are made to discourage sexual interest and as a result there is no latency. Sexual interest is maintained by the children throughout the latency years. Thus, the

Trobriand children support part of Sarnoff's thesis, namely that sexual interests potentially persist through the latency stage. Yet, despite experiencing no sex-free period of latency, children of the Trobriand Islanders certainly become inculcated with their culture's values. So, Sarnoff's example of the Trobriand Islanders seems to disprove his other major point, namely that a latency period is necessary to render children educable about their culture. In other words, the Trobriand children's experience as reported suggests that a period of sexual latency has little to do with acculturation.

To support his ideas about the relative strength of environment over biology in achieving the latency state, Sarnoff cites reports of two experiments in nature: Latency-age children who experience premature puberty nevertheless act like latency children, and adolescent-aged children born without sexual glands do not experience puberty but nonetheless exhibit the outward manifestations of adolescence, at least with respect to behavior, speech, attitudes, manners, and interests.

Sarnoff's conclusions are not significantly at odds with traditional theory. For in her classic paper (1951), Bornstein reiterated Freud's conviction that the task of the child throughout latency is one of "persistent denial of the struggle against the breakthrough of instinctual impulses" (p. 282). Sarnoff, however, emphasizes the role of the environment rather than biology in creating this state.

In sharp contrast, Shapiro and Perry (1976) gathered data from a number of sources outside the purview of psychoanalysis to reach their conclusion that latency occurs because a number of maturational, neurological changes occur between the ages of 6 and 8 (the early latency period). These changes coincide with the end of the oedipal stage and also allow for latency activities. Enhanced cognitive capacities derived from these maturational changes facilitate the resolution of the Oedipus complex in children when they reach 7 years of age.

Specifically, Shapiro and Perry call attention to the facts that the brain achieves 90 percent of its adult size at about age 6, that certain cells in the frontal areas mature, and that the electroencephalogram (EEG) stabilizes with the adult pattern at about age 8. Piaget identified advancement in cognitive capacities from preoperational to concrete operations at this time. Neuropsychological testing demonstrates advances in the perceptual sphere at this time. These maturational changes in the central nervous system led Shapiro and Perry to conclude, as had Freud, that latency is a biologically determined state. It is these neurological advances in cognitive capacities, however, which are the biological changes that give rise to latency, rather than the biphasic character of the sexual drive which accounts for the phenomena of the latency-aged child. This greater neurological stability provides the child with a wider range and depth of ego resources to deal with incestuous and other conflicts.

In support of their conclusions, Shapiro and Perry note that throughout modern history society seems to have recognized 7 as being a significant age in terms of understanding, ability to take responsibility, competence, and so forth. In medieval times children were sent from home to become court pages at age 7, and later children were apprenticed at age 7. Also, English common law held children to be responsible for criminal intent at age 7.

Thus, latency has been considered to arise as a biologically determined, societally reinforced restriction in sexual drive activity which promotes the civilization of the child (Freud). It has been considered as an environmentally induced suppression of sexual drive activity which renders the child tractable for acculturation (Sarnoff). Finally, it has been seen as a biologically determined maturational spurt in ego capacities, importantly including cognitive advances, which offers the child higher level ways of dealing with his inner (drive) and outer (adaptation) realities (Shapiro and Perry).

Despite espousing different origins, these three views are similar in their understanding of the tasks of the latency period. In addition to extinguishing the oedipal conflict, these tasks include the acquisition of formal learning skills. The mechanism by which this learning takes place is understood differently in these different theories. For Freud, learning was the result of displacement of the sexual drive, termed sublimation. It is accomplished by the psychological action of defense mechanisms which neutralize or deinstinctualize the incestuous urges. Sublimation has subsequently come to be thought of as a more comprehensive, broad-based feature of psychic functioning. In this later model greater importance is attached to the exercise of capacities and broadened interests created by neurological maturation. It may be reasonable to expect, as suggested by the empirical infant studies, that children are internally motivated to exercise newly developed abilities as motives in their own right. This phenomenon would be akin to what Bühler (1935) describes as the functional pleasure of play, Hendrick (1942) identifies as the drive for mastery, and Mahlerians describe in the practicing subphase.

With regard to psychopathology, the most common psychiatric referrals for latency-aged children include behavioral problems, often relating to aggression and attention span in boys, and learning disorders. From the traditional psychoanalytic view of the failure of latency development in these areas, one would look for the source of aggressive behavior or learning problems in inadequate defense against incestuous urges and aggressive drive. The intrusion of drive-driven fantasies or the symbolic meaning of learning as knowing in the sexual sense or learning as an aggressive act against another, would be preventing the educational process from taking hold in the child. Such an exploration would be far removed from one which looked for inadequacies in maturation or in the functioning of the ego apparatus itself to explain learning or behavioral problems. These are not mutually exclusive alternatives. We see patients whose difficulties fall into each group, and our task is making certain to apply the correct model to any given case.

Other changes observed in latency children follow from the issue inherent in oedipal resolution, namely disappointment in the child's desires for an intimate relationship with a parent. During latency, children are thought to make their first definitive movement away from parents to peer relationships and the development of a bosom buddy. The maturational view might see this expansion of interpersonal relationships as a function of broadened and shared interests.

In sum, the developmental features of the latency period, basically the years of elementary education, are considered to be: (1) a significant reduction of sexual manifestations; (2) acquisition of the rudiments of precision learning and other skill development; (3) turning from the family toward peers; (4) enhanced control over aggressive drive, particularly through strengthening obsessional defenses of reaction formation, isolation, rationalization as a precursor to intellectualization, and undoing; and this in conjunction with (5) interim consolidation of the superego's function based on accommodation to parental/societal values. This period of ego development, emotional strengthening, and stability of psychological organization then becomes altered by the anticipation and advent of puberty.

SUMMARY

The idea that development is led by ego maturation and adaptation to real experiences, rather than, for example, by libidinal and aggressive drives or by cognitive maturation, has never been accorded the central importance it warrants in dynamic theories of psychological development. Nor has the relevance of this view to clinical theory and technique been illustrated. Nonetheless, as I have and will continue to point out, the writings of a number of psychoanalysts, other authors, and researchers support such a view.

INFANCY

Freud's early model of development (1900, 1911) posits a relatively passive infant, a tabula rasa who is not interested in the outside world and who is primarily interested in gratification of him- or herself. Moreover, the infant is both so self-absorbed and has such limited perceptual capacities that he or she initially perceives only part of mother. These part representations eventually coalesce into an accurate perception of mother as a whole. In this pleasure principle dominated model, judicious frustration of the infant's and child's libidinal and aggressive urges is responsible for ego development (i.e., developmental advance).

That model is much different from the later one suggested by Freud in which the child's overriding consideration, his highest motive, is to please his parents in order to secure his own sense of safety. To do so, the child adopts as his own standard (superego) the standards of his parents and accepts all the factors which had influenced them (1940, p. 206). These latter ideas of Freud are more compatible with an infant actively engaging the parent rather than with the passive, introverted infant of his earlier, more enduring model of development. Freud's later view has been amply confirmed by recent research (see Osofsky, 1987).

THE EGO MATURATIONAL MODEL

In advancing an ego maturation/adaptational model, I assume that something analogous to physical maturation moves psychological development forward. Clinically observable manifestations of inherent, progressive tendencies include efforts by infants, children, and adolescents to extract from their environment what they need to complete their development. They also exhibit self-righting tendencies when foundering in some form of disequilibrium. These adaptive proclivities can be aided or thwarted by the environment. The psychological aspect of this maturational push, "urges" or "strivings to complete development" (Jones, 1922; Bibring, 1937; Deutsch, 1944; A. Freud, 1965, 1968), is a concept that has been largely neglected in psychoanalytic developmental and clinical theory.[10]

Stern's empirical research (1985) demonstrates the clinical concept of strivings to complete development. His findings and those of Emde (1988a, 1991) are also consistent with the idea that adaptation to real experience is the basic mechanism by which psychological development progresses during infancy. Stern finds that neonates are both endowed with a wired-in sense of themselves as separate from others and perceive their mothers as a whole. Stern also observes that infants are inherently motivated to actively engage with their environment above all else and capitalize on extraordinary, built-in capacities like cross-modal perception to learn readily from their experiences.

___

[10]Hendrick's "instinct to master" (1942, 1943), Bühler's functional pleasure of play (1935), and the role Erikson (1956) ascribes to "favored capacities" (p. 116) in ego identity formation all exemplify this concept. Hartmann's (1939) discussion of conflict-free ego functions affords a basis for this view of the developmental process in abstract terms. More recently Harley (Panel, 1980), Sklansky and Rabichow (1980), and Parens (1986) have underscored the importance of strivings to complete development (see chapter 7).

If we can presume that certain organizing principles function continuously from infancy throughout development, then Stern's findings support the model of adolescent development I am presenting. For the appeal of novel, developmentally forward-moving, real experiences is a prominent feature of development during adolescence. I find that adolescents, like infants, have a built-in sense of optimal levels of stimulation. This latter assertion may seem contrary to observations that adolescents tend toward extremes of behavior; however, these extreme behaviors reflect adolescents' experimentation with their own limits and with the limits of their society. In most normal youth these extreme behaviors are confined to relatively safe arenas and are reasonably well modulated. Typically, although not invariably, one finds problematic family relationships in those adolescents who are experimenting far beyond the pale of their own safety.

As Stern has done more recently, Bowlby (1969, 1973) emphasizes the infant's ability to relate to others from the first months of life. He implies a gradual, experientially based relinquishment of the need for physical proximity to the mother, rather than stage theory type incremental advances to higher levels of psychological organization in the early child–parent relationship.

Aspects of Mahler's theory of development (Mahler et al., 1975) are compatible with a model that ascribes central importance to ego maturation or strivings to complete development. For example, a maturational element is important in the process of "hatching" from the state of dual unity. Then in the "practicing subphase" a motor capacity acquired through maturation, namely walking, provides the impetus for a psychological advance toward libidinal object constancy, the condition which renders autonomy possible. For the toddlers' drive to master perambulation motivates them to move physically away from their mothers as they explore the world around them with this newfound ability. This model of a heady, irrepressible, energetic drive to master through repetition could serve as a paradigm for one feature of adolescent development. Also, both maturation and real experiences are important later during the "rapprochement subphase" in creating the toddler's acute awareness of his or her separateness from mother.

EARLY CHILDHOOD

The Oedipus complex, cornerstone of psychoanalytic theory, has probably been the most widely considered developmental issue of early childhood. Although Freud emphasized the internally generated basis of the Oedipus complex in boys, he continued to write about it as if a strong environmental contributant were necessary for it to occur. The latter emphasis on experiences in the genesis of the Oedipus complex is consonant with my own observations. Whenever manifestations of the Oedipus complex (not simply castration anxiety or penis envy) are clinically observable and sustained rather than evanescent, muted, intermittent, and benign to the point of insignificance, then I typically find one of the following conditions: The parent-child experiences are either far from optimal if not abnormal, or else there has been some significant psychic trauma in the child's life.

Even though Freud originally described them as separate and distinct phenomena, he subsequently linked the castration complex inextricably to the Oedipus complex. By contrast I have found clinically that castration anxiety and penis envy arise from children's observations of genital differences without any direct relationship to the Oedipus complex. Dealing successfully with castration anxiety and penis envy are more typical and important features of normal development than resolving the Oedipus complex.

If, as I am suggesting, the Oedipus complex does not play a major role in development, then the child's wish to maintain a positive relationship with parents is not normally interrupted by preordained phases of spontaneously arising, murderous wishes toward them (during the oedipal stage and at puberty). In making this point I do not intend to dismiss sexual and aggressive drives. These urges are present in normal development, but their importance arises in direct proportion to their biological strength in the individual. Thus, sexual and aggressive urges normally become important after puberty, not during the period designated in Freudian theory as the phallic–oedipal phase.

CONSCIENCE (SUPEREGO) FORMATION

I understand conscience function to develop as described in Freud's later writings (1930, 1940), namely, gleaned broadly from experiences with both parents, based on the child's wish to secure parental approval. This view is different from his better known formulation of superego formation as the outcome of resolution of the Oedipus complex (1923).

LATER CHILDHOOD

Shapiro and Perry (1976) summarized evidence that aspects of neurological maturation within the central nervous system occur at around the ages of 6 to 8, the time when the Freudian stage of latency begins. These changes include stabilization of the electroencephalogram (EEG) in the adult pattern and advances in cognitive capabilities. Thus, they find that a maturational thrust in physiological development coincides with a period which is also characterized by progressive psychological development.

THE ROLE OF FANTASY IN DEVELOPMENT

Fantasies may originate from within an individual without any relation to events in which he or she has either been personally involved or has witnessed. Fantasies which have the most telling role in development arise from a synthetic effort of the individual to reconcile his understanding of his experiences with his conscious and unconscious awareness of his developmental needs. These latter are basically to accomplish his goal of completing his development in the context of a positive relationship with his parents.

Part II

Development During Adolescence

CHAPTER 4

The Transition to Adolescence and Puberty

In this chapter I will illustrate the importance of efforts to adapt to one's environment in children who are at the threshold of adolescence. This perspective offers an explanation for current observations that younger children (preadolescents) are exhibiting behaviors which historically have been more typical of adolescents. This perspective on children advancing from childhood into adolescence is contrasted with some influential, long-standing ideas that explain the behavioral patterns of prepubertal/ preadolescent children as attempts to deal with actual or anticipated drive pressures. The chapter concludes with a description of the psychological reactions of children to puberty (biological sexual maturation).

During the middle school/junior high years (ages 11 through 14), children continue to exhibit an unfolding of their strivings to mature. These can be influenced by internal factors like puberty and external factors like parents' attitudes and behaviors. Children most commonly exhibit an accentuation of their preexisting traits and adaptive mechanisms during this transition into adolescence. New or different behaviors can become engrafted onto or substituted for prior patterns. As the following example illustrates, however, striking changes in a preadolescent's and adolescent's behaviors frequently represent a modification of his or her preexisting style rather than a significant alteration in basic ways of adapting:

From his early grade school years, a very bright little boy was looked upon by teachers and other adults as a "Little Professor" because of his precocious vocabulary and penchant for intellectual explanations. This tendency became more pronounced when, as a middle school child, he began contending with teachers. Then, as a young teenager his style of dealing with his parents was relentless argumentation, sometimes specious but often logical and always persistent until he got his way or could accept the logic behind his parents' refusal of his wishes.

As a guitar playing midadolescent, he affected the hair style, dress, language, and manner of admired rock stars. As part of this adolescent rocker persona he became more strident in confrontations with his parents, teachers, and peers. His long-time adaptive mode of intellectual argumentativeness was altered stylistically by his vociferousness and vulgarity. As part of his efforts to emancipate, he did not turn, however, to the drug or alcohol-using ways of rock stars or of his friends who shared his musical interests. Thus, although he now looked and sounded like a very different type of person from his nerdish style prior to adolescence, his basic ways of dealing with the world and with himself, namely intellectually based, argumentative confrontation, had altered more superficially than substantively.

During the period prior to adolescence, imitative behaviors, the basis of identifications, are often practiced with a fervor that resembles the driven quality of toddlers in Mahler's description of the practicing subphase. Adolescents are very much aware of this feature in their confreres. *Wannabe* is the derisive term in the argot of current preadolescents and adolescents for someone whose identification with an admired person or style lacks sufficient authenticity.

Such behavioral practicing can involve experimenting with new identifications, styles, or interests (e.g., music). Some preadolescents and adolescents practice constantly to perfect skills which they have already acquired or for which they have natural ability (e.g., sports). Others, particularly later during adolescence, expose themselves to rigorous challenges (e.g., physical conditioning, rock climbing). In this variation of practicing they work assiduously to acquire inner confidence, which they consider lacking in themselves, but now are able to attempt by virtue of improved coordination and heightened stamina. Their ultimate goal in all of these activities is to be able to progress in their development.

While engaged in such efforts to move forward with confidence and competence, preadolescents and adolescents want to feel secure in their relationships to their family or some other group which assumes that function. This factor helps explain recent sociological data which are a source of anxiety to parents. I refer to reports suggesting that the distinction between preadolescence and adolescence is becoming blurred, at least with respect to overt behaviors; that is, behaviors traditionally associated with teenagers are exhibited by increasing numbers of preteenagers. These include: (1) resistance to the influence and authority of adults; (2) disregard for personal and property rights (e.g., stealing, vandalism), and other forms of overweeningly self-assertive, delinquent, or asocial acts (e.g., cheating in school); (3) experimentation with drugs, alcohol, smoking, and sex.

The developmental perspective I am presenting offers a framework for understanding why these behaviors are occurring earlier: As I have noted, children experience a normative, inner pressure to progress toward adulthood which they view as a state of autonomy. Thus, behaviors they witness in their parents become appealing, especially if the parents seem to enjoy those activities, for example, smoking, drinking. Children are motivated to adopt such activities both because the behaviors must be desirable if parents derive pleasure from them and because children feel that identifying with parents will make them more acceptable to the parents. It is as if children feel that if they're like their parents or do things the parents like, their parents will like them more. Thus, it is not surprising that youngsters who observe that their parents always enjoy a cocktail or two before dinner are going to want to drink. Or in another example, a teacher reported that two mothers of her sixth graders met with her to register great concern that the girls in the class were starting to use makeup; neither mother conveyed any awareness that they themselves wore more makeup than the other mothers of children in that class. Children want to emulate their parents and do so.

On the other hand, children are also acute observers and quick to notice behavior in their parents which is unbecoming. Thus, if a parent seems both to enjoy and to need to smoke, but the parent has a disturbing smoker's cough and a distasteful odor about him or her, then, especially in the presence of the warnings about its dangers, the situation is experienced more ambiguously by a child. And the child's motive for wanting to smoke can stem either from the pleasure the parent derives, or else the child wants to avoid feeling or realizing that the parents' behavior is unbecoming, distasteful, or contemptible. The child does not want to feel sorry for the parent for behavior which he or she observes to be stupid or self-defeating. Children and adolescents do not want to feel critical of or superior to their parents.[1] Adolescents adopt the disquieting parental behaviors in order to retain a positive view of their parents. By appearing as or more profligate than the parent it is as if the youngster is saying, "I'm just like my parents, so if they're bad, I'm worse and certainly can't criticize them."

Behaviors which reflect a sincere effort to be like parents can appear indistinguishable from behaviors which represent the youngster's attempt to master guilt and anxiety engendered by dissatisfaction with one's parents' activities. Identifications which are adopted in an effort to avoid conscious awareness of contemptuous or critical feelings toward parents are termed defensive identifications in this book. They have the additional effect of drawing attention from their parents' unsavory behaviors onto the youngsters themselves; this serves to protect their image of their parents' rectitude. Such precocious adoption of adult behaviors by preteenagers, that is, defensive identifications, plays a central role in the psychology of everyday life as well as in the developmental psychopathology of adolescence (chapter 8). This motive also at times underlies what is frequently considered to simply be adolescent experimentation, as the following example illustrates:

An almost 13-year-old eighth grader was discovered smoking marijuana with some classmates adjacent to the school property, so

---

[1]This observation must seem at great odds with the frequent experience of parents being criticized by their adolescent or preadolescent; however, adolescents criticize, chide, or mock the foibles of parents toward whom they either feel secure or whom they feel are stable. They are much less likely to criticize parents whom they perceive as unstable or in relationship to whom they do not feel secure.

that teachers and fellow students learned about it. This was the first such experience for a lad who had eschewed drug use and was considered an independent thinker and school leader. He was struggling with some courses that year and felt under pressure from teachers and parents to improve his performance. His own initial explanation for trying the marijuana was a combination of "a little curiosity" and a great feeling of frustration from the pressure under which he felt his teachers and his parents had placed him. He interpreted this episode of marijuana smoking as a way of getting back at them and thumbing his nose at them since he could not talk back or swear at them. Thus, the lad's explanation was that he was rebelling against oppressive authority and concomitantly satisfying curiosity.

When asked what else he had been thinking when he decided to smoke with the others, however, he mentioned off-handedly that since his brother and father had used drugs, he couldn't get into too much trouble if he were caught. When asked how he knew his brother and father had used drugs, the lad acknowledged the shock and dismay he had felt when his older brother whom he idolized had told him both that he himself used drugs casually and that their father had revealed to him that he too had tried drugs as a youth. The disbelieving lad asked his father who acknowledged the brother's revelation; the perplexed boy couldn't understand why his father had done so. The lad added candidly, albeit in a tone of rue tinged with defiance, that now teachers and peers whose admiration he had sought were feeling the opposite way toward him; moreover, the boys with whom he had smoked the marijuana were not even his good friends. The interviewer then pointed out that the outcome of the lad's experimenting had been the opposite of what he wanted, namely less rather than more admiration from teachers and peers. Thus, there was perhaps more than experimentation and defiance involved. The interviewer wondered if, under the guise of feeling protected by his father and brother's drug use to go ahead and experiment, the boy had in fact acted to lose the respect of teachers and peers in an effort to deal with his own loss of respect for his father and brother. That is, the interviewer posited that beneath his stated motives of defiance, experimentation, and curiosity the lad's basic motive was to preserve his positive image of the father and brother he idolized by acting like them. For the boy was not comfortable feeling critical of or superior to them, although his shock, disbelief, and dismay upon learning of their drug use suggested those to have been his true attitudes before they quickly succumbed to rationalization. The lad became briefly tearful in response to that interpretation. He then recounted that a couple of weeks earlier he had felt very good about himself after declining to try marijuana with the same peers. This recollection and the boy's tearfulness supported the interviewer's hypothesis that rebelliousness against authority, along with curiosity and experimentation, which can motivate adolescent's behaviors, were nevertheless not the most basic reasons why this lad had tried drugs.

Thus, one reason for the earlier appearance of adult behaviors in preteenagers is that more parents are involved in all the types of behaviors which are being exhibited by preadolescents and early adolescents. Children adopt their parents' activities either to emulate them or to protect the positive image they wish to retain of their parents and other admired people such as older siblings.

In addition to those two motives for adopting adultlike behaviors, children on the way to adolescence can be influenced (against their conservative tendencies) by their peers to adopt adult-type behaviors when their parents do not exhibit sufficient interest in them or are poor role models or are excessively controlling. In the first instance, when the adolescent is unable to secure the parents' interest, he or she adopts the peers' adultlike behaviors to maintain a relationship with that group which now assumes the role of the parents in sponsoring development. In the second situation, disillusionment with the parents' failure sends the preadolescent or adolescent toward peers. In the third circumstance when the parents severely thwart the individual's strivings to become more autonomous, the adolescent adopts the peer group as an ersatz family in order to feel sponsored in his or her efforts to move forward. Thus, adolescent behaviors also arise precociously in conjunction with peer group influences which take hold when parents have either been insufficiently interested, inadequate, or too stifling of the child's development.

The trend toward adolescent behaviors appearing during preadolescence might be explained on the basis that puberty (at least in girls) occurs at a younger age than it did 70 years ago.[2]

---

[2]Katchadourian (1990) has observed that "the second half of the twentieth century has seen the widest separation in human history between the timetables of biological maturation and the socially acceptable expression of sexual behavior" (p. 330).

But physical maturation varies widely in this age group and in my experience does not correlate with behavior. One observes fully developed early adolescents who are dutiful and tractable, and small, physically immature children who are precociously experimenting and acting resistant to parental influence. Thus, it seems more accurate to consider the two issues of responsiveness to parental influence and sexuality as separate matters.

THE TRADITIONAL PSYCHOANALYTIC VIEW: PREPUBERTY AND PREADOLESCENCE

In contrast to what I have just described, traditional psychoanalytic theory has attributed behavior during this preadolescent period largely to children's unconscious anticipation of puberty. Libido theory posits that one change occurs in the sexual drive: At puberty the quality of libido changes from pregenital to genital. Anna Freud (1936) considers the "so-called prepubertal period," the interval between latency and puberty, to be "merely preparatory to physical sexual maturity." The quality of instinctual energy has not yet changed to genital drive; however, the quantity of libido and aggressive energy increases. This predisposes children to more impulsive behavior than they had previously exhibited; for their reaction formation defenses give way to oral, anal, and unruly behaviors. The changeableness of the prepubertal child's behaviors, alternately self-controlled and uncontrolled, reflects the relative success of the child's superego-influenced ego to restore order. Subsequently Helene Deutsch (1944) and Peter Blos (1958) legitimized this period as a discrete phase:

PREADOLESCENCE

Blos (1958), focusing on the psychology of boys, introduced this term for the same period characterized by Deutsch as prepuberty. Like Anna Freud, Blos emphasized the quantitative increase in drive activity, to which boys respond by regressing to pregenital drive cathexes. This represents their efforts to defend against fears of being castrated by the phallic mother. Because the quality of the drive is pregenital, the mother is experienced as a greater threat than the father. The sloppy dress, slovenly appearance and manner, oral greediness, preoccupation with anal language, fascination with odors, skill in producing onomatopoetic sounds, and tendency toward sadism described in middle school/junior high boys all reflect this instinctual regression. The degree of oral and anal drive activity exhibited by these boys led Blos to consider preadolescence as the first stage of adolescence.

PREPUBERTY

In contrast to the regressive behaviors Blos describes in boys, Deutsch (1944) considers that girls strengthen their egos during this period in anticipation of the upsurge of genital drive at puberty. Whereas assertiveness in boys is a manifestation of aggressive drive, assertiveness in girls is a "thrust of activity" which represents the ego's efforts to strengthen itself through mastering the environment. In Deutsch's description prepubertal girls are very busy and intensely involved, though with a play-acting quality. They try on many different identities, based on their observations of others, in a blatant, imitative manner. In this dramatic though unimaginative behavior they exhibit a poverty of fantasy life and introspection.

Deutsch contends that curiosity brings these girls together with boys, not sexual desire. So, although the harbingers of future sexual drives can be discerned in sexual investigations and keeping secrets with girl friends, Deutsch nevertheless considers prepuberty to be the period during which girls experience their greatest freedom from infantile sexuality. The relative lack of drive activity plus the prominence of ego strengthening observed in these girls led Deutsch to conclude that prepuberty is the last stage of latency.

Deutsch considers tomboyishness during prepuberty to be simply another way of shoring up ego strength in anticipation of the obligatory turn toward the active pursuit of passive aims that Freud thought characterizes adult feminine psychological organization. Blos does not offer a dynamic explanation for tomboyish behavior; but, he describes a phallic quality in preadolescent girls which gives rise to a brief period during which they feel unusually adequate and competent; this predisposes them to be the aggressors and "seducers" of boys, though their interest is not sexual.

DISCUSSION

These views of Deutsch and Blos about a discrete transitional stage between latency and adolescence can only be reconciled with each other if we posit sex-related differences in adaptive styles during this period. The following examples are presented to support my contention that maturation of the ego and adaptation are more prominent than features of drive maturation during this period:

1. The difference between the behaviors of boys and girls during this period has been overemphasized by the long-standing psychoanalytic view. We do observe children whose behavioral patterns conform to the descriptions of Blos and Deutsch. But there is sufficient crossover of these behavior patterns between girls and boys who are developing normally, boisterous girls and self-contained boys, to call Blos' and Deutsch's formulations into question. For example, in the following example preadolescent behaviors reported by Blos to characterize development in boys are observed in a normal girl:

> A popular, outspoken, feminine $11^1/2$-year-old sixth-grader developed the ability to belch. She delighted herself and her girl friends with loud burps at every opportunity. A couple of her friends attempted to imitate this girl's facility, and all her friends were tickled by anal jokes and sounds, and acted raucous, squealing loudly and shrieking when together for any activity. While the girl's personal hygiene was usually good, her bedroom was always very messy and even at times littered with uneaten food she had managed to sneak there.

2. A child can exhibit both the behavior patterns which Blos attributes to boys and those which Deutsch attributes to girls.

The following example argues against sex-related differences in behaviors that arise during this period as well as their explanations for the phenomena. This example also illustrates that the individual's efforts to adapt to her real experiences are as evident as efforts to anticipate or defend against puberty in the genesis of preadolescent behaviors. The excerpts which follow are from reports of a psychiatric consultant at a therapeutic-educational day school for emotionally disturbed, learning disabled children:

> Samantha, aged 11 years, 9 months, had an altercation with her foster mother during which she screamed that she didn't love her anymore and didn't want to live there. Her exasperated foster mother called Social Services to have Samantha placed elsewhere. In the immediate aftermath of this experience, Samantha's behavior at school was noteworthy. Dating from an interchange she had with a younger child from another classroom, Samantha began complaining vociferously about the other child's teacher. Specifically, the other teacher "favors her own kids" rather than being even-handed with all the students at this small school.

That complaint mirrored precisely Samantha's contention that her foster mother favored her own (natural) children, particularly a younger son. Thus, Samantha's attitude toward the teacher represented a displacement of her current attitude toward her foster mother.

> Samantha then wanted to work with clay, for the first time since enrolling at this school many months earlier; and she insisted upon using the potting wheel which belonged to the teacher she was condemning. Moreover, Samantha did not feel it was necessary to seek that teacher's permission; she maintained that the wheel belonged to everyone at school, so she could just take and use it.

These expectations also seemed to be a displacement from home, in this case, of her sibling rivalry. From the standpoint of libido theory, her interest in wet clay may represent a regressive pull triggered by the threat to her security engendered by her foster mother's call to the placement social worker. From an ego psychology orientation, the potting wheel conflict reflects Samantha's effort to utilize school personnel to master the anxiety generated in her by the conflict at home.

In addition to these displaced expressions of her anxiety, Samantha also exhibited efforts to deal with her distress in forward moving ways. She acted in a very grown-up fashion toward younger classmates. She encouraged them to stay in control, advised them as an older sister or parent might, and was eager to help them with their schoolwork. Also, she insisted upon sharing her lunches with the staff, literally obliging them to take some of what she offered.

Samantha's overbearing, intrusive, busy, activity-oriented manner conformed to Deutsch's characterization of prepubertal girls. The traumatic circumstances in which these behaviors had arisen, however, namely the threatened disruption of her longtime home placement, suggest that these behaviors are the product of passive into active or identification with the aggressor mechanisms rather than developmental phenomena based on her anticipation of drive maturation. The altruistic aspects of her behavior basically reflected her wishes to be found acceptable by others; she was now managing these wishes by reversing the roles of caretaker and "cared for," that is, turning passive into active.

The most notable aspect of Samantha's behavior pattern at age 12 years, 1 month (4 months later), was the intensity with which she maintained her tomboyishness. She tried more and more to dress like a boy, expressed pleasure when mistaken for a boy, and resisted her foster mother's encouragement to maintain proper hygiene and to wear a brassiere. Once, after having failed to put any of her dirty underwear in the laundry, she had to wear her foster brother's underpants. She reported this enthusiastically to the staff with ostensible pride and pleasure. She was frequently sadistically mean to other children, both verbally and physically, and particularly toward younger boys.

The latter behaviors, Samantha's manner, and her lack of attention to hygiene are all typical of Blos' description of preadolescent boys.

In sharp contrast to these boisterous behaviors and interests, however, during a recent girls' group meeting Samantha expressed an intense desire to have a baby. At the same time, the staff was impressed with how utterly self-centered Samantha had become, demonstrating little compassion or mutuality in relationships.

Deutsch would consider this tomboyish/bisexual position to be a defense against heterosexuality, stimulated by fears of being unable to control urges like her desire for a baby. Her concomitant self-centeredness suggests that this wish for a baby also represented an additional effort to mother herself, in this case by identifying with the mother. Moreover, considered in light of her earlier behaviors, her boyishness seemed as much related to dealing with her sibling rivalry and fear of losing her foster mother's affections to the latter's natural son by identifying with him, as it appears related to her wishes for a baby.

> At age 12 years, 3 months (2 months later), dating from the departure of Tom, the classmate closest to her age and whose boisterous, sadistic behavior had been similar to that of Samantha, she began to lose the brittle toughness and tomboyishness which had characterized her behavior to this point.

Thus, it appears in retrospect that imitation/identification with Tom was involved in her behaviors; she was acting like Tom in an effort to be liked and accepted by him and thus to feel more secure when her relationships at home seemed tenuous. This dynamic is important in the development of preadolescent friendships, which are not more important in themselves than they are earlier in development, but the group of friends becomes more important during this period. The relationship of Samantha's behavior to that of Tom is a good example of how group allegiance via imitative/identificatory behaviors can develop as a means of dealing with insecurity felt in relation to parents. This phenomenon is further clarified by the other elements of Samantha's behavior pattern at that time:

> Samantha began to wear fingernail polish for the first time. She now often chose to stay in during recess and fix her hair with the other girls, rather than rushing out to spend the whole recess in boisterous play with boys. Although she continued to wear her jacket at all times, she was interested in more feminine clothing and generally seemed more passive and settled. She was more friendly and less defensive and hostile toward others. Her responses to questions were now thoughtful, rather than impulsive, nonreflective reactions.
>
> Samantha had been interested in ghost-type stories all year, but during the past six months this interest had changed to a preference for gory, blood-filled, sadistic stories. Recently, for the

first time when she was telling such a story, the protagonist was a girl rather than a boy. She was not yet menarchal, but the staff thought her menarche would occur soon.

The rapid change from identifying with Tom to identifying with her female classmates following his departure underscores the shifting quality of identifications related to Samantha's need to feel secure in relationships with others. As noted, evanescent identifications can occur normally on a developmental basis from the inner pressure to grow up. And there was some sense amongst the staff that Samantha was close to becoming menarchal. Her effort to deal with the insecurity she was feeling in her relationships at home by turning to the peer group during this period was equally as striking. So, this example again suggests that these two factors, adaptation to real experiences and the inner experience of puberty, contribute separately to the individual's behavioral pattern.

Finding the same attitudes and behavioral patterns described by Blos and by Deutsch in the same individual makes it more difficult to understand the differences between prepuberty and preadolescence on a sex-linked basis. It is possible that sex-related differences in behavior patterns were more pronounced a half-century ago when Deutsch described prepuberty than today when society is more indulgent of instinctual expression. If so, that would support my contention that the appearance of any of these behaviors is more accurately understood in relation to the individual's real life experience than in relation to a gender-based difference in dealing with drive pressures. Thus, Samantha's behaviors may well include ego strengthening or regressive efforts to deal with actual or anticipated increases in drive pressure as Blos and Deutsch suggest. When considered in light of other aspects of her life, however, her shifting behaviors seem more accurately understood as efforts to maintain forward momentum to her development in the face of her unique past and present experiences.

To recapitulate, Samantha's developmental pattern during this period was characterized by relatively short-lived behaviors, replaced by others, but all geared toward enhancing her sense of security in the face of threats experienced from without, for example, foster mother's affections, sibling rivalry, and changes she was experiencing from within, such as her pubertal development. Nevertheless, they were all oriented toward developmental advance, since activities aimed at enabling oneself to function with increasing independence represent progression in development.

Most prominent among the mechanisms underlying these behaviors during this period are identification/imitation (in Samantha's case, with Tom and her foster brother, teachers, and fellow girl students), turning passive into active and identification with the aggressor mechanisms which are related to one another, and the need/wish for affiliation with others, that is, to form a group, if only comprising two people.

So, Deutsch is accurate in observing ego-strengthening efforts in these children. In fact, Blos also has a developmentally positive orientation in much of his writing. Children are always trying to adapt; the question is to what are they adapting during this period—anticipated or incipient sexuality, or present and past life? The answer is both; but in focusing exclusively on children's efforts to anticipate unconscious fantasies about puberty as the basis for these behavioral patterns, Deutsch and Blos underplay the more important determinants of these behaviors, namely adaptation to their real experiences as they strive to move ahead developmentally.

PREPUBERTY AS A STAGE CORRELATED WITH PHYSICAL DEVELOPMENT

An alternate view defines prepuberty as the period between the advent of the secondary (i.e., the outward physical changes) and the primary sex characteristics (i.e., menstruation, ejaculation). In linking the evolving behaviors more directly with the biological changes, this theory represents a lesser degree of abstraction than those of Deutsch and Blos. Pubertal children in this alternative view are experiencing genital drive, which by definition accompanies the physiological changes of puberty. Thus, these children are further along developmentally than those described by Deutsch and Blos who are not yet experiencing genital drive.

Kestenberg (1961), writing from this perspective, posits a specific correlation between biological maturation and cognitive style. She observes that prepubertal, that is, premenarchal, girls appear to be in a chronic state of premenstrual tension. This state is characterized by diffuseness and anxiety which pervade their thinking, their emotions, and their behaviors. Menarche and the subsequent, regularly repeating experiences of menstruation potentially bring relief from this state of diffuseness by providing specific points of reference around which girls can organize many of their experiences. This predisposes them to become more focused in their thinking about other matters as well. In this way menstruation can serve as an organizer which has potentially lasting implications for the girl's manner of dealing with discomfort. Girls who use menstruation as a way of focusing and organizing their distress and uncertainty in a mastery of problems mode tend to become more settled and ordered in their thinking. Those who do not will carry over into adulthood the prepubertal tendency toward scattered and disorganized responses to distress and uncertainty as well as a penchant for chronic anxiety.

While this is a fascinating thesis, my own experience underscores another point made by Kestenberg: The mother and the mother's attitudes are an even more important organizer from the outside which provides the model for her daughter's mode of dealing with stimuli emanating from inside herself. In other words, the way any woman deals with menstruation is more likely to be similar to than different from the way she deals with any stress. The latter mechanisms are derived more generally from experiences with parents around stressful issues; and any girl has a long history with her mother which extends much further back than the time of her menarche.

PUBERTY

Puberty refers to the hormonally stimulated, biological changes which eventuate in the completion of physical and sexual maturation. While the sequence of pubertal changes is relatively invariant in girls and boys, there is great variation in the age of onset and pacing of puberty amongst children. For example, some boys have completed their physical maturation before

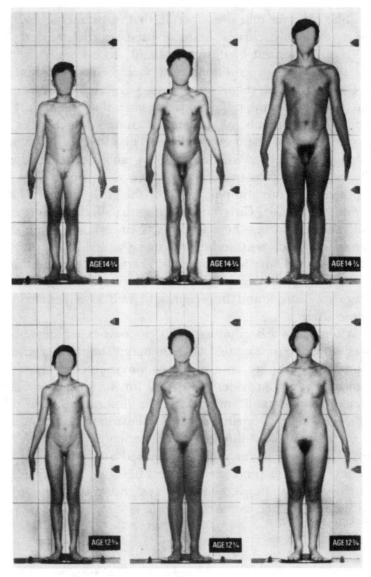

Figure 4.1. Differing degrees of pubertal development at the same chronological age. Upper row three boys all aged 14.75 years. Lower row three girls all aged 12.75 years. (From J. Tanner, 1975. Growth and endocrinology of the adolescent. In: *Endocrine and Genetic Diseases of Childhood and Adolescence*, 2nd ed., ed. L. Gardner. © W. B. Saunders in 1975 Reprinted by permission.)

other age-mates have exhibited any pubertal changes (see Figure 4.1); and in girls the period between the appearance of secondary sex characteristics and menarche can range from 6 months to 6 years.

Girls continue to develop an average of $1^1/_2$ to 2 years earlier than boys. The average age of menarche decreased at a rate of four months each decade during the fifty years prior to the 1960s. That shift has been attributed primarily to improved nutrition. Differences in age of menarche at the present time are thought to reflect genetic rather than environmental factors.

The onset of puberty appears to be related to maturation of certain centers in the central nervous system, particularly the hypothalamus. Stimulation from the hypothalamus causes the anterior pituitary to secrete hormones which in turn stimulate the adrenal glands and the production of gonadal hormones. This results in the formation of mature sperm and eggs. (Brooks-Gunn and Reiter [1990] present a recent, more detailed review of this process.)

In girls the first manifestations of puberty are breast budding and the development of straight pubic hair; these changes occur on the average between ages 10 and 11. This is followed by the maximum physical growth spurt, changes in the pubic hair to a kinky quality, and then menstruation, which now occurs on the average between 11 and 13 years of age. Axillary hair is a later development (Tanner, 1971).

Girls' physical strength peaks about a year before menarche, at which point they stop being able to beat up their brothers. Also, body density, as measured by the thickness of skin folds, increases in girls as they pass through puberty and decreases in boys, whose shoulders broaden and who become leaner and more muscular from the effects of male hormones. Thus, boys seem to need more and more food and eat more and more as puberty progresses yet still become thinner, while girls have a tendency to gain weight. This contributes to the preoccupation of many adolescent girls with their bodies.

In boys the first physical manifestations of puberty are enlargement and changes in the testes and scrotum. These are followed in order by the development of straight pubic hair, enlargement of the penis, first ejaculation, change in the quality of the pubic hair, and maximum physical growth which often occurs later. This process is completed with the development of axillary hair, and marked changes of the voice which along with growth of the beard are late phenomena (Tanner, 1971).

THE PHENOMENOLOGICAL REACTIONS TO PUBERTY

The reactions of individuals to their changing inner feeling states and their outward appearance run a gamut from great interest to great self-consciousness, from avid anticipation to utter denial. During this period youngsters also feel pressure or are drawn toward developmental advance; that is, the more developmentally precocious ones are looked up to or longingly admired by peers, except in cases where the precocious have gone too far beyond the pale of acceptable behavior.

The unsettling bodily feeling states which accompany these physiological changes are often forgotten or recalled with embarrassment in later life; for these were experiences during which one felt an unwelcome lack of self-control. Early adolescents experience waves of unfocused emotions. These unfamiliar, physical sensations create a sense that one's body is a stranger to oneself (Fraiberg, 1955). This can cause the young adolescent to fear for his or her sanity. For example, almost any feeling can cause an erection in early adolescent boys—anxiety, giggling, or anger as well as voluptuous sensations. This causes boys to feel that they cannot control themselves. The interest of prepubertal and early adolescent boys in remote control devices and phenomena like the determined way in which they attempt to master control over skateboards, hacky sax, and musical instruments is thought to represent externalization of this conflict over self-control. Girls exhibit a similar approach to horseback riding, gymnastics, and dancing.

The growth spurt in adolescent boys and girls is thought to be produced by the synergistic action of growth hormone and sex hormones (adrenal androgens and testosterone) (Tanner, 1975); together they account for adolescents' high levels of energy, activity, and aggressiveness. The early adolescent's erratic, impulsive, and radically changing behaviors derive from both the physiological changes and from his or her efforts to control these changes. Feeling either that you cannot control yourself or that you cannot rely on your own senses and perceptions are two of the most anxiety-engendering experiences a person can have. Adolescents whose feeling states are rapidly shifting can find themselves in such positions. Their efforts to avoid this anxiety, especially that associated with feeling that they cannot trust their own senses and judgment, cause some adolescents to maintain vociferously uncompromising attitudes, even when faced with incontrovertible evidence that their view is wrong. Additional contributants to the development of such unwavering inflexibility derive from issues described in the next section.

SIGNIFICANCE OF HEIGHTENED AGGRESSIVENESS

We might ask why the emerging sexuality has been thought to pose the greatest threat to the adolescent, his or her family, and the community. (In chapter 3 [p. 44] I offered an explanation for this in noting that Freud derived his developmental psychology from his theory of neurotic psychopathology.) For what often seems closer to parents' experiences are the manifestations of physical growth[3] and aggressivity. I refer to being faced by a boy or girl who is looking straight at you, not up to you, in an adolescent-at-odds-with-parents scenario that usually involves the issues of autonomy and intention. These are such dominating interpersonal themes as to suggest that the process of adolescence primarily involves the task of consolidating a confident sense of psychological independence from childhood ties to parents, rather than the psychological adaptation to sexual maturation with emancipation being a side effect of that process. In

---

[3]It is not clear whether the rate at which growth hormone is secreted is greater at puberty than in childhood. Growth hormone is not secreted at a constant rate during the day but only episodically in response to some internal rhythm or external stimulus, and thus is difficult to measure. Circulating levels of growth hormone do not correlate with pubertal stage development. Testosterone and adrenal androgens add an additional spurt to the growth rate stimulated by growth hormone. Testosterone in adolescent girls is thought to be produced from adrenal androgens secreted by the adrenal glands and ovaries. The levels of these sex steroids in female adolescents are, of course, lower than those in adolescent males (Tanner, 1975).

other words, much of what is played out between child and parents and the generations is the matter of self-assertion, which often seems closer to aggression than to sexuality. Self-assertion and aggression can have a defense-against-sexuality basis, but probably more often do not in the context of adolescent emancipation.

THE RESPONSES OF GIRLS TO PUBERTY

Breast development remains very important to girls, even in an era which has experienced more casual attitudes toward the exposure of breasts. A 1979 study by Rosenbaum of normal, middle-class adolescent girls revealed that early adolescents thought of breasts as the most important "sexual organ." By age 16 to 17 they were less preoccupied with breast size, and were quoted as saying such things as, "He should like me for what I am." They claimed to be un-self-conscious when not wearing a bra; yet, they were acutely aware of the reactions of others, suggesting more conflict than they acknowledged.

Girls who have experienced intense penis envy may find this abate when their breasts begin to develop, and their breast size becomes a matter of competition with other girls. This contributes to their increasing interest in other parts of the body, including hair and general appearance, and in terms of psychoanalytic theory, they turn from a wish for a penis to the wish for a lovely body.

MENSTRUATION

Menstruation becomes important in integrating mature sexual functioning into a girl's identity as a mature woman. Girls are thought to arrive at puberty with a less complete body image than boys. For children are concrete thinkers, relying on things they can see, touch, and hear rather than on things that they cannot experience with their senses. A girls' hidden body parts cannot be incorporated into her body image until she has had the repetitive experience of a functional activity and that is menstruation. These requirements probably persist despite the high levels of sexual enlightenment currently provided by our schools and communities. For example, a 17-year-old in the study quoted above observed that, "I know scientifically pretty much what happens, how the lining of the uterus sloughs off and all that. I was always curious. I can sort of picture what is happening, like seeing it projected on a screen. In my mind, the uterus seems fairly large—about football-size, I would guess, but it has to fit inside me—it's hard to picture a football fitting. I guess I know generally—I have dissected a cat—I could draw you a picture—but I don't know about *me*" (Rosenbaum, 1979, p. 246).

The quality of and increase in sensations around the vaginal area and the increased secretions all serve to focus girls' attention on what's going on inside them. Ten- to 12-year-old girls who are experiencing these changes become increasingly interested in observing the development of their girl friends. This becomes an age of both curiosity and secrets with peers which can serve as a stimulus for fantasies about what it means to become a woman. Menstruation has a multiplicity of meanings amongst girls. It may be viewed very positively by girls who have been unconflicted about their femininity from earlier in life. A girl's view is probably significantly influenced by her observations and interpretation of her own mother's views and behaviors. Many mothers report that their daughters prefer to be enlightened by friends and sisters. Helene Deutsch (1944) suggested years ago that this is because during the girl's early childhood, her mother's menstruation was associated with cruelty or uncleanliness or bad odors or some reaction of disgust on the girl's part. Such ideas are consistent with anthropological findings that menstruation has been associated in both primitive and modern cultures with ideas of horror, shame, danger, and sin.

The older psychoanalytic literature emphasized negative features associated with early childhood ideas of genital trauma resulting from masturbation and from the reactivation of castration anxiety by menarche. Many girls neither have such recollections nor uncover them in analytic treatment. They trust their mothers but still prefer help from their sisters and friends. Some cite embarrassment in talking to their mothers and feel it is more private to learn from friends. By the time they reach menarche, most girls have been exposed to their mothers' modesty; thus the adolescent daughters in turn feel compunction about exposing their own genitals to their mothers. They feel more comfortable sharing such intimacies with someone closer in age who has just gone through what they are now experiencing. They note that menstruation arises in conversations about sex which is a matter discussed with friends rather than parents. Some feel that menarche indicates that they are now adult and therefore do not or should not need their mothers as much, or that it is important not to have to rely on their mothers. Furthermore, since menarche occurs in most girls after the emancipation process has commenced, most have already begun to pull away from the degree of intimacy they had shared with their mothers. Some may fear that they have lost their perfectibility in the eyes of their mothers, since often their own ideal of a woman and that of their mothers is the asexual mother/woman. In line with this, other girls are reluctant to involve their mothers in their menarche because of emancipatory guilt. These girls anticipate that their own development to womanhood is threatening to their mothers. This typically occurs when the mother has somehow communicated to her daughter either that she prefers that her daughter remain a "little girl" or that she feels competitive with her daughter. But in basically normal mother–daughter pairs such concerns about disappointing the mother are more muted than the optimistic associations to menarche as an important part of the girl's evolution to psychological independence.

SUMMARY

Children's behaviors during the middle school/junior high years often comprise an accentuation or variation of prior adaptive style rather than a dramatic, substantive change in their ways of adapting. The importance of identification and practicing to perfect skills and styles is discussed with respect to the child's behaviors during this transition to adolescence. I find that the sex-linked differences in behavioral styles of boys and girls during this transition posited by psychoanalytic theorists have been overstated (Deutsch, 1944; Blos, 1958). Those views arose because the role of adaptation to drives was emphasized in earlier theories and insufficient consideration was given to the preadolescent's adaptation to his or her real experiences. The role of adolescents' heightened aggressiveness as opposed to sexuality is considered. The utility of another extant view of prepuberty which correlates the prepubertal child's cognitive style directly with the biological changes of puberty is also discussed (Kestenberg, 1961); I concur with that author's view that the mother is an even more important organizer for the girl's way of dealing with anxiety than is menarche.

The appearance of adolescent behaviors and attitudes in the current generation of preadolescents is explained on the basis of children's efforts to secure approval of parents by identifying with their behaviors or to retain the positive view of their parents that they wish to maintain. The latter is accomplished by adopting parental attitudes or behaviors which the children find foolish, distressing, or contemptible; this phenomenon is termed defensive identification in this book. When parents are either too neglectful (uninterested), inadequate, or too controlling of their child's efforts to move forward developmentally, the preadolescent is more inclined to turn to a peer group which serves a substitute parental role in the process of emancipating. This turn to peers also predisposes to precocious involvement in behaviors which have more typically been observed in adolescents.

CHAPTER 5

The Onset of Adolescence

RELATIONSHIP TO PUBERTY

Common wisdom has long associated the onset of adolescence with puberty. Psychoanalytic theory links the onset of adolescents' efforts to emancipate and their adult-mimicking behaviors to sexual maturation in a specific manner: Puberty is accompanied by a resurgence of incestuous desires. These yearnings impel children to emancipate from their childhood attachments to their parents; their motivation for emancipating is to avoid anxiety associated with the oedipal conflict (Freud, 1905b). The urgency in this process is attributed to the fact that unlike the child, the genitally mature adolescent is a true oedipal competitor (A. Freud, 1958). Thus, emancipation is basically a defense against regressive urges, motivated by self-preservative wishes, namely to escape punishment for oedipal desires.

With all other aspects of development moving forward, rendering the adolescent bigger, stronger, smarter, and more sexually mature, it becomes difficult logically to accept the premise that personality development is occurring on an opposite, defensive, basis. For that would suggest that the psyche is impelled in the opposite direction from the soma. Common sense suggests that the adolescent experiences some innate pressure to spread and try out the wings of his or her enhanced capacities. Nor does a defensive motive for emancipation seem congruent with the robust attitude of eager anticipation, intensity, and energy exhibited by many if not most adolescents as they strive for greater independence and adult prerogatives. While counterphobic elements are certainly observed in their behaviors, the predominant tone of this emancipatory effort seems neither compulsive, defensive, nor highly conflicted.

Since the resurgent oedipal urges normally remain repressed (unconscious), the psychoanalytic theory becomes difficult to test. However, by focusing on: behaviors and attitudes which are commonly considered to be derivatives of oedipal yearnings; plus objective evidence that puberty has occurred; and conventionally accepted evidences of inner and overt efforts to emancipate, we can clinically investigate the relationship between puberty and emancipation.

EXAMPLE 1: EMANCIPATORY PHENOMENA APPEAR TO COINCIDE WITH PUBERTY, AS POSITED BY TRADITIONAL PSYCHOANALYTIC THEORY

> The youngest of four children had always maintained a close, dependent relationship on her mother and a warm tie with her father. Then, late in seventh grade at age $12^1/_2$, her behavior changed over a relatively short period of time from affectionate and open to bristling, rejecting, rude, and withdrawn from her parents. Friendships with girls which had always been important to her now became even more so, and she expanded this group to include girls who were a year older.
>
> Her menarche occurred six months later. During the remainder of her thirteenth year she expressed a conviction that she was different from all other members of her family. She often scornfully advised her parents to "get a life" so they would not have to be so interested in hers. She objected to any restrictions they placed on her activities. But she always ultimately accepted their limits. In fact, none of her behaviors was objectively self-defeating, save for a lack of interest in schoolwork.
>
> Two years after her menarche, her parents found her "somewhat easier to live with," in terms of being more reasonable, though she could quickly revert to her rejecting, shrewish behaviors when not allowed her own way. She was performing well academically, was active in social and extracurricular activities, and was not involved in drugs, drinking, or sexual activity.

The change in this girl's behavior occurred in the months before sexual maturation was objectively confirmed. Psychoanalytic theory does not maintain that menarche or first ejaculation per se motivates emancipation, but rather that the period of puberty does. My more specific focus in this chapter on the relationship between first menstruation or ejaculation and emancipatory behaviors is simply to provide incontrovertible evidence that puberty has occurred in the individuals being described. The coincidence of emancipatory phenomena and puberty does not prove a causal relationship between them. The phenomena observed in the previous example are consistent with the relationship posited by psychoanalysis.

EXAMPLE 2: SEXUAL MATURATION COEXISTS WITH OVERT OEDIPAL BEHAVIORS AND NO MOVEMENT TOWARD EMANCIPATION

An 11-year-old boy experienced his first nocturnal emission during a heterosexual dream. He was distressed by the experience, thinking that he had wet the bed. At that time he and a male friend were talking a lot about sex, though he seemed afraid of girls and was acting aggressively toward them.

In the months following that wet dream, he made no effort to become more independent from his parents. Quite the contrary, he still attempted to monopolize their attention in immature ways. Also, he exhibited blatant oedipal attitudes and behaviors. He continued to hug and kiss his mother, offered to share her bed when his physician father was on call at the hospital, and was keen to race and beat his father in their swimming pool.

A year later (age 12), he was no longer asking to take his father's place in bed and claimed to prefer and idolize his father. He exhibited little, if any, evidence though of having moved psychologically away from his childhood dependency on either parent. He had some different male friends, but was developing no closer bonds to them than he had formed with his previous buddies. He was no longer fighting with girls as he had been a year earlier. His daydreams, which distracted him from studying, were now of the aggressive/heroic rather than sexual variety.

At age 13 he was consolidating political views different from those of his parents, though he remained closely allied to their religious beliefs. He was observing, with an attitude of supercilious amusement, both parents' feet of clay and their idiosyncrasies. He often thought about which girls he liked and which of them might like him, and he had many heterosexual fantasies.

This boy matured sexually at the relatively early age of 11 years. He did not exhibit evidence of pulling away from his childhood attachment to parents until two years after that time; and even then, his emancipatory moves were more evident in his attitudes than in his behaviors. In fact, for much of the period described, sexual maturation coexisted with overt oedipal attitudes. Psychoanalytic theory maintains that the incestuous urges normally remain repressed (unconscious); the emancipation process is the means by which the adolescent avoids awareness of these oedipal yearnings. Psychoanalytic theory would consider that this boy did not commence emancipatory efforts at the time of puberty because he was experiencing overt oedipal behaviors. That is, he is held in this childhood, nonemancipated position by the compelling neurotic gratification derived from these regressive oedipal behaviors. So, the traditional psychoanalytic view becomes circular and difficult to disprove; that is, if the child is not emancipating in the manner prescribed by psychoanalysis, it is because he or she is abnormal. This lad did begin to exhibit emancipatory attitudes and behaviors, but at the same time that his peers were exhibiting similar behaviors rather than at the time of his early-onset puberty. Thus, factors other than and/or in addition to sexual maturation influence the timing of emancipatory attitudes and behaviors.

The next example further illustrates that the processes of sexual maturation and emancipation can occur independently of one another.

EXAMPLE 3: PREEXISTING OEDIPAL ATTITUDES PERSIST AFTER PUBERTY, WITH EMANCIPATORY PHENOMENA ARISING LATER

From the age of 9 this girl began to resent her mother intensely; this was the point at which the latter went to work so that the girl's older brother could attend a private university. During the next two years the girl began to favor and idealize her father; she felt he was more available than her mother when she needed assistance. At age 11 she herself began to work and achieved a reputation of being a very reliable mother's helper. At ages 12 and 13, in junior high school, she tried to establish intense, possessive, "exclusive" relationships with other girls, and frequently found herself embroiled in female triangles in which she feared being rejected.

Menarche occurred at age 13 and had no discernible impact on these interpersonal patterns of thinly suppressed hatred of her mother, idolization of her father, and intense relationships with girl friends. She was less interested in boys than were her girl friends. This pattern continued during her freshman high school year, two years postmenarche.

At age 15 her parents considered her behavior rebellious. She was fighting with them, staying out late, not concentrating on her studies, and flaunting a preference for junk food (to the consternation of her dietitian mother).

At age 15¹/₂ she had her first boyfriend. Although flattered by his interest, she felt dissatisfied with him and was sure that she could only fall in love with someone just like her father. Also, she was still much more emotionally invested in her girl friends than in her boyfriend.

Then, three years postmenarche, between ages 15¹/₂ and 16, her masturbatory fantasies evolved from ones involving women to ones involving men, and she began to feel sexually aroused with her boyfriend.

As her seventeenth birthday approached she was making more decisions independently. She felt less angry toward her mother and more critical of her father, though observed that changing her idealized view of him threatened her sense of security. And she thought that her dependency on her girl friends persisted because she did not feel secure in her mother's or father's love.

The behaviors and attitudes described by psychoanalysis are observed in this girl's relationship to her parents and peers, but these elements did not occur in a progression which is consistent with psychoanalytic theory: The resurgent oedipal attitudes were prompted by experiences with her parents during latency, not by puberty. Her movement toward triangular involvements with girls (Deutsch, 1944) may have been influenced by puberty; however, the more important determinant of her dependent relationships with girl friends was her effort to compensate for her mother's withdrawal from parenting at home.

Moveover, this girl did not exhibit further, meaningful emancipatory movement until several years after puberty and months after the psychological maturation of her masturbatory fantasies, from images involving women's bodies to those of men. Even then, while moving toward psychological independence, as evidenced by her more balanced view of both parents and her autonomous decision making, a remnant of her early adolescent pattern of jealous attachment to girl friends persisted.

Since these phenomena did not occur as prescribed by psychoanalysis, I conclude that the psychoanalytic explanation is not accurate or sufficient. This example illustrates the influence that real experiences can have in determining the onset of the adolescent emancipatory process. It also suggests that a distinction can be made between biological sexual maturation, psychological sexual maturation, and psychological maturation.

This girl's persisting, relative reliance on peers and parents for making her decisions conveys the impression that she was relatively psychologically immature. Nonetheless she had been a reliable, sought-after worker in several jobs which she had held from before the time she became adolescent, and in that area she exhibited relative maturity compared to many peers. Thus, features of psychological maturity can carry through from childhood without being significantly influenced for better or worse by adolescent development.

The next example continues to illustrate the variations which exist between puberty and the appearance of attitudes/behaviors which reflect adolescents' efforts to emancipate themselves.

EXAMPLE 4: PUBERTY SEEMS TO HAVE NO IMPACT ON THE EMANCIPATION PROCESS WHICH OCCURS GRADUALLY AND SILENTLY

A girl who had always moved through her life with relative ease looked forward to growing up; she wanted to become a mother and had less clear plans about other careers. She was a conscientious student, was liked and respected by peers, and maintained good friendships with girls during latency while managing to avoid cliques. She was considered responsible by all who knew her. Between ages 12 and 13 she was proud of her developing figure and greeted her menarche at $13^1/2$ with a little apprehension but considerable pleasure as an important milestone. Her attitude and behavior toward her parents changed little before or after this event. She was casually affectionate with both parents. She continued to confide in them about matters which were of particular concern to her, and kept her own counsel and that of her friends about other matters. She remained primarily occupied with her school and after-school activities and her girl friends.

During the next two years (ages 14 and 15), she was interested in boys; however, much of that interest centered around talking with girl friends about guys. Frequently she found herself sharing an interest in the same boy with her best girl friend at the time.

Between ages 15 and 16 she wished to have a boyfriend and did for short periods of time, while concurrently retaining close, noncliquish friendships with girls. During this period she participated with her girl friends and several boys in social activities without pairing; thus, they functioned as a heterosexual gang. She wished for more romance and wondered when she should have intercourse, but made no movement toward sexual involvement; in fact, she withdrew from girl friends who had become sexually active.

At 16 she secured her long-awaited driver's license. She looked upon this in the same way that she had her menarche—an important milestone in growing up. Subsequently she would at times become impatient with her parents, accusing them of not trusting her when they refused to allow her free rein with the family car. But in fact, as the Offers (1975) suggest in their studies of boys who exhibit "continuous growth," this adolescent's behaviors and trustworthiness made it easy for her parents to allow her much of the leeway she requested.

This gradual transition to adulthood continued during her seventeenth year. She was more involved in activities outside her home, working part time, spending time with friends, and particularly her boyfriend with whom she shared ego interests as well as romantic feelings. She still maintained a strong, positive relationship toward her parents, and would eventually (i.e., often after the fact) share important issues in her life with them. Gradually and almost imperceptibly she was growing away from doing so, however, whilst exhibiting increasing independence of thought and action. During her seventeenth and eighteenth years she demonstrated a more incisive analytic ability in her schoolwork than she had exhibited prior to her seventeenth year.

Sexual maturation seemed to have little impact on this girl's emancipatory behaviors or attitudes. Sexual development, evidenced by secondary and primary sex characteristics, just as her later acquisition of a driver's license, seemed less a propellant toward emancipation than simply a reassuring indicator to herself that the process of developing to maturity was occurring. Cognitive maturation became apparent relatively late in the process.

SELF PSYCHOLOGY AND COGNITIVE PSYCHOLOGY

In both these theories adolescent development is instigated by cognitively influenced changes in ideals and values. Self psychology theorists have posited that adolescence is initiated by a disintegration of the ideal self (Wolf, Gedo, and Terman, 1972). New values offered by the peer group prompt the youngster to become disillusioned with his parents. This disenchantment can occur at any time during the adolescent years, and it does not necessarily arise in conjunction with puberty.

Piagetians emphasize an incremental advance to the capacity to think abstractly (formal operational thinking). This enhanced cognitive capacity motivates the adolescent to develop his own moral code and ways of dealing with the world (Kagan, 1971; Kohlberg and Gilligan, 1971). Thus, cognitive changes precipitate the movement toward psychological independence.

The onset of adolescence in some individuals may conform to the models presented by these theories. However, descriptive and empirical studies of nonpatient populations of adolescents raise questions about the universal applicability of each of these theories. Writing from a libido theory perspective in the 1930s, Bernfeld (1935) described adolescents who seemed to have always been striving for independence and adulthood. His observations seem similar in several respects to conclusions of the Offers (1975) who wrote from an adaptive perspective about adolescents in the late 1960s and 1970s. They describe a group of normal adolescents who exhibit what they call "continuous growth." Even if not striving in the way Bernfeld described, this subgroup of the Offers' subjects seemed to approach emancipation without great internal conflict.

Bernfeld states and the Offers (1975) imply if not state[1] that the ego ideal from childhood is not shattered by disillusionment following exposure to the ideas of peers; rather, it remains relatively unchanged throughout adolescence. The Offers find that

---

[1]The Offers observe with tongue in cheek that "if we want to change our society, clearly we must become social engineers and intervene before children accept parental values, as is seen the most characteristically in our first [continuous growth] group" (p. 48).

the views and values of their subjects' parents were invariably more closely adhered to than those of peers. These individuals do not seriously question parental values. These findings are not compatible with the self psychology view that adolescent development/emancipation requires disillusionment with parents as ideals.

Bernfeld states that this type of adolescence gives rise to a coarse, simple character structure. Bernfeld maintains that this group is least creative and the Offers' findings imply that these individuals are most likely to emerge as adults very similar to their parents (1975, p. 48). The Offers' continuous growth group was a subgroup of a research population of average students. This plus the fact that this subgroup seemed to be turning out more like their parents than the other research subjects suggests that the capacity to use formal operational thinking would not be a prominent characteristic of these individuals. Formal operational thinking is probably necessary in order to develop a new ego ideal or ideal self in the self psychologists' view; and the ego ideal is intimately related to conscience and morality (Kohlberg and Gilligan, 1971). Thus, the Bernfeld observations and the Offer studies on normal adolescent males, while not ruling out a contribution from Piagetian and self psychology, support a broader view of the initiation of adolescent development than those theories provide.

The individual described in the next example exhibits several features consistent with the cognitive and self psychologists' views of how adolescence is initiated. In my experience, however, such individuals have been intellectually precocious prior to adolescence; and this feature of their endowment seems to be a crucial determinant of the form taken by their adolescent development. Quotations from the autobiographies of Havelock Ellis (1939) and Albert Schweitzer (1949) in chapter 6 are additional examples of this phenomenon in which cognitive changes appear more prominent than sexual ones in initiating adolescent emancipatory behaviors and attitudes.

EXAMPLE 5: EMANCIPATORY EFFORTS ANTEDATE AND OVERSHADOW FEATURES OF SEXUAL MATURATION

During his eleventh year, the long-standing, headstrong ways of an intellectually precocious boy became more pronounced. He pressed his parents to do only what he pleased, to be the master of his destiny, and to have minimal responsibility for anything else. He also pulled away from his long-time friends and took up with others who were less stable but shared his newfound interest in theater. He was experiencing pubertal changes at the time and his growth spurt began that year.

He became more contentious and withdrawn from his family during his thirteenth year. His parents were unable to induce a better school performance from him; he achieved mediocre grades though learned much about subjects which interested him. By his fourteenth year he was espousing and living without apparent compunction by a moral code which differed in important respects from that of his parents. He lied with impunity to parents who did not lie and who actively espoused honesty. He wrote school papers for schoolmates for money and was willing to give other students answers on tests. He also developed and sustained political beliefs which differed from those of his parents. He could not be persuaded to change his views or behaviors in any matter unless the opposing view was logically convincing to him.

As a 15-year-old he claimed to be interested in girls, but had no female friends, much less a girl friend. Nevertheless, because he was traveling with a crowd that included sexually active adolescents, the lad's father provided him with condoms when he was 16. He used them early in his seventeenth year, thus functioning responsibly when he joined the ranks of the sexually initiated. During these years before he left home, however, he showed no inclination or willingness to assume responsibility for any household chores or to secure a part-time job to contribute to school or pocket expenses.

At age 18 he functioned independently with ease at a distant college. Yet, he remained unwilling to work to contribute to college expenses even though such assistance would have been helpful to his parents. His interest in girls remained focused on sexual experiences. That is, in psychoanalytic terms he was still consolidating his sexual identity; he had not yet made the transition to psychological independence which is represented by "object removal" (Katan, 1937) to a love relationship with a nonincestuous object.

This boy's struggles for the prerogatives of independence antedated puberty. Moreover, for several years this drive toward independence was much more pronounced than evidence of psychological sexual maturation. He was functioning with a world view more akin to that of his new friends than that of his parents;

this seems consistent with the self psychology theory of how adolescent emancipation is initiated. The moral code with which he functioned was of his own construction and logic; this seems compatible with the importance cognitive psychology theory attaches to the acquisition of formal operational thinking in framing one's own philosophy of life.

In terms of psychoanalytic theory, the delay in this boy's psychosexual maturation to heterosexual object finding would be attributed to sublimation of his sexual drive in theatrical and intellectual interests and the development of his personal moral code. Adolescence is thought to be prolonged in such individuals because the developmental issue of sexuality is avoided. This is one typical progression described by psychoanalysts (Bernfeld, 1923). However, this lad's sublimations were not associated with inhibition in his heterosexual development or in his ability to function apart from his family.

The difficulties in demonstrating the disjunction between emancipatory strivings and puberty are twofold: One is definitional—adolescence has traditionally been defined by puberty; the other is that the ubiquity of puberty renders it difficult to document that these two features of development can evolve independently. When we consider examples like this boy and the girls in example 3, whose preexisting oedipal attitudes coexisted with emancipatory behaviors, and example 4, whose development seemed to proceed as if puberty were a sign rather than motivator of adolescence, the evolution of strivings for independence seems to proceed without any consistent relationship to the physiology or psychology of sexual maturation. Each seems to follow a course of its own.

Examples 3 and 5 also illustrate continuity from before or early in puberty of behaviors and attitudes of independence which have traditionally been associated with the ending of adolescence. The youth in example 5 exhibited a personal moral code and self-definition regarding schoolwork and personal behavior from early in adolescence. At the same time he demonstrated a notable absence of other of the features of adolescence associated with emancipation; for example, assuming greater responsibility for his own care. By comparison, the girl in example

3 exhibited the opposite pattern of emancipatory traits. She demonstrated a high degree of financial responsibility and self-care, but remained dependent on her parents and friends for her values, moral standards, and approval of her actions. Note also that in both individuals the features of maturity had been evident prior to adolescence. The Offers (1975) have stressed the stability of the adolescent's character from childhood through adolescence. Lichtenberg (1982) has identified continuities and transformations between infancy and adolescence from clinical material. Also, the empirical longitudinal research (chapter 2) bears on this issue. Those studies have shown patterns of continuity and of change between early childhood and adolescence (Kagan and Moss, 1962), and in the traits of distinct personality types of boys and girls followed from early adolescence to young adulthood (Block and Haan, 1971) and into midlife (Eichorn, Clausen, Haan, Honzik, and Mussen, 1981). The examples I have presented support the idea that some traits are percolating along without much relationship to sexual development or other features of the adolescent developmental process. Thus, the motive force for this continuous and progressive development seems broader-based than either sexual or cognitive maturation, though it includes both.

Individuals who do not experience puberty represent one end of the spectrum I have been documenting and potentially provide an avenue for determining whether emancipation can exist in the absence of sexual maturation.

EXAMPLE 6: EMANCIPATORY BEHAVIOR DURING ADOLESCENT YEARS IN THE ABSENCE OF PUBERTY

The following data are from a study published in the 1950s of an early adolescent who had been born with the external genitals of a normal female and thus raised as a girl. It was subsequently determined that she had no sex glands (gonads) and had a male chromosomal pattern (Hampson, Hampson, and Money, 1955). Lacking gonads she could not experience puberty, for the hormones from the pituitary, which initiate puberty by stimulating the ovaries or testes to produce estrogens and androgens, would have no effect. Her appearance was quite typical of such individuals; her growth was moderately stunted, she was overweight, and had a short, broad neck. She clearly felt herself to be a girl, however, despite being genetically male.

At age 14 years, 5 months, pubertal changes were artificially induced by treatment with estrogen. Our interest is in determining whether she experienced inner attitudes and outer behaviors which would represent emancipatory efforts before that time. Assessment of this is complicated by the fact that this was not the theme of the study in which the case was reported so all data relevant to the question I am addressing were not included.

At age 11 she had occasionally engaged in sex play with a friend who was already beginning puberty. They would unclothe, get in bed together, and tickle each other's genitals. The girl did not comprehend the enjoyment her friend experienced when having her breasts fondled. When she was 11½ her mother reported feeling that the child must be unhappy because she seemed at times irritable, complaining, and ungrateful. Her usual behaviors seemed more similar to than different from those of her age-mates. She seemed to exhibit features of both relative maturity and relative immaturity compared to peers. For example, she was a leader at school, but still played with paper dolls and enjoyed playing house. There were suggestions of emancipatory movement; at age 12 she admired an 18-year-old girl in the neighborhood and basked in the attention shown her by that older girl; at the same time she had a best friend of her own age. At 14 she entered junior high school and functioned well there socially. Her mother reported that her tastes, clothes preferences, and mannerisms changed in line with those of her peers.

Apparently prior to hormone therapy she reported both heroic daydreams and sexual fantasies which were typical of pre- and early adolescents. The former included fantasies of becoming an opera singer and being successfully married. The sexual fantasies were masochistic in nature, often involving murder, torture, or beatings, usually by a group of men. Typically she was taken out of the earshot of others against her will, her clothes were torn off, and she was cut with knives, beaten with a club, or had objects like knives or penises stuck into her vagina. Sometimes these fantasies, which usually occurred at bedtime, were accompanied by feelings of excitement, primarily in her genitals. Genital penetration fantasies were less exciting than ones in which she was tortured/hurt. Manual or thigh-pressing masturbatory activity usually accompanied these fantasies. She also masturbated at times without fantasies. In addition, she reported conventional daydreams of romance, courtship, and marriage.

Estrogen treatment was begun at age 14½ and by age 15 she had begun to have normal breast development, which pleased her greatly. From then on her fantasies were exclusively of a romantic and erotic nature, with pleasure and excitement anticipated at the thought of the boy touching her breasts and compunction at the thought of him touching her genitals.

The authors of this study emphasized the difficulty that such girls have in negotiating adolescence because of their juvenile appearance—short stature (usually less than 4 feet, 10 inches tall), and lack of secondary sex characteristics. While reporting that she was not infantile psychologically despite having been so physically, they concluded that the appearance of a physically mature body is an essential ingredient for the advancement of psychological maturation in adolescence. Those authors suggest that individuals who do not experience puberty nevertheless become emancipated adults, albeit with some inhibitions in their personalities related to the fact of their physical immaturity.

The points I want to make here are that these girls do make emancipatory moves regardless of whether they experience puberty. This girl (example 6) had masturbatory fantasies with a strong pregenital quality prior to the inception of estrogen treatment and she had developed a relationship with an older girl whom she idolized. Thus, she exhibited sexual and emancipatory phenomena respectively which are traditionally considered to be motivated by pubertal urges. Moreover, she was a leader amongst her peers, suggesting independence of action and spirit. The latter emancipatory trait antedated but continued after her artificially induced puberty; similar phenomena were reported in examples 3 and 5.

EXAMPLE 7: PUBERTY HAS NO IMPACT ON DEVELOPMENT (PUBERTY IS EXPERIENCED AS SEXUAL/AGGRESSIVE EXCITEMENT WITHOUT OEDIPAL-TYPE OBJECT RELATIONSHIPS AND WITHOUT EMANCIPATORY PHENOMENA)

To continue this consideration of the relationship between puberty and emancipation and cognitive development and emancipation, I will turn from the last example, an experiment in nature (genetic/biological insufficiency), to the opposite situation, an experiment in nurture (environmental insufficiency).

Itard (1802) described the reaction of puberty in Victor, the Wild Boy of Aveyron, a feral child, seven years after becoming his caretaker:

I have seen . . . puberty arrive or rather burst forth, and our young savage consumed by desire of an extreme violence and of startling constancy and this without any presentment of its purpose or the slightest feeling of preference for any woman. Instead of that expansive impulse which precipitates one sex towards the other, I have observed in him only a sort of blind and slightly pronounced instinct which, as a matter of fact, does make him prefer the society of women to that of men without in any way involving his heart. Thus, I have seen him in a company of women attempting to relieve his uneasiness by sitting beside one of them and gently taking hold of her hand, her arms and her knees until, feeling his restless desires increased instead of calmed by these odd caresses, and seeing no relief from his painful emotions in sight, he suddenly changed his attitude and petulantly pushed away the woman whom he had sought with a kind of eagerness. Then he addressed himself without interruption to another woman with whom he behaved in the same way. One day, nevertheless, he became a little more enterprising. After first employing the same caresses, he took the lady by her hands and drew her, without violence, however, into the depths of an alcove. There, very much out of countenance, and showing in his manners and in his extraordinary facial expression an indescribable mixture of gaiety and sadness, of boldness and uncertainty, he several times solicited the lady's caresses by offering her his cheeks and walked slowly around her with a meditative air, finally flinging his arms about her shoulders and holding her closely by the neck. This was all, and these amorous demonstrations ended, as did all the others with a movement of annoyance which made him repulse the object of his transitory inclinations [pp. 97–98].

I have added this example to make two points. Its significance for our consideration is that a human can experience puberty without developing sexual maturity in the sense of being able to perform sexual acts, and without any movement toward emancipation from more infantile object ties. It can be argued that this youth's cognitive functioning was subnormal, on either a constitutional or environmentally induced basis, so this example can form no basis for talking about adolescence in normal humans. There had been a deficit in his early human object relatedness since he had apparently been raised by animals. He experienced puberty, to Itard's satisfaction; but the only change wrought by puberty was an awareness that his inner tension would be relieved through some relation to women. There was no natural understanding of the way in which this would occur; this has also been suggested by the Harlows' studies of monkeys raised by surrogates (Harlow and Harlow, 1962).

Gagnon (1971) suggests that mature sexual functioning itself involves much more learned gender-specific, socially taught behavior than a model of development which emphasizes biologically based drive pressures would imply is necessary. Freedman (1983) writes that previously established object relationships are a prerequisite for the process of mature sexual functioning to develop; that is, drives cannot develop, at least to fruition, in vacuo. And again, the individual's real experiences prior to puberty profoundly affect his response or lack of same to sexual urges and the development of adolescent attitudes and behaviors. The idea that biological sexual maturation, psychological sexual maturation, and psychological maturation for that matter are all different phenomena is borne out by the following example.

EXAMPLE 8: EXPERIMENTS IN NATURE IN WHICH THERE IS A DISJUNCTION BETWEEN THE TIMING OF SEXUAL MATURATION AND CURRENT SOCIETY'S EXPECTATION OF EMANCIPATION

To round out this examination of the relationship between puberty and the onset of adolescence, I will now switch back from an experiment in nurture described in the last example to another experiment in nature (as was example 6). Girls and boys who become pubertal before ages 9 and 11 respectively are considered to experience precocious puberty. While it can commence in the first year of life, precocious puberty frequently begins in early childhood (e.g., ages 2–6 years). The condition is diagnosed as idiopathic or true precocious puberty when a physical cause, such as a tumor in the brain, adrenal glands, or ovaries is not found. The physiological process and bodily changes which occur are essentially normal in all respects; puberty simply occurs prematurely or precociously.[2]

The outcome is young children who have fully developed and functioning sexual organs and breasts, axillary, pubic, and

---

[2]For example, a 5-year, 8-month-old girl has given birth to a full-term, healthy infant by Caesarean section (Tanner, 1975).

facial hair, and voice changes. Because sex hormones, particularly testosterone, contribute to growth, children who experience precocious puberty are usually the size of youngsters a couple of years older than themselves. Some children with precocious puberty, especially those who are also intellectually precocious, migrate to peers who are closer to their physical height and intellectual abilities; nevertheless, psychologically most are closer to age mates than children of their physical size. Their larger size, energy, and strength incline adults to inappropriately expect them to behave and be as physically well coordinated as children of their size rather than of their age. Sex hormones are also involved in closure of the growth plates of the long bones. Thus, children who have experienced precocious puberty end up shorter as adults than their peers (Tanner, 1975). This condition presents another opportunity to study the relationship between biological (sexual) maturation, and psychological and psychosexual development.

Case studies and reports have described difficulties these children (Noshpitz, 1991) and their parents (Krims, 1962) experience in adjusting to the child's precocious puberty. Krims (1962) observed that the children themselves evince little curiosity about their sexual maturation and, if anything, are more concerned about their height than their mature secondary sex characteristics. The psychoanalysis of a girl with precocious puberty conducted from ages 3 to 10 years revealed unconscious conflicts that may not be elicited in research interviews and longitudinal studies (Thomas, Folkart, and Model, 1963). In that particular case, however, it is difficult to differentiate between the contributions of her reaction to precocious puberty, to frequent hospitalizations at an early age, and to interactions with troubled parents in the genesis of her problematic conflicts. More important for our purposes, those authors conclude that precocious puberty is not accompanied by an increase in sexual drive associated with puberty. Nor did the child show any features of adolescence at age 10.

Money and Hampson (1955) had found that the content of sexual dreams and fantasies described by a boy with precocious puberty who acknowledged having them, and the romantic fantasies of girls who described them, are typical of their chronological level of development, not their level of biological sexual maturation. Since children are acute observers of differences, it stands to reason that their own and their peers' observations of them would arouse some anxiety and fantasies in the child. However, the overriding impression has been that the psychological adjustment of these children encompasses the same spectrum as that of their chronological age mates.

In more recent, controlled questionnaire studies, the parents of girls who had experienced true precocious puberty report their daughters to have exhibited a much higher prevalence of behavioral problems, including social withdrawal, depression, and aggression, than is expected from norms. Yet, these girls exhibit less social competence than their peers. We might anticipate greater social competence if their psychosexual development paralleled their biological sexual development. (The longitudinal study cited in chapter 2 did suggest that normal, early maturing girls seem less socially confident than late maturers.) The behavioral problems of girls and boys do not correlate with the level of sexual maturation, as measured by stage of breast and pubic hair development (Sonis, Comite, Pescovitz, Hench, Rahn, Cutler, Loriaux, and Klein, 1986). These authors also find that most children with precocious puberty fall within the range of age-appropriate psychological development. Another study reported that some girls with idiopathic precocious puberty may exhibit greater interest in boys than do age mates, as well as a type of interest in their own appearance that is typical of older pubertal girls. The girls with precocious puberty are, if anything though, more emotionally shy and constricted than age mates, and not psychosexually precocious. The conclusion of this study also is that the biological changes of precocious puberty do not usher in adolescent development; that is, their psychological development follows their chronological age rather than their biological sexual stage (Solyom, Austad, Sherick, and Bacon, 1980).

When interviewed during their late teens and early adult years, some girls who had experienced precocious puberty report periods of moodiness, depression and withdrawal (Money and Walker, 1971). A retrospective parent questionnaire study of a small cohort comprised predominantly of black American girls (mean age $17^1/_2$ years) was conducted. Girls who had experienced idiopathic precocious puberty were reported to have had more conduct problems (not otherwise specified), antisocial problems, socialized delinquency, and psychosomatic complaints than matched controls (Erhardt, Meyer-Bahlburg, Bell, Cohen, Healey, Stiel, Feldman, Morishima, and New, 1984). In each of these areas the statistical differences were mild, being characterized only as either a tendency or a weak tendency. The subject girls also exhibit more problems with inadequacy and immaturity than the controls; those behavioral traits are probably the opposite of what one would expect if the conduct problems were manifestations of adolescent efforts to emancipate. The same research group reported that those who experience idiopathic precocious puberty reall having experienced several psychosexual milestones a year to two before the matched controls; these milestones include first boyfriend, falling in love, kissing, petting, and intercourse. However, these differences were reported to be modest at best and far narrower than the disparity in the ages when puberty commenced in each group (Meyer-Bahlburg, Ehrhardt, Bell, Cohen, Healey, Feldman, Morishima, Baker, and New, 1985).

Thus, the prevailing concensus from clinical, descriptive, empirical, controlled, and longitudinal research is that children who experience idiopathic precocious puberty exhibit the same spectrum of psychological functioning as their age mates. Also, they may experience behavioral difficulties but their condition does not seem to be accompanied or followed by serious psychiatric symptomatology, especially if the children and their parents are counselled appropriately by professionals (Money and Hampson, 1955; Hampson and Money, 1955; Thomas et al., 1963). And most important for our purposes, these children exhibit no tendency toward precocious adolescence, that is, to emancipate prematurely to greater psychological autonomy; nor do they typically exhibit precocious psychosexual interests or behaviors (Thomas et al., 1963; Money and Walker, 1971; Solyom, Austad, Sherick, and Bacon, 1980; Krims, 1962; Sarnoff, 1976). Barring future research findings to the contrary, this experiment in nature provides additional evidence that the adolescent imperative to emancipate is not inextricably related to puberty.

SUMMARY

These eight examples illustrate a spectrum of relationships between puberty (psychoanalytic theory), cognitive development (Piagetian psychology), and disillusionment with parental values (self psychology) on the one hand, and emancipatory attitudes and behaviors associated with adolescent development on the other hand. Emancipatory phenomena are considered in psychoanalytic theory to arise as a direct response to fantasies associated with puberty; in cognitive and self psychology emancipatory phenomena are thought to develop respectively from cognitive advances and from shattering of the parents as ideals.

The spectrum of examples presented includes individuals who seem to conform to those models (at least in some respects) and others who do not. The latter include individuals in whom:

1. Puberty is associated with overt oedipal-type behaviors without movement away from childhood attachment to parents;
2. Emancipatory phenomena exist in the absence of puberty;
3. Emancipatory phenomena seem more closely associated with preexisting intellectual precocity than with puberty;
4. Maturation of sexuality and emancipatory phenomena seem to follow independent courses;
5. Puberty is experienced as an indicator that a silent process of emancipation is occurring;
6. Puberty itself is not experienced as a maturational phenomenon.

The existence of these variations calls for a broader-based explanation for the onset of emancipation in adolescents than the existing theories offer.

CHAPTER 6

The Developmental Process During Adolescence

Those contributions from psychoanalysis, self psychology, and cognitive psychology which are important to adolescent development can be incorporated into a more comprehensive thesis which emphasizes the motivation to advance. Contributions from those fields to the new theory will be elaborated upon and critiqued in this chapter. Three different clinical observations support my thesis about the progressive thrust in adolescent development: (1) behavioral patterns which can only be explained by such a thesis; (2) phenomena which seem better or more completely understood by a theory different from the existing ones; (3) evidence of self-generated, self-righting, or self-regulating tendencies toward accomplishing developmental goals (see Emde, 1988a; Lichtenberg, 1989).

The concept that adolescents are motivated to progress can be inferred from two mechanisms they utilize prominently in the developmental process, namely, identification and forms of learning. Individual adolescents vary in the degree to which they are consciously aware of their use of these mechanisms: (1) Adolescents identify in order to experiment with newly acquired abilities, enhanced potentialities, and tastes as described in chapter 4. (2) They identify in order to maintain their sense of security as they become increasingly independent. Younger children are motivated to identify with parents for the same reasons of love and admiration for their parents. (3) Adolescents identify with their parents' worst traits in order to ward off conscious awareness of justifiable contempt and severe criticism of parents, so as to retain a positive view of them (chapter 4). (4) Adolescents identify in order to reverse the effects of previous traumatic experiences with parents. This involves identifying with the unhealthy behaviors which the parent has exhibited toward the adolescent (turning passive into active). The operative mechanism when an adolescent's behavior seems dramatically different from his or her prior conduct is frequently turning passive into active.

In addition to identification, there are various ways in which adolescents learn that demonstrate this motive to progress. These forms of learning include: (1) capitalizing on one's natural proclivities and abilities (Erikson [1956] considers "favored capacities" to be one ingredient of identity formation); (2) age-appropriate practicing. People of all ages practice skills in order to perfect them; however, this activity seems especially prominent in adolescents. They passionately practice pursuits they enjoy, either of an individual (e.g., athletics, skateboarding, horseback riding, dance, music, reading, writing) or of a group nature (e.g., team sports, music group rehearsals). Compared to younger children, adolescents are much more frequently self-motivated to practice skill development. In these activities the energy of adolescents is boundless, their manner earnest and upbeat, and their satisfaction abundantly evident to any observer. They do not seem to be forcing themselves to undertake these endeavors in a defensive, compensatory manner.

In traditional psychoanalytic theory such activities involving skill acquisition are considered sublimations of the drives. That conceptualization recognizes the social appropriateness of the activity, but does not give sufficient credence to its basically non-defensive motivation. As noted in chapter 3 (p. 86), sublimation has come to be considered different from other defense mechanisms of the ego. Its original meaning of defense by displacement has been modified to imply a more complicated process involving conflict-free ego resources and the synthetic function of the ego. This modification of the basis of sublimation has allowed psychoanalysis to incorporate the very type of progressive activities I am describing without having to abandon the implication of libido theory that all psychic activities include a significant element of defense against regressive urges. My point is that many activities in adolescents which psychoanalysis characterizes as sublimations do not seem to have any significant basis in defense activity and represent strivings to complete development rather than strivings to modulate sexual or aggressive drive.

SEXUAL DEVELOPMENT DURING ADOLESCENCE

The integration of genital sexuality into the adolescent's soma and psyche is one important component of adolescent development. Along with the completion of physical growth it represents the last area of biological maturation. The primary psychological importance of puberty is not to drive the adolescent away from his or her family out of fear of incestuous desires; rather, its major import lies in confirming to the adolescent that emancipation to adulthood is possible.

Psychoanalytic theory maintains that the adolescent strives to become independent because of sexual maturation. I illustrated in the last chapter that this is not invariably the case. The adolescent's efforts to become more independent and the integration of genital sexuality are separate matters which occur during the same period but are not necessarily causally related. They are both features of a more encompassing process of ego maturation termed strivings to complete development. And in fact, in my clinical experience, the adolescent's fear of being held by parents in a nonemancipated state is much more prevalent than fears of incestuous longings as the motivation for adolescent–parental turmoil. (My reasons for considering the effects of physical growth to be as important in the process of adolescent emancipation as the effects of sexual maturity are presented in chapter 4 [pp. 113–114]). The rationale for a broader-based understanding of the emancipation process is further elaborated in the section on "Adolescent Turmoil" (p. 172).

I will consider the integration of genital sexuality separately, because it has been emphasized in theorizing about adolescence.

This reflects the sway of psychoanalysis which has had the greatest influence on our understanding of sexual development during adolescence. But psychoanalytic theory has overemphasized the role of sexual maturation in the emancipation process of adolescence. In this section I will illustrate that psychoanalysts have accurately described many features of the developmental process, including patterns of behavior, types of object relations sought, reaction patterns, and fantasies; but the psychoanalytic explanation for these phenomena is neither complete nor totally accurate.

According to psychoanalytic theory, two interrelated tasks become integrated into the developing personality during adolescence. The first of these is to consolidate one's heterosexual identity, which has traditionally been thought to occur in the earlier years, and then to find (nonincestuous) partners in later adolescence. Actually aspects of both features occur concomitantly throughout the process. For experimentation with the new role or identity of an adult heterosexual invariably involves an element of the impression one is making on others; so this dimension of relatedness to others is present long before the adolescent is truly interested in engaging in heterosexual activity. Making a distinction between consolidating one's heterosexual identity and object finding (i.e., seeking partners) is worthwhile. For it implies that in arriving at psychological maturity with respect to sexuality an adolescent can have difficulty either in accepting his or her role as sexually mature or in choosing a suitable partner with whom heterosexual activity will be part of the relationship; these are related but to an extent separate issues.

CONSOLIDATING ONE'S IDENTITY AS A FUNCTIONING HETEROSEXUAL

This involves becoming relatively comfortable with both the genital and social roles of a sexual partner. It includes coming to grips with both the new physical sensations and the ideational concomitants (i.e., sexual, romantic, or heroic fantasies) of adult heterosexuality. The importance to adolescents of securing a sense of self-control over inner urges was illustrated in chapter 4 by the unpredictable occurrence of erections in boys and menstrual periods in girls. Masturbation is another phenomenon which helps the adolescent adjust to the changed sexual circumstances of his or her inner life.

MASTURBATION

Masturbation can serve either progressive or regressive developmental purposes. In the progressive direction, it allows the adolescent to experiment in fantasy with voluptuous sensations and with different situations, roles, and identities for fit, while protecting him- or herself from action. This process enables sexual feelings and fantasies to become organized together with an object in mind, namely, another person's body. Such fantasies involving another person can enhance the individual's empathy and thus increase his or her capacity for object relatedness.[1] Finally, masturbation affords the adolescent an opportunity to increase his or her capacity to bear inner tension; thus, it can enhance the youngster's capacity for self-control.

The regressive potential of masturbation derives from the fact that it is objectless. It can become an exclusively narcissistic experience by serving as an avenue for immediate discharge. Used this way masturbation can function solely for immediate relief of tension rather than for strengthening the adolescent's internal resources for dealing with tension.

Such repetitive and ceaseless activities as scratching, nose picking, cuticle-tearing, fingernail biting, hair twisting, pencil chewing, and endless playing with rubber bands have been reported to be equivalents, that is, displaced, ego-filtered, and de-erotized expressions of masturbation (Blos, 1962). However, I am unaware of studies which have clarified how frequently masturbatory conflicts rather than other sources of anxiety have been confirmed to underlie either these behaviors or gambling, reckless driving, or certain forms of procrastination which have

---

[1]Deutsch (1944) considered this stimulation and elaboration of fantasy very important for developing intuition, enriching the personalities of girls, and heightening their capacity for foreplay.

also been considered displaced masturbatory conflicts (Blos, 1962).

HETEROSEXUAL OBJECT SEEKING

Traditionally it has been considered that when masturbatory fantasies become boring and repetitive, consequent to consolidating their heterosexual identity, adolescents seek experiences to confirm their sexual maturity. Early sexual experiences involve more preoccupation, curiosity, and experimentation than emotional involvement. In fact, strong admixtures of aggression and a lack of tenderness are the more typical emotional concomitants, especially on the part of boys. These attitudes suggest that early adolescents are still more involved in the task of consolidating their sexual identity than truly involved in finding new love objects.

The foregoing descriptions convey the impression that a large element of practicing and experimenting with newly acquired feelings, interests, attitudes, and potentials is involved in these activities. My emphasis on such motives compared to defensive ones might be questioned when thinking about such phenomena as the early adolescent girl's masturbatory fantasies which have frequently been reported in the psychoanalytic literature to involve being forced by the superior power of a man or older woman and being watched by others. I find that such fantasies often stem from the girls' efforts to relieve guilt engendered by the pleasure they derive in fantasy and that they anticipate from sexual experiences. They are curious but feel that such interests are considered improper by their parents, unacceptable to their ego ideal of the asexual mother, and are at odds with their own natural conservatism regarding coitus. To be able to enjoy the sexual excitement associated with masturbation, they relieve their guilt by fantasizing that they are being forced into the act by someone else. So, the underlying driving force is often not masochism or exhibitionism, but a wish to enjoy, to anticipate, and to experiment in fantasy with a newly acquired interest and capacity.

THE ROLE OF COITUS

There are regressive and progressive aspects to coital experience among adolescents. Recourse to actual sexual experiences at this stage can predispose an adolescent to abandoning him- or herself to sensation-seeking, rather than enhancing the development of mutuality, tenderness, and affection in heterosexual relationships. Bernfeld (1935) considered that early recourse to heterosexual experience by boys coarsens their personality structure and their sexuality. Deutsch (1944) concluded that early recourse to coitus reduces girls' capacity for creativity, particularly if it occurs in lieu of an initial close relationship with a same-sexed peer; that is because important stages of identification with same-sexed peers may be inhibited. This is felt to curtail the development of intimacy, including sharing ideas and ideals, which develop from relationships with members of one's own sex. This can lead to the establishment of lasting, latent homosexual conflicts.

Also, at least until recently, intercourse had been considered the prerogative of adulthood, that is, of emotional maturity and responsibility.[2] The persistence of that idea in our culture will often engender guilt, which can inhibit rather than foster the very consolidation of independence which is being attempted. Even in this era when cultural situations dictate that sex is permissible without guilt, boys who become sexually involved with their girl friends can become paranoidally jealous, suggesting that they have not reconciled the prostitute–Madonna split; or, they can become very disappointed, feeling that the good friendship they had with the girl friend has changed. Girls, too, can become depressed and disappointed after their first sexual experiences. This is not just because the pleasure is often less than they had anticipated, but because they have failed their earlier ego ideal which was of the asexual mother.

The foregoing psychoanalytic formulations seem apt for

---

[2]The facts that the incidence of sexual intercourse amongst adolescents has burgeoned during the past 20 years and that, according to a recent study, the majority of those adolescents who initiate intercourse earlier in adolescence wish they had waited, are discussed in the section on "Adolescent Turmoil" (p. 172).

some cases. I have found though that just as oedipal guilt represents a special case of separation–survivor guilt, adolescents' attitudes about early sexual experiences often reflect emancipatory guilt. Their concerns are about arrogating experiences in fantasy (masturbation) as well as reality (coitus) which they consider the prerogatives of adults. Despite protestations that they don't care about what their parents think, adolescents feel that it is not all right in the eyes of parents for them to enjoy this pleasure; so, they punish themselves with jealousy, disappointment, or depression. This differs from the traditional psychoanalytic formulation which considers such responses to reflect incestuous desires.

That notwithstanding, this area (sexual intercourse), perhaps more than others, is one for which peer attitudes and social norms can have greater influence on the adolescent's behavior than do his or her parents' wishes, expectations, and practices (see Katchadourian, 1990). This reflects the continuing dynamic state that exists between parental, societal, and peer societal influence on the individual. In early childhood the child forsakes immediate gratification in favor of gratifying the wishes of parents to retain their love. In a somewhat paradoxical manner, some adolescents who feel secure in their parents' love allow themselves to experiment in ways they realize their parents would disapprove of, because they do not at base truly fear losing their parents' support. Thus, peer group influences can outstrip parental proscriptions, even in well structured families.[3]

---

[3]Writing in 1957, Blos (1957) observed that female delinquency during that era was almost exclusively sexual delinquency. He reported that these girls' recourse to genital sexuality was undertaken as an effort to defend against a strong pregenital, regressive pull to their mothers. He termed this "pseudoheterosexuality." Some twenty years later (1976) Blos reflected on those earlier ideas at a time when involvement in sexual intercourse had become more prevalent than abstention amongst young adolescent girls and blatantly so. Since it was tolerated even if not completely accepted by the social order, this sexual activity could no longer be characterized as delinquent behavior. Blos identified three different patterns amongst adolescent girls who engaged in sexual intercourse. Some girls went along with peer influences and participated in relatively casual sex until they developed sufficient inner strength to make their own personal decisions independent of peer pressure regarding their sexual activity and desired level of intimacy with partners. Sexual activity was serving the emancipation process, which Blos characterizes as "an adolescent severance conflict in relation to childhood dependencies" (p. 250). A second group of adolescent girls was also conforming to the liberalized sexual mores with the aim of achieving psychological independence from parents. However, the often

VICISSITUDES OF OBJECT CHOICE DURING ADOLESCENCE

Psychoanalysis identifies specific types and progressions of object choice (i.e., the recipient of the adolescent's love or emotional interest) during the process of emancipation: The reactivation of oedipal urges at puberty impels the adolescent away from his childhood attachment to his parents, the incestuous objects. This process involves withdrawal of libido from his mental representations of his parents into the self. This creates the sense of isolation and loneliness reported by some adolescents. That sense of aloneness motivates the adolescent to cathect (i.e., to invest libido in) mental representations of new objects, such as peers. Lurching back and forth between cathecting self and cathecting parents and others in an effort to avoid either pole of incest or loneliness, accounts for the mood swings, erratic interpersonal behaviors, and moodiness observed in adolescents.

In trying to reconcile this dilemma by finding nonincestuous objects, the first choice of new object is typically someone of the same sex who is either much like the adolescent or the way the adolescent would like to be. This attachment to an individual of the same sex basically involves love of the self and is undertaken as a way station toward heterosexual object finding. Thus, it is considered to be a narcissistic rather than a bona fide homosexual object choice. The following example demonstrates the

---

promiscuous sexual behavior of these girls lost its developmental reason for being and took on the quality of a lifestyle which continued into young adulthood, potentially compromising the ability of these girls to experience commitment, fidelity, and intimacy as adults. Nonetheless, the basic motive underlying these girls' sexual involvements was also developmentally progressive. By contrast, in a third group of adolescent girls Blos identified motives similar to those he had described in the sexually delinquent girls during the 1950s. These girls undertook sexual activity either to ward off a regressive pull to their mothers, or to gratify an infantile desire for physical contact (cuddling) while remaining genitally anesthetic themselves, or as a way of identifying with an idealized, caring mother by acquiesing to the sexual demands of their partners. I explain throughout this book the differences between my understanding of the psychodynamics of adolescent psychology and those of Blos, particularly as they would apply to the third group. His point about the first two groups is of interest. I refer to his observation that there is an effort on the part of these adolescent girls to accommodate the intensity of extrafamilial pressures on their developmental progress; this can in some cases be achieved with success but in other cases may leave a lasting scar regarding the consolidation of some important features of interdependence in adulthood.

emergence of this phenomenon, but not in the sequence which would be required for the psychoanalytic explanation to be tenable.

EXAMPLE 1: THE NARCISSISTIC-TYPE OBJECT RELATIONSHIP DESCRIBED BY PSYCHOANALYSIS IS FORMED LATE IN ADOLESCENCE FOLLOWING CONSOLIDATION OF HETEROSEXUALITY AND EMANCIPATION

In the sixth and seventh grades, a 12- to 13-year-old pubertal boy drifted away from his two long-time, very close buddies, nor did he replace them during the next couple of years of junior high school. Rather, he became more casually involved with several other boys who shared his particular interest in music. During his freshman year in high school he developed an admiring, though casual relationship with a senior, but he formed nothing resembling the close tie he had enjoyed with each of his two earlier childhood friends.

During his high school years he became sexually mature, evidenced by occasional, casual sexual intercourse with willing girls. He also achieved age-appropriate psychological autonomy, evidenced by his functioning without difficulty at a university distant from his family. Thus, he appeared to be well on his way to psychological emancipation.

Then, during the summer between his freshman and sophomore college years, at age 18, he and a former, casual, male friend became much closer, and in a specific manner. They spent much time together and shared an inclination to be intellectual; and they began to use each other's phrases and manner of speaking to a degree that was noticed by new girls they would meet together. At summer's end, each returned to his respective college but maintained frequent contact.

Psychoanalysis may be correct that such relationships help adolescents to integrate intimacy, intuition, empathy, and altruism in the process of defining and finding out what they are like. Such friendships may even be important antecedents for forming meaningful relationships with members of the opposite sex. For this lad had not yet had a true girl friend in whom his emotional investment included more than sexual interest. The development of a close male friendship in this youth bore little relationship, however, to consolidating a confident sense of his sexual maturity or the emergence of age-appropriate independence from his family. Again, such same-sex friendships may be an important feature of adolescent development, but their formation does not bear any invariable, causal relationship to achieving adult heterosexual identity or emancipating from childhood attachments to parents.

EXAMPLE 2: HETEROSEXUAL OBJECT CHOICES OF THE TYPE THOUGHT TO REPRESENT DEFENSE AGAINST INCESTUOUS URGES HAVE A DIFFERENT DYNAMIC BASIS

Psychoanalysis observes that boys move quickly through the oedipal stage into latency and girls take a longer time. This is because girls have no motivating force equivalent to castration anxiety. In adolescence the opposite occurs; girls go through adolescence quickly while boys take a vacillating course. This plus their earlier sexual maturation puts girls out of phase with boys. Girls yearn for opportunities to meet older boys, and generally consider their male age-mates to be immature until later adolescence. Adolescent girls have to be able to accommodate the pressures of incestuous feelings and still make their eventual heterosexual object choice, that is, choice of marital partner, on the basis of ego compatibility. Thus, the expected sequence is that relationships based on defense against incestuous motives are formed during earlier adolescence and followed later by relationships based on ego compatibility.

An example that demonstrates object choices based on defense against oedipal conflicts is that of the young, pretty, intelligent, college-oriented high school girl who takes the dumbest athlete or musician for her boyfriend—someone who seems to bear no resemblance to her erudite college professor father. Psychoanalysts often conclude that she is either avoiding awareness of her incestuous wishes with this choice of boyfriend, or else she perceives subtle similarities between him and her father, or tries to change him to be like her father, or becomes domineering over him as she felt her own mother infantilized her father. Her motives are at one and the same time to gratify incestuous urges while denying their existence.

Or, as much as examples can be axiomatic, it has been thought that choosing a boy or girl friend from another racial or ethnic group reflects the adolescent's efforts to escape the pressure of oedipal yearnings; to wit, by choosing someone whose background or appearance is so different from her or his own, there is less danger of the incestuous desire becoming conscious. While that dynamic may apply to some individuals, the following example suggests a different motive and process in operation. We observe the adolescent experimenting with different identities in boyfriends for fit, rather than avoiding incestuous drives:

> A pretty, popular, and psychologically well-structured 14-year-old white girl from a stable, middle class, suburban family looked forward eagerly to high school and having a boyfriend. During her freshman year, after several months of casual friendships with senior boys who showed interest in her, she had her first boyfriend. He was a couple of years older and the scion of a very wealthy, prominent family. Within a few months she lost interest in this ardent boyfriend. She considered him too tied to his family and found herself wanting to feel freer to do things with her girl friends and meet more boys. So, she broke off that friendship and enjoyed her "freedom" for several months.
>
> She then felt discontented because she wished that more boys were interested in her. Shortly thereafter a handsome, charming, new boy transferred to her school where he immediately became the object of many girls' interest. He took an immediate liking to the young lady in question. His background was a bit offbeat compared to that of many of their peers. She spent some time with him, perhaps as much flattered by his preference for her when so many others desired him, as by any great interest in him. As he began to press her for more time and attention, she realized she found him too passive for her liking, and pulled away.
>
> She continued on her active way, but was again feeling disenchanted during the latter part of her sophomore year because no boys whom she considered desirable were showing any interest in her; and she fretted at moments that her high school life was passing her by without romance. Then a handsome, charming, black youth, a couple of years older, began to pursue her. She was quite taken by him and excited by his interest. As she began to see more of him, she realized that his values and hers were very different; and soon both of them became aware that she spent much time exhorting him to "straighten-up and fly right," just as his own mother was also doing. So, as he sought a closer relationship with her, although conflicted, she told him as she had the last boy that she preferred to be "just friends."

In each of these choices, the girl's initial interest was in the handsome appearance of these boys, or their physiques or their wit, or studiousness or athletic ability or popularity, and their interest in her. In a matter of months, while still appreciating the features which had attracted her to them, she would find ego incompatibilities that caused her interest in each one to wane. The last boy's values deviated too much from her own, the second was too passive, and the first too dependent. None of these traits characterized her father. The traits she objected to placed her squarely in the camp of her own parents' style and values. Thus, there was little evidence that she was attempting to escape oedipal pressures in her choice of boyfriends. Rather, she was experimenting with different sizes, shapes, styles, colors, manners, and identities in boyfriends, to see what she did and did not like and want in a man. We see, then, the young adolescent girl selecting for features of ego compatibility from the beginning of her dating career, not toward the end of it when she should, according to psychoanalytic developmental psychology, make her ultimate choice of marital partner on an ego compatibility rather than an incestuous basis.

At age $16^{1}/_{2}$ our young protagonist became more romantically interested in a classmate with whom she had been friendly for some time, after this young man began to reveal his crush on her. They shared many interests in common and were of like dispositions—serious about their responsibilities but easy-going, friendly, popular, respected, and close to their families. After several weeks of having him for a boyfriend, the young woman again found herself wanting more freedom. She broke up with him, but during the next couple of months as they remained friends, she came to feel that she wanted to remain his girl friend. So, the two of them became closer again and remained increasingly so for the duration of her junior and senior high school years. Despite the compatibility of their interests, temperament, and values, she always realized and anticipated that they would break up when they went off to different colleges.

This example suggests that struggles with incestuous conflicts are not necessarily an important feature of object choice during adolescence. It also suggests that adolescents can have an unconscious sense of what they want and what they are doing throughout the emancipatory process of adolescence. In this case, even though she and her last boyfriend were very compatible, she realized implicitly that it was not in their best developmental interests to consider making their adolescent romance permanent.

This example has addressed the prototypic developmental conflict that psychoanalytic theory maintains the adolescent girl faces regarding object choice. She must make her ultimate choice of partner on an ego compatibility basis rather than on an incestuous basis. Psychoanalytic theory maintains that in resolving the equivalent incestuous conflicts of adolescence, the boy must eventually bring together into one the image of the Madonna, or asexual woman, and of the sexual, devalued woman, so that he can trust and respect the same woman with whom he can share sexual passion. The next example suggests that girls can experience the same conflict.

EXAMPLE 3: FEMALE EQUIVALENT OF THE PROSTITUTE-MADONNA DILEMMA WHICH IN PSYCHOANALYTIC THEORY IS CONSIDERED THE NORMATIVE CONFLICT OF ADOLESCENT BOYS

A 19-year-old infantryman from a rural, Midwestern area was brought to an evacuation hospital in Vietnam from the field because of intense bladder pain. Following surgical removal of a glass rod from his bladder, he was referred to a psychiatrist at the hospital, to whom he told the following: He had been enamored of a girl in his home town. Upon professing his sentiments in asking her to be his girl friend, however, she had responded that he was "too nice." Filled with self-loathing and humiliation in response to that specific form of her rejection, he had forced the glass rod up his penis into his bladder and lived silently with the pain for a year and half until it became unbearable.

While these data are sketchy and the history is from the boy not the girl, her observation and his response together suggest that the young woman was in conflict about the kind of issue which has traditionally been ascribed to boys. This likely fact does not discount the possible accuracy of psychoanalytic clinical theory on this point. It does raise the possibility though that there is more commonality in the issues faced by adolescent boys and girls than traditional psychoanalytic theory has considered because of the differences and emphasis it places on sexuality in adolescent development. The next example is a further illustration of this point.

EXAMPLE 4: HOMOSEXUAL CONCERNS WHICH IN TRADITIONAL PSYCHOANALYTIC THEORY ARE CONSIDERED TO BE PRIMARILY A SOURCE OF ANXIETY FOR ADOLESCENT BOYS ARE OBSERVED IN NORMAL GIRLS

Traditional analytic thinking, based on clinical observation, holds that adolescent boys harbor intense concerns about homosexuality which their female counterparts do not. This difference is attributed to the unique impact of castration anxiety on boys. The following example illustrates similar concerns in adolescent girls, suggesting either that girls experience equivalent castration anxiety or that some other motive is responsible for these concerns.

> Two attractive, clearly heterosexual, best girl friends in their middle teens found themselves without anything interesting to do one summer evening, having left a dull party but not feeling ready to return home. One suggested that they drive to a hilltop which overlooked their city and talk about boys. They did so and found a romantic spot under a full moon. Each talked about returning there some time with her favorite boyfriend. They were enjoying their conversation until another car drove up—presumably carrying a boy and girl. Both girls became immediately concerned that the new arrivals would think them lesbian, and they crouched down in their car seats and drove away.

EXAMPLES 5 AND 6: CURRENT HETEROSEXUAL "DATING" PATTERNS IN PREADOLESCENTS AND ADOLESCENTS

As evidenced by liberalization of abortion laws, markedly reduced censorship of sexual material in the media, and the more ready availability of contraception, the current parental generation has sanctioned relaxed social controls against sexual expression. In this environment of adult tolerance of sexual expression by adolescents, evidence of conservative trends in preadolescents and adolescents which serve to protect themselves from premature sexual involvement have emerged alongside evidence of earlier and more ready recourse to sexual intercourse. The conservative trends, illustrated in the following examples, suggest that adolescents understand their developmental needs even if they cannot always consciously articulate them; and they try to find ways to accommodate these needs when society does not help. These are examples of adolescents' unconscious, self-righting, and self-regulating efforts to preserve a normal course to their development.

EXAMPLE 5: HETEROSEXUAL PAIRING ("GOING") IN PRE- AND EARLY ADOLESCENTS

Some fifth and sixth graders become preoccupied with "going" (i.e., being boyfriend and girl friend). Much time and talk, and mental, if not scribbled-out charts, are kept of who is paired with whom. Nevertheless, when one inquires of such youngsters what it means to be "going" and how this affects their social relations, the response is often puzzling. For they are never quite sure what "going" means, other than connoting that they are special boy and girl friend. Furthermore, the effect of such a liaison is that these two individuals forsake communicating directly with one another in favor of doing so through intermediary friends or by phone. Thus, formally acknowledging the special interest that the pre- or early adolescent boy and girl have for each other results in having less personal involvement, except at the protective distance of the telephone line.

Preadolescents fifty years ago acted similarly with regard to the lists of pairings, whisperings, and gossiping. At that time, however, short-lived as the relationship might prove to be, the pair would spend more time together, and, for example, steal a few moments of hand-holding, rather than moving further away from each other upon recognizing their mutual attraction.

EXAMPLE 6: A NEW TYPE OF GROUP FORMATION IN MIDDLE ADOLESCENTS— THE HETEROSEXUAL "GANG"

Esman (1979) suggested that the rise of organizations such as Hare Krishna in the late 1960s which espoused ascetic practices, might be predicated on the need of some adolescents for such external social controls to help them modulate impulses. A less dramatic but more prevalent example involves middle teenagers, whose wishes to be away from home throw them together.

A new type of group formation has emerged. It is the heterosexual gang, a group of boys and girls who spend much time doing things together, without romantic attachments or pairings amongst them. This appears quite different from the pattern of double dating fifty years ago, when groups of identified couples spent time together. In double dating, couples were helped to withstand the intensity of their impulses by the presence of other couples, in addition to the greater societal proscription against intercourse at that time, the illegality of abortion, the inaccessibility of contraceptives, and thus objectively greater risks of pregnancy. Today, with less ostensible need to be concerned about pregnancy and less social pressure against intercourse, the lack of pairing in the heterosexual gang reduces the likelihood of sexual involvement; at the same time, it affords adolescents the opportunity to develop other aspects of boy–girl friendships, and in some cases, to offset homosexual anxieties, until the adolescents are ready for more intimate involvements. Often parents, particularly mothers, seem more worried about the lack of romance in their children's lives than do the adolescents themselves.

As in the previous example, it is as if these young people are functioning with an underlying, unconscious awareness of their developmental needs, and are adapting to the social order in such a way as to protect their development and advance it at the same time.

CHANGES IN SENSIBILITY DURING ADOLESCENCE

We have just considered the developmental psychology associated with sexual maturation and group formation. I will now consider other changes observed in adolescents that psychoanalysis attributes to sublimation of sexual drives and cognitive psychology attributes to the newly acquired capacity for formal operational thinking. These changes often seem better understood on a broader basis than those theories posit, as the illustrations will demonstrate.

Many teenagers experience changes which are difficult both for the youth themselves and for observers to describe. Adolescents are experiencing their inner lives intensely at a time when their observing egos (capacities for self-observation) are strongly colored by self-consciousness and concerns about self-control.

(The term *self-consciousness* basically refers to consciousness of the impression they are making on others.) It is always difficult for an observer to know what another person experiences, particularly when the other is in a state of flux. Yet, characterizations by talented authors and autobiographers strike a resonant chord of familiarity in many readers. This suggests a universal quality to the inner changes being described in such literature. Two passages from fiction and a song lyric illustrate some of these changes and their timeless quality, at least across a span of 200 years.

The first passage is from Goethe's *The Sorrows of Young Werther* written in 1774. Werther, a late adolescent, had fallen deeply in love with a young woman who was betrothed to another man. Werther is writing a letter to his friend, William:

> Oh, how wildly my blood courses through my veins when, by chance, my hand touches hers or our feet touch under the table! I start away as if from a fire, a mysterious power draws me back, and I become dizzy ... and in her artlessness and innocence she has no idea how much such little intimacies torment me. When she puts her hand in mine in the course of a conversation and, absorbed by what we are talking about, draws closer to me, and the heavenly breath from her lips touches mine ... then I feel I must sink to the ground as if struck by lightning. William, if ever I should presume to take advantage of this heaven on earth, this trust in me ... you know what I mean. But I am not depraved. Weak, yes, weak God knows I am ... and can this not be called depraved?
>
> She is sacred to me. All lust is stilled in her presence. I can't explain how I feel when I am with her. It is as if every nerve in my body were possessed by my soul. There is a certain melody ... she plays it on the piano like an angel, so simply yet with so much spirit. It is her favorite song, and I am restored from all pain, confusion, and vagaries with the first note.
>
> Nothing that has ever been said about the magic power of music seems improbable to me now. How that simple melody touches me! And how well she knows when she should play it, often at moments when I feel like blowing my brains out! Then all delusion and darkness within me are dispelled, and I breathe freely again [p. 51].

In the next passage, 16-year-old Holden Caulfield, Salinger's "Catcher in the Rye," is describing an experience to the book's readers in 1945:

I don't want you to get the idea she was a goddam *icicle* or something, just because we never necked or horsed around much. She wasn't. I held hands with her all the time, for instance. That doesn't sound like much, I realize, but she was terrific to hold hands with. Most girls if you hold hands with them, their goddam hand *dies* on you, or else they think they have to keep *moving* their hand all the time, as if they were afraid they'd bore you or something. Jane was different. We'd get into a goddam movie or something, and right away we'd start holding hands, and we wouldn't quit till the movie was over. And without changing the position or making a big deal out of it. You never even worried, with Jane, whether your hand was sweaty or not. All you knew was, you were happy. You really were.

One other thing I just thought of. One time, in this movie, Jane did something that just about knocked me out. The newsreel was on or something, and all of a sudden I felt this hand on the back of my neck, and it was Jane's. It was a funny thing to do. I mean she was quite young and all, and most girls if you see them putting their hand on the back of somebody's neck, they're around twenty-five or thirty and usually they're doing it to their husband or their little kid—I do it to my kid sister Phoebe once in a while, for instance. But if a girl's quite young and all and she does it, it's so pretty it just about kills you [pp. 62–63].

The following lyric from a Beatles' song in the late 1960s relates similar pleasure in hand-holding and touching:

Oh yeh, I'll tell you something,
I think you'll understand.
Then I'll say that something
I want to hold your hand
I want to hold your hand
I want to hold your hand.

Oh please, say to me,
And let me be your man.
And please, say to me,
You'll let me hold your hand,
Now let me hold your hand.
I want to hold your hand.

And when I touch you I feel happy inside
It's such a feeling that my love I can't hide,
I can't hide
I can't hide.
I can't hide.

Yeh, you got that something I think you'll understand
When I feel that something
I want to hold your hand,
I want to hold your hand
I want to hold your hand
Oh yeh I want to hold your hand.
I want to hold your hand.

Each of these works and their authors enjoyed immediate and immense popularity in their eras—1770s, 1940s, 1960s. Thus, something about what they were describing resonated with many people's sensibilities. The experiences being described are ones of intense pleasure, if not passion. Each embodied a sensual element that was satisfying in itself without impelling the experiencer toward sexual excitation. This is a different emotional experience from that of younger children who experience a greater sense of security from having their hand held, at least until they want to walk alone.

To explore the developmental changes underlying such phenomena, and to illustrate the existing theories, consider the following two poems which were written by a girl when she was 11 and 16 respectively:

Home

The fire was glowing all golden and bright
It kept us warm through that cold winter's night
The family together, a symbol of love
Love for each other and God up above.

Salacious Sea

The roaring, surging waves
    seduce the beach.
Their foamy lips
   tickling,
   teasing
   the palpitating shores.
The fingers of seaweed entwine
   and constrict the helpless,
   relenting shores.
   Incessantly the
    thrust-ing

```
thrust-ing
thrust-ing
    of the sea
separates the continguous grains of sand.
But, as each docile wave recoils
        it gently strokes
and smooths the golden, yielding
        flesh of the shore [Quoted in Werkman, 1966].
```

From the perspective of psychoanalytic developmental theory, the second poem, especially when contrasted to the first, exemplifies successfully sublimated pubertal, sexual drives. It also illustrates the unique, evanescent spurt of creativity which waxes and wanes mysteriously in midadolescence and will be discussed in the next section. Can the multitude of differences between these two poems be adequately understood as the outcome of successful efforts to avoid conscious awareness of newfound sexual desire or simply a reflection of greater cognitive capacities or both? The differences between the poems are dramatic, and encompass everything from the themes which interest the poet (from religious and conventional to secular with thinly veiled erotic yearning), to style and meter, choice of words, and even visual depiction on the printed page. In the second poem she exhibits greater intellectual sophistication, greater freedom of expression, more imaginative use of metaphor, and a more erotic theme. Her mode of expression, however, namely poetry writing, is one for which she had exhibited a predilection prior to adolescence. Now, as an adolescent, she is practicing this ability, developing her skill, and whatever talent she may have.

The next example suggests that this "opening up" of the developing personality, these alterations in the individual's sensibility, might not always require the presence of hormonal changes, but can be prompted by an interpersonal experience. The following excerpt is from the autobiography of Havelock Ellis, the English psychologist, who died in 1939, and from whom Freud adopted the terms *autoerotism* and *narcissism.* Ellis described an experience at 12 years of age:

My mother, though on occasion hospitable, cared little to have strangers staying in the house; a girl or boy cousin would sometimes be invited to spend a week, and left no impress on my imagination. The first stranger not of my kin to stay in the house was a girl of sixteen, the only daughter of my mother's stepbrother, who was in a well-to-do position. Agnes, then, for that was her name, was invited to spend a summer week or two with us at Wimbledon in 1871. She was a dark, pretty, vivacious girl, with long black ringlets. . . . Old enough to be a woman in my eyes, and yet young enough to be a comrade and equal, she adapted herself instinctively to the relationship and won my heart immediately. I took not the slightest liberty with her, and never had the slightest impulse to do so, but she, on her part, treated me with an easy familiarity which no woman had ever used with me before, and that fact, certainly, though its significance was then beyond me, undoubtedly had its influence. She would play and romp with me in all innocent unreserve, and when we went out together for long walks, as often happened, she would sometimes make me offer her my arm and treat her as a lady, then again asserting her superiority by treating me to lemonade and at the best places she could find. One day, as we strolled arm in arm through the poppied cornfields which then lay between Merton Station and the college—it was in these fields that I first knew the beauty of poppies—my severe little school master suddenly came round the corner onto us. Timid though I habitually seemed, I raised my cap without flinching and withdrawing my arm under my master's stern eye, and have ever since prided myself on that early little act of moral courage. He doubtless smiled to himself at thus seeing a handsome girl hanging on his quiet pupil's arm and he subsequently asked my father who she was, but without, I think, mentioning that detail. Agnes returned home, and strangely enough, I have never seen her since . . . we exchanged a few notes, but our correspondence speedily withered, without protest on my part. . . .

I never saw Agnes again; I never made any effort to see her; I never mentioned her name; no one knew that I even thought of her. But for four years her image moved and lived within me, revealing myself to myself. I had no physical desires and no voluptuous emotions; I never pictured to myself any joy of bodily contact with her or cherished any sensuous dreams. Yet I was devoured by a boy's pure passion. That she should become my wife—though I never tried to imagine what that meant—was a wild and constant aspiration. I would lie awake in bed with streaming eyes praying to God to grant that this might some day be. I have often felt thankful since that our prayers are not heard.

Under the stress of this passion I became a person, and, moreover, in temper a poet. I discovered the beauty of the world, and I discovered a new vein of emotion within myself. I began to write verse. I began to enjoy art, and at the same time, Nature. In a still vague and rudimentary way, all my literary activities slowly took on a new character. Hitherto they had been impersonal, displaying indeed a certain research, a certain orderly and systematic spirit, perhaps inborn, yet not definitely personal. Now the personal element took shape. The touch of the careless vivacious girl had placed within me a new ferment which began to work through every fibre of my being. It was an epoch-making event in my life . . . [pp. 87–89; quoted in Kiell, 1964].

Ellis specifically disavows awareness of any pubertal urges at the time, attributing these changes in his sensibility, the capacity for and interest in emotional expression—changes which have been attributed to falling in love in adolescence—to a nonsexual experience with another person. Ellis stresses an interpersonally precipitated romanticism, in contrast to the last poem, which appeared to be internally precipitated. While there is little data in this passage alone to help us understand the operative mechanism in these changes, the most telling clue is Ellis' description of his mother as basically unfriendly, inhospitable, readily offended, and the only female with whom Havelock had had extended contact. Agnes, by contrast, treated him with "an easy familiarity which no woman had ever used with me before, and that fact, certainly, though its significance was then beyond me, undoubtedly had its influence." Her positive attitude toward him freed up latent abilities and sensitivities which had been squelched in his mother's care. This is an example of how adolescents unconsciously try to capitalize upon and extract from their environments what they need to complete and maximize their development.

In the next passage, Albert Schweitzer describes a period during his adolescence. He reports a burgeoning of his intellectual capacity and interests which he exercises with a passion, rather than a passion that enhances cognitive and emotional interests as Havelock Ellis described. Schweitzer portrays his behavior as if he were practicing indefatigably with his newfound ability. This proclivity to master newfound abilities through repetition is a crucial part of the developmental process which is not adequately encompassed by the concept of sublimating a drive.

Between my fourteenth and sixteenth years I passed through an unpleasant phase of development, becoming an intolerable nuisance to everybody, especially to my father, through a passion for discussion. On everyone who met me in the street I wanted to inflict thorough-going and closely reasoned considerations on all the questions that were then being generally discussed, in order to expose the errors of the conventional views and get the correct view recognized and appreciated. The joy of seeking for what was true and serviceable had come upon me like a kind of intoxication, and every conversation in which I took part had to go back to fundamentals. Thus I emerged from the shell of reserve in which I had hitherto concealed myself, and became the disturber of every conversation which was meant to be merely conversation. What a number of times . . . did I bring the conversation at meals into stormy water! My aunt scolded me as being insolent, because I wanted to argue out my ideas with grown-up people as though they were of my own age. If we went to pay a visit anywhere, I had to promise my father not to spoil the day for him by "stupid behavior during conversations."

I must confess to having been as intolerable as a well-brought up young man, half-way through his education, ever can be, but it was not in the least any egotistic disputatiousness which made me so; it was a passionate need of thinking, and of seeking with the help of others for the true and the serviceable [pp. 54–55; quoted in Kiell, 1964].

Piagetian psychology could point to Schweitzer's description as an example of the incremental advance to formal operational thinking which occurs in adolescence. Schweitzer's "passion for discussion," that is, practicing this newly acquired faculty, however, seems as striking, if not more so, in his description than his development of the capacity for "closely reasoned argument."

At the least, the foregoing examples suggest that significant changes in sexuality and in cognitive capacities influence the sensibility of the adolescent. I have not discovered any clinical evidence that one of these factors is more important than the other in the development of these changes in the sensibility of adolescents. Thus, it may be most accurate to consider that both changes, at the psychological level, are part of a natural unfolding of the individual's potential during these years. Does every adolescent exhibit these changes? My clinical impression is that all do experience these substrate changes, but the degree to which they are stifled or brought to fullest expression reflects the influence of environmental factors. One of the most common, popular, and appealing themes in movies, plays, and literature involves a tough girl or guy whose keen perceptiveness and sensitivity emerge in the throes of a newly formed relationship, revealing a noncynical sensitivity toward others, and sometimes a 'heart of gold' as well.

From the standpoint of psychoanalytic libido theory, Schweitzer's behavior would be considered an example of intellectualization as defense against sexual drive—one of the prototypic defense mechanisms utilized by adolescents.[4] When considered together with the previous examples, I conclude that

---

[4]Anna Freud (1936) identified intellectualization and asceticism as the two defense mechanisms of the ego which gain ascendance during adolescence. This is because both are suited for defense against quantity of drive as opposed to a specific drive quality. It is the intensity of the drives which makes the adolescent's experience uniquely different from that of children and adults.

Intellectualization represents an effort to control instinctual processes by connecting them with ideas which can be dealt with at a conscious level. Efforts to control feelings with thoughts, to substitute thought for action, and to use thought as trial action, begin in infancy and develop throughout childhood. Nevertheless, this capacity seems to flower in adolescence, aided by the adolescent's expanded cognitive capacities. Examples of intellectualization are college students' interminable dorm room arguments over such topics as free drug use versus legal control, free speech, the draft, the existence of God, the best form of government. These can be seen as fairly transparent displacements of instinctual conflicts, which are being considered in a setting where no conclusion or constructive outcome to the argument is anticipated. Rather, this activity serves a defensive function in the form of "thinking over of the instinctual conflict" (A. Freud, 1936, p. 161). Intellectualization as defense then differs from intellectuality in being an end in itself, having little influence on behavior, and not being used for any reality-oriented, task-fulfilling purpose.

While the foregoing, traditional psychoanalytic description may accurately characterize the use of intellectualization on some occasions, I think it misses the more important aspect, namely, that intellectualization is an effort to begin rigorously to bring to bear one's newly increasing intellectual capacities on an issue of immediate interest, and to arrive at and support a conclusion. This form of practicing is very goal-directed in the sense of developing a process which will become the basis for decision making and value formation for the rest of the individual's life. So, if we focus on this process rather than on the goal of any specific discussion in which the adolescent is utilizing intellectualization, I find that this phenomenon is being used to achieve much more than "merely to minister to daydreams" (A. Freud, 1936, p. 161).

Also, the following example illustrates that intellectualization can be the symptomatic expression of conflicts which do not involve sexuality:

A 19-year-old college freshman felt himself alienated from his peers because he was preoccupied with philosophical questions. These involved such matters as what is the right thing to do and how do things work. While he preferred his thoughts to the more mundane interests of his fraternity brothers, he yearned for someone with whom to discuss his ideas. And he feared that if

this is too limited a view of the developmental process during adolescence. Rather than representing a restructuring undertaken to integrate genital sexuality and to avoid awareness of incestuous libidinal objects, the adolescent developmental process seems more comprehensively understood as an augmentation of

---

he did not engage in discussions of subjects which interested his peers, he would be left standing alone, and thus unbearably lonely. As he became indecisive about the direction in which he wanted his life to go, he became immobilized in his course work and his grades plummeted.

At first glance this adolescent seemed to be utilizing intellectualization as described by Anna Freud. Further exploration revealed, however, that he was a highly intelligent young man who harbored intense survivor guilt conflicts about his own intellectual endowment compared to that of a mildly retarded older sister whom he thought his parents had favored. He himself felt it wasn't right to capitalize upon intelligence which he had acquired simply through "the luck of the draw." So, on the verge of a successful college career, his immobilizing preoccupation with such questions as "What is the right thing to do?" both bespoke and represented an accession to his survivor guilt.

His own compunction about his superior intelligence was compounded by his feeling that their parents favored his sister because she had to struggle with the handicap. In his efforts not to take advantage of his intelligence, so as not to offend or make his parents feel worse about the sister's difficulties, this young man was doing what I have typically observed in such situations; he demonstrated to himself and the world that he was no better off than she. The rejection he anticipated from his peers if he capitalized on his intelligence was a displacement from that which he anticipated and feared from his parents. For he had experienced their favoring of his sister as disapproval of his taking advantage of his superior ability when she had less. This is an example of a typical maladaptive resolution of the basic conflict of adolescence based on emancipatory and survivor guilt. The adolescent needs to be able to move ahead with confidence that in doing so he still retains a positive relationship with his parents. Parental sponsorship of his forward movement reduces ambiguity experienced by the adolescent about what truly pleases his parents. Adolescents tend to sacrifice their forward movement if they feel this is necessary to retain a positive relationship with their parents.

Asceticism is the other defense mechanism which Anna Freud considers to be specifically suited to adolescents. Asceticism differs from other defense mechanisms in being a wholesale, primitive renunciation of all instinctual gratification, rather than being a defense mechanism deployed against a single impulse. For example, one can repress a sexual impulse but enjoy oral gratification, either as a substitute or a compromise formation, or as an instinctual gratification acceptable to the ego. The other defense mechanisms predispose to compromise formation which gives rise to symptom formation. By contrast, aceticism alternates with instinctual excess rather than compromise formation and symptoms. This form of behavior may be less commonly observed in normal development than when it was described fifty years ago. Yet, it is prominent in the psychopathology of anorexia nervosa and bulimia, conditions which have been described more frequently in recent years.

existing capacities by newly accrued abilities, of which sexuality represents one, a deepening capacity for emotional expression is another, a capacity for self-observation is a third, enhanced cognitive abilities represent a fourth, increased physical capacities, strength, stamina, and coordination represent a fifth, all monitored by heightened self-awareness and self-consciousness.

THE ADOLESCENT SELF-OBSERVATION/SELF-CONSCIOUSNESS AXIS

The passages by Ellis and Schweitzer quoted above illustrate heightened self-awareness which, along with its interpersonal concomitant, self-consciousness, is another feature of the altered sensibility of adolescents. Whether adolescents are actually more self-conscious and prone to feeling embarrassed or humiliated than younger children remains an open question. At any rate, more attention is focused on it during adolescence because adolescents are supposed to be more independent, and self-consciousness implies dependence. Psychoanalytic theory attributes self-consciousness primarily to the heightened narcissism experienced by the adolescent when, as part of the emancipatory process, libido is withdrawn from mental representations of parents into his or her self. Piagetian psychologists would attribute this heightened self-awareness to the incremental advance they posit in the cognitive ability to think about one's thoughts (i.e., abstract thinking).

At first blush, the increase in the intrapsychic element during adolescence, self-awareness, and the interpersonal component, self-consciousness, seem to derive from the inner and outer experiences of puberty. This state has been characterized as feeling one's body is alien to oneself: "The stranger inside is the tenant of a house which does not seem to be his own" (Fraiberg, 1955, p. 265). The anxiety engendered within young adolescents about understanding and controlling these new urges and thoughts naturally leads to concerns about what they will unwittingly reveal to others (i.e., self-consciousness). Also, since adolescents wish to feel and be older, they watch themselves more closely. Evidence of the phenomena is legion, from the overt embarrassment of some adolescents to the defensive, studied indifference of others, to the endless and precise attention to details of clothing, hair combing, and appearance which preoccupy still others, to feeling tongue-tied in the presence of some peers and adults. Their ostensible concern is the reception they will receive from others, which correlates with their dual motives of maintaining ties to others while forging their individuality. Especially when it is intense, there is, however, often a significant contribution to the development of self-consciousness from the environment (family):

> For example, an 18-year-old was aware of feeling so concerned about the reaction of other people to him that he could not "be myself," that is, act naturally around employers (toward whom he was overly responsive and eager to please), with coworkers (too quiet), and customers (too ingratiating). He was sure that he would be better off and found more appealing by others if he acted relaxed and natural. He also observed his tendency to feel ashamed about things he did for which there was no objective reason to feel that way.
>
> In thinking about this condition two recollections came to his mind. Once, when he was an eighth-grader, he tried to shave his upper lip with his father's razor. As he was doing so, his father came into the adjoining bedroom and asked crossly what was going on. The lad hurriedly wiped away the shaving cream, replaced the razor, never said what he had been doing, but felt ashamed, as if he had done something wrong. He could now see that this reflected his feeling that his father disapproved of his growing up (i.e., emancipatory guilt).
>
> His other recollection was that he had grown up never being certain how his parents would respond to any of his actions. He could not feel sure when they would or would not punish him for the same action. As a child he would insist that they write down rules for his behavior and sign them. But even when they did, he recalled that they would still not consistently abide by their own written rules. So, he lived with a chronic sense of never being sure how he would be responded to, and this was an important source, even if not the sole cause, of his extreme adolescent self-consciousness.

In this example we see another vicissitude of the basic adolescent developmental conflict I have posited, albeit now displaced from parents onto others. I refer to the conflict which is experienced when an adolescent wishes to assert himself but does not feel parental approval for his self-assertion and autonomy.

THE EVANESCENT SURGE OF CREATIVITY DURING ADOLESCENCE

This creativity, which typically waxes and then wanes as mysteriously as it had arisen during the middle years of adolescence, only rarely gives rise to objectively superior works. Rather, it refers primarily to a different form of expression than the adolescent has heretofore exhibited. It can be observed in poems, diaries, and artwork. Thirty years ago it could be observed in the ingenuity with which some adolescent boys worked on automobiles. The productions of self-taught rock musicians are more recent expressions of this phenomenon, along with several aspects of adolescents' use of language. The latter includes their ability to trenchantly and evocatively convey the essence of an experience; an example is the term *rip-off* which began as an expression of adolescents some twenty-plus years ago and found its way into the lexicon of adults. Other examples are their keen ability to incisively capture some feature of a confrere's style in nicknaming and their phraseology, which reflects the heightened perceptiveness and synthetic function of the ego associated with creativity.

The original explanations for this creative surge were psychodynamically oriented, focusing on the individual's efforts to integrate mature sexual capacities into the developing personality during the emancipation process. The withdrawal of libidinal cathexis from parents into the self renders the individual more self-absorbed and more aware of his inner state of aloneness. The fluidity of these cathexes, between self and other people, reflects a proclivity for regression which contributes to the creative ability of this period. The creative activity illustrates the ego's efforts to utilize sublimation and the synthetic function of the ego to resolve these instinctually based developmental conflicts while they are rife. After "object removal" (Katan, 1937) has been accomplished, that is, emancipation from the conflict over incestuous object choice, the pressure from these conflicts is eliminated and the creativity wanes.

That formulation may account for some expressions of the evanescent spurt of creativity, and the poem quoted earlier, "Salacious Sea" (pp. 158–159), may be a representative example. But current-day expressions of this creative surge by teenage rock and rap musicians who are notoriously sexually active and whose creative productions (their lyrics) are replete with references to and encouragement of direct sexual expression, suggest that more than defense against sexuality is or can be involved in the evanescent spurt of creativity in midadolescence.

Furthermore, the following poem and its author's circumstances suggest a different motive from that which gave rise to "Salacious Sea." It illustrates my point that developing and mastering enhanced capacities of self-expression may be more important or universal motives for this creative surge. This creative capacity can then be utilized by individual adolescents to deal with whatever area presents significant conflict for them. This poem was written by a 17-year-old boy a month after he underwent surgery for cancer:

Yea!!!

Well, here I am! Seventeen years
   old today,
boy the years are going by too
   quick!
Birthdays are very special to me,
a day to celebrate your existence,
a day to look back.

Well, here I am! Seventeen years
   old today,
boy the clock's ticking fast.
Birthdays are a special time,
a day to celebrate your existence
and cherish the ones around you.

Life is so full,
abounding with wonders to be seen
and emotions to be experienced.
If we all just open our eyes and gaze
upon the subtleties and finer shadings

of life
greater worlds unfold.
Worlds we rarely find time to look
    at.
But they're here and always will be
when we choose to find them.

I'm grateful to be a leaf
in the ever growing tree of life
and this leaf's not falling off
for nothing [Garver, 1982].

This young man died some months after he wrote the poem, and the poem certainly demonstrates denial. But, much more important for our understanding of development and the creative surge is the fact that the poem reflected self-preservative trends within the author which he used to deal with a threat imposed upon him from inside himself. This particular creative expression was being used to manage psychic trauma, relating to basic issues of survival and existence, rather than sexual or aggressive drives.

"STRUCTURAL" EXPLANATIONS FOR THE MIDADOLESCENT SURGE OF CREATIVITY

In recent years formulations of the surge of creativity in adolescence have shifted from psychodynamic to "structural" explanations. In structural theory, mental representations of objects rather than objects themselves are cathected. Freud's structural theory (id, ego, superego) has been augmented by more recent theorists to include ideas of self and object mental representations (Sandler and Rosenblatt, 1962; Hartmann, 1964; Jacobson, 1964; Blos, 1967; Kernberg 1976), and internal objects and internal object relationships (Klein, 1934, 1975; Fairbairn, 1952, 1963; Winnicott, 1958, 1965; see also Sutherland, 1980; Ogden, 1983). These additions have been introduced basically to explain how objects influence the drive-driven individual. In the explanation for the surge of creativity which follows, Blos' idea is that one's attitudes and behaviors are dominated by internal object representations, rather than, for example, by dynamic features of one's interactions with the objects themselves, or by pathogenic beliefs which are ideas based on experiences with important objects (Weiss, Sampson, and the Mount Zion Psychotherapy Group, 1986).

Blos posits that the creative surge arises as an effort to "accomplish urgent tasks of internal transformations" (Blos, 1962, p. 126). Blos (1967) hypothesizes a second individuation process in adolescence. He contrasts this with the first individuation process (Mahler, Pine, and Bergman, 1975) during which the toddler achieves psychological separateness from objects by integrating internal representations of himself and his mother. The second individuation during adolescence allows for the opposite condition to occur, namely finding new external love and hate objects. This is accomplished by a normal regression in the service of development to an approximation of the early childhood level of self and object representations; the latter are decathected, freeing up the adolescent to form new, nonincestuous self and object representations. Blos attributes adolescent turmoil to this process.

Schemata like Blos' second individuation may be necessitated by a theory in which drive gratification is basically antagonistic to object relationships. By contrast, I am advancing a different view of development, which is in line with Freud's later ideas about development of superego. Drive activity is not necessarily antithetical to object relatedness, but it can become a source of conflict owing to the child's strong need to maintain the relationship with his parents. This is sought from early in life to insure the child's sense of security. The features of development described in this chapter conspire during adolescence to lead to potential conflict. The conflict is between adolescents' underlying urges to allow complete unfurling of their capabilities and residual apprehension that breaches in their important object relationships (with parents or their surrogates) will deprive them of their needed sense of security.

VICISSITUDES OF MEDIOCRITY: RELATIVE "FAILURE" IN ADOLESCENCE

The midadolescent evanescent surge of creativity is not thought to bear any relationship to more substantial creativity in adult life; however, it may be instructive to consider the significance of those who appear quite the opposite during adolescence. In his study of adolescence published in 1904, G. Stanley Hall illustrated that not all individuals who prove to be creative, independent, and successful adults, exhibit this ego synthetic capacity during adolescence, at least as judged by their teachers and families:

> Byron was so poor a scholar that he only stood at the head of the class when, as was the custom, it was inverted, and the bantering master repeatedly said to him, "Now, George, man, let me see how soon you'll be at the foot." Schiller's negligence and lack of alertness called for repeated reproof, and his final school thesis was unsatisfactory. Hegel was a poor scholar, and at the university it was stated "that he was of middling industry and knowledge but especially deficient in philosophy." . . . Swift was refused his degree because of "dullness and insufficiency," but given it later as a special favor. General Grant was never above mediocrity, and was dropped as corporal in the junior class and served the last year as a private. W. H. Seward was called "too stupid to learn." Napoleon graduated forty-second in his class. "Who," asks Swift, "were the forty-one above him?" Darwin was "singularly incapable of mastering any language." When he left school, he says, "I was considered by all my masters and by my father as a very ordinary boy, rather below the common standard in intellect. To my deep mortification, my father once said to me, 'You care for nothing but shooting, dogs and rat-catching, and you will be a disgrace to yourself and to all your family' " [Hall, 1904, pp. 541–542].

These examples illustrate Hall's point that the developmental course for some capable and gifted individuals does not fit well into the standard institutions society uses to facilitate development in adolescence. This passage also demonstrates the great variation in the pacing of the development of the ego's synthetic capacities. These individuals were apparently not performing well academically during adolescence, at least by conventional standards. So, they were either stuck or the emancipatory process was moving them forward silently during this period.

With Hall's observations in mind and in anticipation of the consideration of adolescent turmoil which follows, an observation of Anna Freud is of interest. She wrote:

[I]t has always struck me as unfortunate that the period of adolescent upheaval coincides with such major demands on the individual as those for academic achievement in school and university, for a choice of career, for increased social and financial responsibility in general. Many failures, often with tragic consequences, in these respects are due not to the individual's incapacity as such but merely to the demands being presented to him at a time of life when all his energies are engaged in solving other major problems, namely, those created for him by sexual growth and development [1966, pp. 46–47].

As I will discuss shortly, there are other developmental issues in addition to sexual growth on which adolescents can founder. But Anna Freud's basic point is very well taken in my experience. That is, some adolescents are struggling so much with developmental issues that their ability to perform in the arenas expected by society is severely compromised; sometimes the results are devastating and lasting, especially if the environment does not respond to the adolescent's struggles in development-promoting ways.

ADOLESCENT TURMOIL

This concept has been a cornerstone of the psychoanalytic theory of adolescence. As enunciated by Anna Freud (1958), "adolescence is by its nature an interruption of peaceful growth" and the converse, "the upholding of a steady equilibrium during the adolescent process is in itself abnormal" (p. 275). For adolescent turmoil, in all its forms, basically represents the outward manifestations of the process by which the adolescent's capacity for adult sexuality is being integrated into his or her developing personality structure. Anna Freud further elaborated that "few situations in life . . . are more difficult to cope with than an adolescent son or daughter during the attempts to liberate themselves" (p. 276). She also suggested that "perhaps more than any others . . . [that group which shows no evidence of turmoil] . . . is in need of therapeutic help to remove the inner restrictions and clear the path for normal development, however 'upsetting' the latter may prove to be" (p. 265). For those adolescents who show no outer evidence of inner unrest are exhibiting excessive supergeo defenses against their drive activities, and their normal psychosexual maturation is being severely compromised.

Anna Freud also noted that while adolescent turmoil is inevitable, its manifestations are not predictable. This is because the signs and symptoms depend largely on the quantitative relationships between the strength of the drive and the strength of the ego's attempts to deal with the anxiety generated by this upheaval of drive. The signs and symptoms of adolescent turmoil can be the same as those of psychopathology. Differentiation between normality and abnormality is also based on quantitative rather than qualitative factors. Specifically, shifting behaviors, symptoms, and attitudes are more normal than single, unwavering attitudes, behaviors, or mechanisms for dealing with inner stress. Unpredictability of reaction is more normal than predictability. For example, to act embarrassed or ashamed of acknowledging one's mother in the presence of others, but then wanting to have intimate talks with her, or alternating love and hate for parents, are more normal reactions than maintaining either one of those attitudes exclusively (A. Freud, 1958).

THE NORMALITY OF ADOLESCENT TURMOIL

The major and most publicized challenges to the concept of adolescent turmoil have been studies which dispute the normality and the inevitability of this phenomenon. Based on a study (1956–1962) in which 70 of 101 consecutive admissions to an outpatient clinic were followed throughout the full five years, Masterson (1967) concluded that adolescent turmoil is more often a symptom of illness than of normality and we too often err by passing it off as normal and self-limited. The danger of considering adolescent turmoil as normal and of undertaking treatment with the idea that turmoil is expected, is that therapists will be inclined to treat adolescent patients less definitively than is necessary. The result is that they do not get better.

Masterson's caveat is well taken. We should not be lulled into complacency because of the idea that adolescents' symptoms are self-limited, and thus fail to approach diagnosis assiduously. But Masterson's study and conclusions warrant a couple of qualifications. One is that few experienced clinicians reading his case reports would conclude that many of his subjects were simply experiencing adolescent turmoil (Masterson, 1969). The other qualification is that Masterson approaches diagnosis from a psychodynamic but not from a developmental perspective (Mogul, 1969). That is, his diagnoses are based on symptoms and defenses, without consideration of their relationship to the developmental tasks that the adolescent is striving to accomplish during this period. If normal and psychopathological adolescent turmoil can have similar manifestations, then a clinician's ability to differentiate between the two will be limited if consideration is not given to both the developmental tasks facing the adolescent and his current and earlier relationship to his family (Mogul, 1969). This point will be clarified in chapter 9.

THE INEVITABILITY/UNIVERSALITY OF ADOLESCENT TURMOIL

In 1962 the Offers selected 103 14-year-old high school freshman boys from a Midwestern suburb, on the basis of average as representing what is normal. That is, the boys they chose were closest to the mean on all screening questionnaire instruments administered to themselves, their parents, and their teachers. Seventy-three of these boys were followed through high school and sixty through the second post–high school year with questionnaires, interviews, and interviews of collaterals (Offer, 1969; Offer and Offer, 1975).

The Offers identified three routes through adolescence, all of which are normal, in the sense of being successfully adaptive and not associated with any specific psychopathology. But each differed in the degree of stress or strain the individual experienced. One group experienced continuous psychological growth, without manifest difficulties or turmoil. The second exhibited periods of growth like the first group, but these occurred in surges interspersed with periods during which they seemed stuck and unable to move forward. The progress of the third group was characterized by more ongoing tumult and their pattern conformed most closely to the psychoanalytic view of adolescent turmoil.

The Offers reported differences in the family environments of the three groups. The family backgrounds and home life of the continuous growth group were most stable, and historically free from disruptive events, either between parents or involving individual parents. By contrast the family backgrounds of the surgent group contained more histories of parental differences in opinions and attitudes, severe illness, and traumatic life events. The family lives of the tumultuous growth group were characterized by even more traumatic life events, like mental illness, separation, and death. These latter findings underscore the importance of real experiences in the developmental process of individual adolescents.

From the standpoint of psychoanalytic theory, this study is important because, on the basis of prospective, longitudinal research on nonpatient adolescents, it challenges the notion that turmoil is more normal than lack of such unrest. That is, adolescent turmoil is not inevitable for normal development to occur. The Offers' findings are more compatible with my thesis about the crucial role of real experiences in the adolescent's behaviors than they are with the psychoanalytic view that instinctual conflicts involving the integration of sexuality are the source of adolescent turmoil.

On the other hand, the Offers' data may be consistent with one of Anna Freud's premises about those children who do not experience adolescent turmoil. She observed that children who basically remain "good" during adolescence, without evidence of rebelliousness against their parents and their parents' standards, are basically restrained from moving ahead in their adolescent development by a crippling, overly strong identification with their parents' superegos. The Offers conclude that the youths in their continuous growth group, who exhibited no evidence of turmoil, retained strong identifications with their fathers and were going to turn out most like their parents. So, this group is least likely to provide new directions for the next generation. If this is what Anna Freud meant by being constrained in one's development by retaining and carrying over from childhood the supergeo attitudes of one's parents, then the Offers' findings may support her conclusion. I will mention shortly some additional, less pathological explanations for the absence of overt turmoil in adolescents.

A SYNTHETIC VIEW OF TURMOIL IN ADOLESCENCE

In a sense, the term *adolescent turmoil* is unfortunate. By not differentiating an inner process from external manifestations of the process, the traditional view does not do itself justice, and allows its detractors to imprudently dismiss it (e.g., Oldham, 1978). Inner turmoil, from mild unsettlement to severe tempest, is usually reflected in behavior. The absence of outward manifestations does not necessarily reflect though either the absence of inner unrest or the presence of overweening defenses. The absence of overt turmoil can also reflect adequate and appropriate defenses and adaptive mechanisms, which enable the individual to integrate unsettling circumstances without manifest upset. Much work on important developmental conflicts is undertaken and resolved silently to the observer, even during adolescence; this supposition is supported by recent empirical research (Offer and Schonert-Reichl, 1992). Also, whether and particularly how turmoil shows itself behaviorally depends to a certain degree on the attitude and reaction of the individual's immediate environment. This is another reason why adolescent turmoil is not predictable. When viewed in this way, both Anna Freud and the Offers are correct. There is always inner unrest, if not from sexuality, then from other sources or from the experimenting that adolescents are prone to do with newfound capacities.

Considering even the dramatic issue of sexual maturation, these unsettling sensations can be displaced into a variety of activities. These range from the exercise of cognitive functions (daydreams, fantasies) and creative endeavors as discussed in the last section (including journal writing), through physical activities conducted privately (masturbation), and in public (sports, theatricals, participating in or attending musical events), to discussions with close friends. These experiences are being utilized to integrate (in the sense of becoming more familiar with, in control of, and accepting of) new sensations, attributes, and potentialities. These activities might enable an adolescent to adapt sufficiently to his or her unsettled sexuality so that more dramatic, behavioral manifestations of inner unrest would not be observed by parents or teachers.

Thus, it may be easy for adults to overlook turmoil, even in adolescents they know well. In a study directed toward proving the resiliency of adolescents to permanent emotional scarring, Perun and Erkut (1986) quoted epidemiological studies which demonstrated that while the incidence of psychiatric disturbance was low in a population of 14-year-olds, almost half of the sample reported feelings of misery and uncertainty. Those authors commented, "Curiously, in most cases these feelings had not been recognized by parents or teachers who were also interviewed in this study" (p. 266). Furthermore, twenty-eight of thirty college women they interviewed reported having felt confused, miserable, lacking in self-confidence, or unhappy at least some time during their adolescence. My point is that the misery of those adolescents who suffer in silence represents one subspecies of adolescent turmoil if that misery involves developmental issues; and this is why the term *adolescent turmoil*, which implies blatant manifestations, is misleading about a common feature of the adolescent developmental process.

As I have implied, researchers and others who write about this issue now tend to minimize if not discredit the concept, prevalence, and significance of adolescent turmoil. The prevailing view is exemplified in a succinct review of a volume on recent research on early adolescents. The reviewer devoted two of his four paragraphs to significant points raised in the volume. In the first of these paragraphs he focused on the consensus that adolescent development is less fraught with stormy and serious behavioral difficulties than is generally accepted. In the next paragraph, he emphasized the distressing relationship between psychosocial factors and morbidity and mortality in adolescents (Volkmar, 1994). While commentary is perhaps not expected in a brief review, I think it is instructive that neither the reviewer nor the book pondered a relationship between these two findings. The prevailing view seems to be that there are two groups, the majority who move relatively smoothly through adolescence with no more than "temporary periods of perturbation"and "disequilibrium" developing in the adolescent–parent relationship (Steinberg, 1990), and a relatively small group of psychosocially deprived youth who suffer the morbidity and mortality.

Disturbances in adolescents are linked to psychosocial, environmental phenomena. That formulation may or may not be accurate. I suspect that there is more of a continuum between "temporary perturbation" and morbidity than current research is suggesting. What seems missing is any significant consideration of a dynamic, developmental perspective on the genesis of the morbidity in current-day adolescents. In fact, the editors of that volume do observe that the field currently lacks a unitary theory which can draw together the disparate research findings (Feldman and Elliott, 1990). As I will discuss shortly, I consider that the thesis I have proposed to explain adolescent development provides such an avenue for relating adolescent turmoil to normality and pathology. That notwithstanding, current epidemiological data justify continuing to investigate adolescent turmoil on the basis of the traditional psychoanalytic explanation which emphasizes the adolescents' efforts to integrate mature sexuality into their developing personality structures.

For the consensus of epidemiological studies is that sexual activity amongst American adolescents has increased markedly during the past 20 years to the point that the majority of males have had intercourse by 16 to 17 years of age and females by age 17 to 18 (Seidman and Rieder, 1994). Acting upon sexual urges is now more societally permissible than it was in 1958 when Anna Freud elaborated the concept of adolescent turmoil. Nevertheless, the epidemiological findings leave us with unanswered questions: Has adolescent turmoil been eliminated by the dramatic increase in socially accepted, overt sexual activity, even though the act of sexual intercourse represents only one aspect of the psychological experience of integrating adult sexuality into one's personality? Or, is the more prevalent sexual activity an expression of adolescent turmoil? For early age at first sexual intercourse correlates with using drugs, with not using contraception at first intercourse, with having intercourse more frequently and with more partners, with sexually transmitted diseases, with unplanned pregnancies, and with cervical cancer (Seidman and Rieder, 1994). The latter problematic, dangerous, self-defeating, and probably self-punishing behaviors almost certainly reflect inner turmoil, be it about sexuality or something else. The results of a national poll conducted in April 1994 support this supposition that adolescents initiating sexual intercourse are experiencing inner conflict. According to the Roper Starch Worldwide nationwide telephone survey of 503 high school students conducted for Rolanda in association with the Sexual Information and Education Council of the United States (SIECUS), the majority of sexually active teenagers wish they had waited until they were older to initiate sexual activity. On average, they identified 17 as the "best age" to begin sexual intercourse; that was two years older than the average age at which the sexually active adolescents reported having begun to have intercourse (Roper Starch, 1994). I think it is reasonable to infer that if the adolescents acknowledged regret a couple of years later, it is likely that they were in conflict unconsciously when they initiated sexual activity. The alternative explanation for the correlation between early onset of sexual activity and the other problematic behaviors is that there is a greater level of psychological disturbance in that subgroup of adolescents which initiates sexual activity. It is difficult to reach the latter conclusion since the numbers of adolescents engaging in intercourse are so great. Obviously, from the clinician's standpoint, each youth must be assessed individually. But, as I said, the distinction between pathological and normal is probably difficult to ascertain at times; thus, it is important in thinking about the psychology of current adolescents not to just ride the pendulum of current fashion, which seems to have swung further away from the traditional view of the relevance of adolescent turmoil to development than the current data warrant.

The following example illustrates other contributants to adolescent turmoil, which as I noted, is best explained in some cases by a combination of the individual's maturation, his environment, and certain developmental phenomena:

A 15-year-old had begun to "goof-off" toward the end of his freshman high school year, and in doing so, jeopardized his class standing and his good relationships with teachers and school administrators. Referred to a therapist for this mildly disruptive but certainly self-defeating behavior, he gingerly began to describe his frustration—he felt and wanted to be independent of adult strictures. Not only was he unable to be independent, but he couldn't even express to anyone the frustration which had built up in him during the year—certainly not to teachers or peers in class. Moreover, his father would not tolerate expressions of anger toward him, and his mother felt guilty whenever he got angry at her, and that in turn made him feel guilty. So, the lad had found himself having elaborate, compelling daydreams of perpetrating intense aggression on those who frustrated him and fantasies of having control over everyone at school (i.e., in contrast to feeling so controlled there). At times, from out of the blue, he would find himself overtaken and intensely immersed in fantasies which left him oblivious to what was going on in class. Sometimes they seemed so real that he was actually living them. But, he hastened to add, with a questioning expression toward the therapist, that he always knew they were just fantasies and that he would never act upon them. The lad was clearly more anxious than he had represented himself as being to the therapist. The latter pointed out to him that his daydreams sounded like compensatory efforts to deal with pent-up frustration for which he felt he had no other outlet. And the therapist asked the lad what was so bad about having such harmless fantasies, since he was aware that he would never act upon them. The boy seemed only partially relieved. But then, because the therapist had reduced the lad's anxiety by indicating that the fantasies were not so bad, rather than heightening it by indicating that they were bad, the youth was able to ask the therapist about his underlying concern—"I'm not crazy am I?" The therapist elaborated in more detail his reasons for feeling confident that the boy was not crazy. The lad expressed great relief and told the therapist he had been worried about that for some time.

The development in an otherwise well-functioning lad of disruptiveness at school and inability to concentrate on one's studies would seem to qualify as adolescent turmoil. But in this example it represented the adolescent's efforts to deal with fears that he was crazy because of aggressive, sadistic, and megalomaniacal fantasies which engendered guilt and confusion about why they were occurring. Psychoanalysts often report that this fear of being or going crazy, that is commonly harbored by adolescent boys particularly, stems from difficulties controlling masturbatory urges and fantasies. In this case, the fear of being crazy was related to the intensity of aggressive fantasies. These in turn stemmed primarily from an inability to express anger to the sources of his frustration—parents, teachers, administrators, and certain peers. Drive activity may well have contributed to the development of his fantasies. Certainly, more imaginative cognitive capacities contributed as did the particular environmental context in which he found himself, namely, feeling controlled without recourse at a time in life when he felt and yearned to feel more independent.

This example illustrates that in addition to maturing sexuality and the incestuous and the parricidal, there are other physical and emotional maturational phenomena which adolescents must integrate psychologically. The latter include nonincestuously based aggression. Adolescents are generally more aggressive than children or adults; this is related to the effects of male hormones which are also secreted in greater amounts in adolescent girls. They must, therefore, find ways to achieve confidence in their ability to modulate these urges and the fantasies which accompany them. Adolescent risk taking, which can have several motives, including reality testing and omnipotence testing, sometimes involves aggressive or destructive behavior. For some individuals this may represent a greater source of turmoil than integrating sexuality.

Adolescents are better thinkers than younger children. As the passage from Schweitzer's autobiography indicated (pp. 161–162), these cognitive capacities must also be integrated and can themselves be a source of turmoil. Their more sophisticated thinking, coupled with an awareness that they are becoming more independent, causes adolescents to consider, consciously or unconsciously, the way in which they will bind themselves to their society. That is, to what degree will they uphold society's laws as opposed to acting as a law unto themselves? Turmoil experienced in this area can be expressed in driving offenses, violations of property rights, underage drinking, and other minor or major delinquent activities. Thus, the process of defining or fine-tuning one's conscience can become an important source of turmoil for some adolescents as they experiment to temper vestiges of omnipotence fantasies and narcissism with reality.

In other adolescents a need to test the limits of their abilities may become a source of turmoil, driving them to dangerous feats and exploits. Such activities may include a counterphobic effort to deal with resurgent castration anxiety, but such exploits can also stem from the need to test their sense of reality and enhance their self-confidence. Natural abilities are often capitalized upon in such behaviors.

> For example, a boy who had grown up the smallest in his class, shy and overtly lacking in self-confidence, had adapted by becoming the protected mascot of peers. Although mortified by that role, he felt that he had no alternative during his grade school years. His pubertal development was late, but he reached close to an average height.
>
> In his late teens he did a couple of things. He successfully developed a very muscular physique. Also, probably aided by inborn abilities, he became a superb and fearless driver of cars and motorcycles. He would drive very fast, under difficult conditions, over challenging streets and suburban country roads. He would usually only do this late at night when he was alone, not wanting to risk anyone else's safety; but he always felt confidently in control of himself and the vehicle. He never had an accident and rarely received traffic citations. There was an element of proving his "manliness" to himself which he had not been able to do during childhood. His primary motive was not to compensate for his earlier mascot status by showing off to his friends, since he usually performed these feats alone. Rather, he was both increasing and demonstrating his competence to himself, enhancing his self-confidence in this way, and reality-testing the limits of his abilities.

Lastly, and perhaps most importantly, if, as I have maintained, the issues of integrating mature sexuality and emancipating from childhood attachments to parents should be considered separate issues rather than causally interrelated, a prime source of adolescent turmoil can involve the need to feel confidently more independent from one's childhood attachment to one's parents. In my clinical experience the adolescent's fear of being held by parents in a nonemancipated state is an infinitely more common source of adolescent–parental turmoil than anxiety associated with incestuous longings. When adolescent–parental turmoil is based on the adolescent's fears that he or she will not be able to emancipate, this is often an effort to resolve conflicts involving childhood relationships to parents; or, it is an attempt to master prior traumata by turning passive into active and by trying on new identities for fit. The following examples illustrate turmoil during adolescence based on efforts to deal with unresolved issues from earlier childhood relationships to parents:

> After a shy and insecure entry into high school, a midadolescent found herself not rebelling in the more conventional ways that she had anticipated she might, like letting her grades suffer or cutting classes. Rather, she became "wild," involving herself sexually and pursuing to great lengths some rejecting boys, to whom she subordinated herself, while realizing that they were more interested in drinking than in her. She envinced no sexual interest in them nor enjoyed any part of her sexual experiences or the wild life she was leading. She was often aware that she would rather be home at her curfew than out with her boyfriend all night. She realized with rue one day that her mother, to whom she had lied about her whereabouts, had not even been aware that she failed to return home the previous night. She also realized one day that throughout her life her father would unpredictably disengage himself emotionally and literally become unavailable to her, and that her mother had always been critical and disapproving of her. Those rejecting attitudes on the part of her parents toward her had contributed to the development in this girl of the idea that there was something wrong with her. And she entered high school with the sense she was not really acceptable to others.

This girl's adolescent rebellion was hardly that. It was a desperate, albeit misguided, effort to resolve her feeling of being unwanted by others—desperate because as a midadolescent she knew she had to become more independent, and feeling unacceptable to others made it very difficult to emancipate with confidence. Her effort was misguided because, as is so often the case, she chose individuals with whom to work out this conflict who replicated her parents' attitudes of indifference toward her. She was attracted to such individuals because their attitudes were familiar to her and the known is more comfortable than the unknown, especially to one who questions her acceptability to others. By choosing the partners she did, her efforts to resolve her conflict about being unwanted were repeated rather than resolved. She was trying to secure the love of uninterested partners. The fact that both of her parents had also drunk heavily in her presence during her childhood supports the idea that she was trying to reconcile her feeling of being unacceptable to her parents by involving herself with people who acted toward her like they had. If her adolescent turmoil had been based on integrating sexuality, we should have been able to ferret out some evidence of sexual interest or sexual desire during intensive therapy with this perceptive patient, and as I noted, no such evidence was uncovered.

The next example also illustrates the relationship between earlier childhood experiences and adolescent turmoil:

> A girl's behavior changed from affectionate and open with her parents to rude and scornful around the time of menarche, which she otherwise seemed to experience with ease. She agitated for independence, but except for her haughty rudeness toward her parents, she was well controlled, not using drugs nor becoming sexually involved, though very involved with her friends and secretive with respect to her parents.
>
> Her parents were at a loss to understand her contumely, because they did not consider themselves like that. Then one day her father began to hear himself in his daughter's tone, and realized that on occasion when she had been younger, he had dealt with her and her sibling in the same peremptory, dismissive, intense, demanding, demeaning manner in which she was now addressing him and her mother. As a child she had occasionally been upset and frightened by his manner, but as she approached adolescence, she seemed more amused and indifferent than traumatized by it. It now appeared that she had been more traumatized earlier than was apparent, because she was utilizing the mechanism of turning passive into active to resolve the trauma by repeating it in reverse. She felt emboldened to give her parents these doses of what she had experienced by the developmental imperative to grow up, and by her increasing capacity to function independently.

The magnitude of the changes which occur during the adolescent period, both generated from within the individual and expected by the environment, would augur for the likelihood of some inner turmoil, even if the developmental process is one which evolves gradually. The absence of overt turmoil does not necessarily mean that there is no inner turmoil. And the sources of adolescent turmoil differ amongst adolescents depending on their real experiences prior to and during adolescence as well as on their reaction to the physiological changes they are experiencing.

ADOLESCENCE AS MOURNING

The centrality of mourning is frequently stressed in discussions of the developmental process of adolescence. From the standpoint of libido theory this mourning is for the relinquishment forevermore of the childhood oedipal yearnings. From the standpoint of object relations theory the loss of old ties to parents which represented security in dependency or the fantasy of union with the mother are what is being mourned. These concepts have been derived from a combination of clinical experience with adolescent patients and ideas that no libidinal position is given up easily (libido theory); or, as enunciated by Spielman (personal communication, 1991), a central issue in development with which one is always dealing is how to exist both separately and with others.

In the latter conceptualizations of development, any tendency of adolescents to capitalize upon the new surge in their egos' capacities to function is counterbalanced by the assumption that such activities will cause the adolescent to feel sad and anxious about losing old ties to parents. Things are no longer going to be the way they were. Thus, relinquishing old ties is done with real grief over a significant loss.

Certainly moments of nostalgia do overtake at least some adolescents. Often these arise in response to some specific, fond memory from childhood. For others a sense of well-being experienced within the proverbial bosom of one's family is recalled rather than specific experiences. But I do find that this idea about mourning has been overemphasized in considerations of the developmental process in normal adolescents. While the issue of living together and separately may be a lifelong one, I have found a developmental ebb and flow to the desire for attachments and separations more characteristic of development. For example, as common sense might dictate, in observing normal soldiers of different age groups serving in Vietnam, unmarried late teenagers did not exhibit the same difficulty in being separated from their families as did married soldiers several years older who had started their own families. Separation was more in-phase for the younger men (Bloch, 1970). I find that the same holds for adolescents who are not experiencing forced separations from their families or who do not feel held back by their families.

In my experience those adolescents in whom such lugubrious tendencies outweigh or even vie significantly with their eagerness to move ahead, invariably come from families in which the libidinal objects were hardly gratifying or in which there had occurred some significant breach in the family's stability. So, if anything, these adolescents are mourning what they never had rather than what they are giving up; or else, they are adopting the attitude of a parent who is having difficulty tolerating the adolescent's emancipation (this phenomenon will be illustrated in chapter 8). A good analogy is to the termination process in the analysis of adults, where the issues are those of adolescent development—overvaluing the analyst as an ideal figure, devaluing the analyst, and emancipating from a psychologically induced object tie with a regressive quality. When the patient's reaction to termination is more like severe grieving than a more ego-filtered experience of missing (Bloch, 1981), then the analyst considers the likelihood that something has gone awry in the treatment.

IDENTITY FORMATION AND IDENTITY

The concept of identity and its related terms, identity seeking, identity formation, and ego identity, have been developed by Erikson in his psychosocial framework. I find their relevance to clinical work difficult to ascertain; like a wisp of smoke, they exist but are difficult to grasp and work with.[5] From the clinical standpoint of adolescent development, identity and identity seeking can be understood as efforts to retain a sense of security as one becomes increasingly autonomous. By imparting both the sense of one's individuality and of implicit alliance with others, identity

---

[5]Efforts have been made to codify and submit Erikson's ideas to research verification and to incorporate concepts like identity status into clinical work (Marcia, 1980; Josselson, 1989). On the other hand, a commentator writing from outside the field has archly characterized identity as "the artificial flower on the compost heap of time" and a "sea on which many philosophers have lost their way" (Menand, 1994).

formation contributes to the adolescent's attempts to reconcile the basic developmental conflict between autonomy and dependency.

At least two types of activity are involved in this feature of development: One involves trying on identifications which enable the adolescent to feel that he or she is affiliated with others. Elsewhere I have used the term *identities* in referring to the adolescent's experimentation with different styles and roles (e.g., see pp. 18, 40, 102, 150, 151, and 182); these identities are basically identifications. Those new identities being tried on for fit that are obvious to the observer gradually become selectively winnowed. These in turn become amalgamated with other identifications derived from security-engendering experiences during the adolescent's life which have been evolving less conspicuously (see p. 227). In contrast to this more unconsciously conducted process of identification, the second type of activity involved in identity formation is undertaken consciously by some adolescents. These are attempts by adolescents to identify their uniqueness within the confines of character traits they share with others. Efforts at self-definition address the existential question, "Who am I?" and are observed in such disparate exercises as writing lists of personal characteristics that can include everything from one's physical features and character traits, to sources of anxieties, to dressing in a unique style.

These two processes, the more un-self-conscious absorption of identifications and the more self-conscious definition of one's evolving traits and desires, become the adolescent's vehicle for exploring and consolidating his expanded potentialities and interests. The coalescence of these two types of activity help the adolescent achieve a sense of him- or herself as unique but functioning with a sense of security. Individuals vary in the degree to which they derive a sense of security from knowing confidently that they see themselves in a certain way or from having an underlying sense of association with others. This remains a dynamic, changing condition rather than a static state throughout life.

For Erikson (1956), identity implies more than identification; it is a confluence and selective synthesis of multiple identifications into a gestalt that is more than the sum of the individual identifications. Ego identity is the level of identity formation which must be achieved at the end of adolescence if the individual is to undertake the tasks of adulthood. Ego identity refers to a mutual recognition of "something in the individual's core with an essential aspect of a group's inner coherence" (p. 102); "it connotes both a persistent sameness within oneself (self-sameness) and a persistent sharing of some kind of essential character with others" (p. 102). Erikson's focus seems to be on binding ties which link the youth and his society. These represent the age-appropriate reflections of mutuality which he considers necessary for psychosocial development to occur. My focus implies less mutuality and is more clinically directed to the manner in which the adolescent attempts to achieve maximum autonomy in completing his development.

The formation of a negative identity is one way Erikson describes development going awry. Negative identity is much like what have been termed defensive identifications in this book. Erikson's formulation of identity though makes negative identity a more comprehensive, fixed, and integrated type of psychic phenomenon than I have found the case to be in adolescents (chapter 8). Erikson (1956) writes that a negative identity is one "perversely based on all those identifications and roles which, at critical stages of development, had been presented to the individual as most undesirable or dangerous, and yet also most real" (p. 131). He cites as an example a mother, "filled with unconscious ambivalence" toward an alcoholic brother, who repeatedly responds "selectively only to those traits in her son which seem to point to a repetition of her brother's fate," leading her son in a futile effort to become a drunkard. Erikson suggests in this and other examples that the individual derives no satisfaction from the behaviors associated with the negative identity and senses somewhere in his sensibility that he is different in himself from the way he is acting. I often find in such cases that defensive identifications do not so much arise from roles which have been presented as most undesirable or dangerous; rather, defensive identifications stem from the adolescent's conclusion that these behaviors hold out the hope of satisfying his mother's underlying urge to condemn (in Erikson's just-quoted example); and by gratifying her in this way the son can secure her love. Thus, in my experience a negative identity resembles a defensive identification; both are more like a foreign body engrafted upon the individual's more accurate, underlying sense of himself and his strivings to complete development, rather than a well-integrated conviction about what he is truly like. While there may be other explanations for such cases, I have found these dynamics to be the source of such reactions much more frequently than is recognized.

THE REACTIONS OF PARENTS TO THE DEVELOPMENTAL PROCESS OF ADOLESCENTS

At the risk of oversimplifying, my experience has been that most people's first recourse in attempting to work out their own unresolved difficulties is to expose someone else to the same conditions. This is the basis for the universally used mechanism of turning passive into active. One's children become the prime targets upon which parents attempt to deal with their own unresolved developmental conflicts. In general, parents tend either to expose their children to what they themselves had experienced at the hands of their own parents; or else, parents specifically attempt to spare their children from traumatic conflicts that they had experienced with their own parents. In the latter situation, the parental motive is to shield children from both the pain the parents had endured and from the likelihood of developing maladaptive traits that they themselves acquired from their own unhappy childhood experiences. The latter position is clearly more ego filtered, benign, reasonable, and potentially forward moving for their child. In many such cases, though, this parental stance of sparing their child from their own childhood traumata proves to be only half of a constellation of the parents' attitudes. The other half involves the child fulfilling the parents' unrealized dreams—which may not correspond to the child's wishes for him- or herself. So, this parental stance can also prove problematic for the child.

Since most adults' behaviors are characterologically based, it stands to reason that basic features of parents' behaviors toward their children will be similar during their progeny's childhood and adolescence. Certain conditions unique to the adolescent period predispose parents to react in a different way quantitatively if not qualitatively. Foremost amongst these differences are the developing maturity (size, sexuality, and intellectuality) of the adolescent. It is difficult for a parent to not feel his sway more threatened by someone who has now become an equal in size, strength, sexual appeal, and ability to think clearly. For most people it is easier to maintain one's adult cool in dealing with a recalcitrant child who is looking up at you than with someone who is looking down at you. This represents in reality a kind of threat that is not presented by someone whom the parent can still pick up and carry to his or her bedroom. Especially if the parents feel that their powers and potential are waning while those of their adolescent sons and daughters are waxing, the parents' own earlier conflicts with aggression, sexuality, intelligence, competence, or competition can become reactivated. These reactions in turn require greater efforts on the part of parents to deal with their own impulses at the same time they are attempting to deal with and help their adolescents deal with their impulses.

Thus, there is a multiplicity of potential reactions which may not differ at base in their motivation with respect to the parents' manner of approaching his or her child. Greater anxiety is likely to be aroused in the parent by the potential physical threat or threat of basic disobedience to which the adult can respond either by capitulating or by attempting to clamp down even harder on the adolescent. There seems to be greater potential for the parent to become seductively titillated by the adolescent's burgeoning sexuality, and as a result, to either become inappropriately interested, involved, and stimulated, or to have to go to the opposite extreme of defending against this even more assiduously. Or, the parent may feel greater impetus to either competitively match wits with the adolescent or act submissively toward the teenager's impressively logical arguments (Bell, 1961; Anthony, 1970).

Lastly, the following examples illustrate that parents often do not readily recall certain similarities between their adolescent's behaviors and tastes and their own adolescent experience:

> A reasonably tolerant father found himself becoming quietly fretful as his adolescent son's hair reached shoulder length, at a time

when most of his peers were wearing their hair short. Then one day he spontaneously recalled that during his own adolescence he had been alone in letting his hair grow, albeit not to nearly this length, but longer than that of his peers and sufficient for his friends to have dubbed him "Nature Boy."

Another father was frustrated by his son's interest in an avant-garde form of popular music which held absolutely no appeal to this music-loving father. He was equally frustrated by his son's complete lack of interest in the music that he preferred. Then one day, the father recalled that his own musical interests had been very different from those of his own parents, and that he had exhibited similar indifference to his own father's efforts to get him to appreciate the music his father loved.

SUMMARY

This chapter has examined many features of development during adolescence. Behavior patterns and changes which occur in adolescents described by existing theories are illustrated. They are compared with my observations and those of others (including writers and autobiographers) in an effort to suggest that a more encompassing theoretical framework than that of the extant theories provides a better working model for these alterations. The prominence of vicissitudes of identification and of learning during adolescence represents evidence of a strong, underlying progressive current in the developmental process. Features of development during adolescence which are specifically discussed include sexual development; changes in the sensibility; the self-observation/self-consciousness axis; the evanescent spurt of creativity during midadolescence; the question of adolescent turmoil; the idea of mourning in adolescent development; identity formation and identity; and the reactions of parents to the developmental process of their adolescent children.

CHAPTER 7

The Transition to Adulthood and a Theory of Adolescent Development

THE TRANSITION FROM ADOLESCENCE TO ADULTHOOD

The nature of this transition is most accurately explained by viewing development as a gradually evolving process, the timing and pacing of which can be significantly influenced by the adolescent's unique past and present real experiences. This approach depicts the developmental process as more dynamic and ongoing than stage bound.[1] It is consistent with observations that no clear border exists between adolescence and adulthood (Scharfman in Panel, 1987), that the transition to adulthood is often imperceptible (Fountain, 1961), and that all features are not consolidated at the same time (Kaplan, 1980, 1989; Arnstein, 1989). It is also compatible with the conclusions of psychoanalytic authors who characterize this transition as one involving consolidating, integrating and restructuring, stabilizing and harmonizing the psychic processes or the personality (Adatto, 1980; Staples and Smarr,

---

[1]The gathering evidence that development is not completed at the end of adolescence but continues to evolve during adult life is consistent with this view of the developmental process (Erikson, 1950; Block and Haan, 1971; Vaillant, 1977; Levinson, Darrow, Klein, Levinson, and McKee, 1978; Eichorn, Clausen, Haan, Honzik, and Mussen, 1981; Emde, 1985).

193

1980; Brockman, 1984; Coppolillo, 1984). Such evolving changes do not lend themselves to delineating stages in a criterion-based manner.

From the perspective I am recommending, the issue becomes whether an adolescent's movement toward completing his or her development is on track, or is hindered or stalled, rather than whether adolescence has been completed. This focus obviates the problems of the criteria-bound approaches which have been used to mark the transition from adolescence to adulthood. The problems which are inherent in these traditional approaches will be illustrated shortly. They center around the observation that the variation amongst adolescents and within individual adolescents in the time-frame when different criteria are attained is too great to demarcate a transition between adolescence and adulthood. Morever, some criteria do not typically end with adolescence and others have been present in many individuals since childhood. In addition, the existence of other criteria which are defined in terms of inner processes is difficult to confirm.

In my view the transition to adulthood is best explained in terms of the ongoing developmental issue of reconciling strivings to complete development with the need for parental sponsorship. This concept implies that the transition must be considered in a case specific manner. The end of adolescence is usually considered to have a psychosocial precipitant, namely, expectations placed on the late adolescent by the society (Group for the Advancement of Psychiatry [GAP] Report, 1968; Isay, 1980; Staples and Smarr, 1980). That conclusion is compatible with my point that the adolescent's unique environment can significantly influence this transition.

DIFFERENCES BETWEEN ADOLESCENTS AND ADULTS

Even though this transition between adolescence and adulthood does not fit a stage theory model, there are descriptive differences between average expectable adolescents and adults. I will illustrate these as part of my exposition of adolescent development. These characteristics are not useful as criteria for measuring a transition to adulthood, for some individuals exhibit one or more of these traits from earlier in their development rather than at the end of adolescence. Yet, such individuals are neither adult during their childhoods nor radically changing as they reach chronological adulthood.[2] Examples of these descriptive changes include the return of adolescents to a friendlier or more considerate relationship with their parents and comporting themselves in a more emotionally settled manner. Another example is the emergence of seriousness of purpose regarding important aspects of their lives which some late adolescents had not evinced to that point. This shift is not always as dramatic as Joseph Conrad's characterization of it as "the change from youth, carefree and fervent, to the more self-conscious and more poignant period of maturer life" (Conrad, 1927, quoted in Krasnow, 1989, p. 203).

Fountain (1961) observed that adolescents yearn for experiences. I understand this trait to reflect an aspect of the adolescent's urge to practice with his or her expanded sensibility, competence, and ability to handle new situations without parental assistance (chapter 6). Rock concerts, which are so popular with adolescents, provide opportunities for gratifying their yearning for experiences and emotional intensity. The audience members experiment with feeling and losing control of intense emotion; and they share that intensity with other adolescents in a setting that expands their experience. At the same time the experience is usually impersonal enough to be safe from compromising involvement. There are risks involved on occasion; and risk taking, finding out more about one's own limits in an effort to enhance one's sense of reality, is another feature of adolescence which can occur in conjunction with the hunger for experiences.

Relative self-absorption or self-centeredness and an orientation toward immediacy have also been characterized as typical of adolescents but not of adults (Adatto, 1958, 1966; Fountain,

---

[2]Identity researchers reconcile these phenomena by positing the development of different identity statuses (identity achievement, foreclosure, moratorium, diffusion). This basically amounts to a way of describing an individual's current modus operandi and relating it to his past history (Marcia, 1980; Josselson, 1989).

1961). By remaining preoccupied with the urgency of the moment, adolescents exhibit different priorities than many adults evince in similar circumstances. I think that their seeming omnipotent lack of concern about longer-term consequences often reflects the expectation of many adolescents that their parents will ultimately assume responsibility for assuring their welfare. This mind-set is often the basis for what has been characterized as a relative failure of self-criticism which reflects less effective reality testing in adolescents compared to adults (Fountain, 1961). The reality testing of such adolescents seems defective only in the broadest sense of that term, as it applies to judgment and a sense of responsibility for self and others.

> A 19-year-old returned for vacation from an out-of-state college to his home in a drought-crippled area during the height of water rationing. A native of that area, he had lived through the last drought as a little boy. He was concerned about the environment, particularly the plight of the wild life on the hill next to his home. He staunchly favored rationing and had righteous, scathing things to say about a long-time, water-squandering neighbor. He realized that his family's allotment was not increased during his two-week visit and certainly wanted to do his share. But when his parents approached him on the second day of his vacation about the amount of water used in his daily, 15-minute shower, he responded that there was no alternative. They surely recalled that he had always needed to take long showers to wake up, and there was no other way of getting the shampoo and conditioner out of his thick mane of below shoulder-length hair. Any inconsistency he could see in his position was quickly washed away by his conviction about the lack of alternatives. And his parents could think of it this way, he'd try to catch some of the water and they could put it on their prized fruit trees, so his showers were really helping them out. In any event, it wasn't "a big deal" and he was sure his parents could "work it out."

His grandparents, hearing this story, felt smugly confirmed in their long-standing conviction that he was nothing but a spoiled brat. Clinicians, hearing this tale, would tend to agree with his parents, who shook their heads in frustrated resignation, considering him adolescent, and hoping that he'd soon grow up and start thinking about someone besides himself. If the same clinicians were to hear this story about a 23-year-old, they would find themselves considering a character or character assassination diagnosis, like "narcissistic."

As the foregoing illustrates, what is accepted in common wisdom and clinically as immaturity risks being labeled as character pathology in young adulthood. Vaillant (1987), who followed a cohort of men from age 18 to 50, has called attention to this phenomenon and also observed that the men eventually mature out of a number of these adolescent traits. Also, Vaillant (1977) and Levinson, Darrow, Klein, Levinson, and McKee (1978) found that men seek "mentor" relationships until midlife. This suggests that, as noted earlier, the hallmark of adulthood, namely, psychological independence from parental-type influence, occurs more gradually than is compatible with a stage theory of development.

The use of developmental task criteria (Staples and Smarr, 1980; Arnstein, 1989) for marking the transition between adolescence and adulthood presents the same problem as was just noted with respect to the matter of psychological independence. Some of the following developmental task criteria do not end with adolescence (the second part of 1, 2, 3, sometimes 4 and 5). Others are often not attained until far enough into adult life as to render them meaningless for demarcating a transition to adulthood (second part of 1, 3, 6). Developmental tasks that have been considered requisite for crossing the threshold of adulthood include:

1. Consolidation of adult (genital) sexuality, with the further proviso of having reconciled sexual and tender feelings toward one's partner.
2. Disengagement from childhood dependency on one's parents and replacement of this by a relationship of mutuality with them.
3. Establishment of a sense of conscience and a moral code independent from those of one's parents.
4. Selection of a realistic occupational choice based on probability of success rather than on possibilities and wishes of parents.
5. Achievement of a sense of confidence that one can control and express unconscious impulses in socially acceptable ways.

6. The establishment of a coherent sense of one's self, a cohesive
self (Weissman, Cohen, Boxer, and Cohler, 1989), or the consolidation of identity (Josselson, 1989).

Blos (1977) considers several internal, psychological criteria
more reliable and crucial than developmental tasks in demarcating the end of adolescence. These criteria seem at base to be
derived more from theory than from clinical observation. His
criteria are: (1) a second individuation (1967) which allows the
adolescent to form stable relationships with other people; (2)
ego continuity which affords a realistic perspective on one's past
and future (1977); (3) formation of a mature ego ideal which
congeals one's sexual identity (1985); (4) adaptive mastery of
residual traumata from childhood into ego syntonic personality
traits which contribute to the uniqueness of the individual's character (1977).

I find these postulated criteria for the transition to adulthood inadequate and difficult both to comprehend and to apply
in any practical manner. The concept of a "second individuation" is so abstract, ego continuity so complex and amorphous,
and the establishment of sexual identity through ego ideal formation so theoretical that it is difficult to recognize their appearance.[3] Moreover, if they do exist, none necessarily seems to occur
within a time frame which renders them useful for marking a
transition to adulthood. For example, in my experience childhood traumas that have impeded development are not usually

---

[3]Blos explains these concepts as follows: (1) He observes that "the adolescent has to come into emotional contact with the passions of his infancy and
early childhood, in order for them to surrender their original cathexes" (1967,
p. 178). This is accomplished by an obligatory regression during adolescence
of ego and drives to an approximation rather than a consummation of the early
childhood, undifferentiated state of object relatedness. The disengagement
from these "internalized" "love and hate objects" frees the adolescent to find
new, nonincestuous love and hate objects. He terms this process the "second
individuation" of adolescence. (2) Ego continuity involves the development
of the ability to subject one's personal history to mature reality testing. This
development of a historical sense of oneself is based on self-consciousness, improved reality testing, advanced cognitive functioning, and physical maturity; it
is evidenced in the capacity for existential thought. (3) "Sexual identity formation is predicated on the transmutation of the gender-inadequate [Ed. note:
i.e., homosexual] component of the sexual drive into a new psychic structure,
the ego ideal" (Blos, 1977, p. 419).

rendered ego syntonic at the end of adolescence. Rather, they are continually repeated for purposes of mastery in the lives of people who have presumably reached adulthood.

Given the difficulties in applying all criteria that have been used to demarcate this period, I have concluded that the best approach to understanding the transition to adulthood is through examining factors which cause the adolescent's development to become stuck in this transition. This is because it may be easier to derive understanding of the normal developmental process by extrapolation from impediments to it in situations of this sort. The latter refers to situations in which changes normally occur very gradually and imperceptibly, and where there is great variation between and within individuals in the age when the changes are completed.

FAILURE TO TRANSCEND ADOLESCENCE

THE ROLE OF CHANCE

A premise of this book is that adolescents' needs to adapt to their environment have crucial impact on their efforts to complete any feature of their development. Their "environment" was originally their parents. Some aspects of completing development, for example, movement toward a vocation or toward self-sufficiency, can now be profoundly influenced by people other than parents and by circumstances over which adolescents have little control (Blaine and Farnsworth, 1980). Thus, chance can play a significant role in the timing, pacing, and success of completing developmental objectives. This powerful influence of real experiences on progress in development contributes significantly to the great variation between individuals and within any individual adolescent in the time when he or she achieves different objectives or internal changes that are considered to signal the advent of adulthood. Military service provides numerous examples of this phenomenon since many adolescents enlist when they are at the chronological threshold of adulthood. The particular officers assigned to any enlistee can have a profound, sponsoring effect or a devastating impact on his or her development. And while the

vast majority of enlistees fare well, there is too much chance involved in the assignment of leaders to these youth to predict the
outcome for a number of individuals (Bloch, 1970).

WORKING ON ONE DEVELOPMENTAL ISSUE AT A TIME

Another factor often becomes more evident as the youth progresses into adulthood; namely, late adolescents/young adults often tend to work on one developmental issue at a time.[4] For
example, they may strive either consciously or unconsciously to
accomplish vocational goals before facing the matter of choosing
an appropriate marital partner.

IMPEDIMENTS TO MAKING THE TRANSITION FROM ADOLESCENCE TO ADULTHOOD

I will now describe an individual who had been unable to make
the transition from adolescence to adulthood as indicated by traditionally used criteria. The basic impediment to his progress
proved to be his inability to reconcile his strivings to complete
development and his need to please and feel sponsored by his
parents.

> An intense, 24-year-old presented in the throes of distressing, self-
> diagnosed "paranoid" fears that he would be accused of a series
> of unsolved rapes on the university campus where he still lived
> with his father, an administrator, and his mother. Closer ques-
> tioning revealed that he did not believe that anyone would truly
> think he had committed the crimes. Rather, he was convinced
> that people wanted to accuse him in spiteful retaliation for his
> outspoken, critical attitudes toward militant feminists and other
> strident "liberation" groups on that campus; however, this dis-
> tinction afforded him no relief. For he recounted stories of inno-
> cent people who had served long prison terms, and he was

---

[4]This idea about development finds support in empirical research on the
therapeutic process in psychoanalysis and psychotherapy. Weiss, Sampson, and
the Mt. Zion Psychotherapy Research Group (1986) have found that patients
work to resolve or master problems sequentially, one at a time. Thus, it may be
reasonable to surmise that individuals can address some developmental issues
in the same manner.

panicked about being falsely accused. Then, in the next breath, he would reverse that attitude and intimate that he deserved to be censured because of his contemptuous attitudes toward others.

He had been unable to complete college despite good intelligence, because he couldn't decide whether he wanted to become a professional or a semiskilled laborer. His heterosexual identity was well established, but he avowed contempt for women and interest only in sexual relations, in which he had engaged, though he had never had a girl friend. He maintained an intensely contentious relationship with his parents, who reciprocated the antagonism. He had few stable friendships at that point.

So, although he was chronologically an adult, this young man had not resolved issues which have been used to define the offset of adolescence, namely disengagement from a dependent relationship on parents; reconciliation of sexual and tender feelings toward heterosexual partners; movement toward a realistic occupational goal.

The high level of this man's anxiety prompted the therapist to immediately establish four weekly sessions. Within a few weeks the young man lost concern that other people would suspect him; however, he became increasingly obsessed with the idea that the therapist would become suspicious and turn him over to the authorities. He now felt himself in a Catch-22 situation. He had to tell the analyst more in order to be helped and to experience relief; but, the more he revealed, particularly about his angry, deprecating attitudes toward women, the greater became his worry that the therapist would suspect that he was the rapist. The very relationship he was attempting to form for help had now become his nemesis, causing him to lose sleep and his condition to deteriorate.

At this juncture, with the patient at an impasse because of what appeared to be an intense transference reaction, the therapist reflected back to his patient that he, the therapist, was now the tormentor of the patient, and the cause for his emotional deterioration. The therapist then asked if such a circumstance was familiar. Had the patient ever been tormented in this manner by anyone else (i.e., was this straight transference); or had anyone else ever accused him as he was now accusing the therapist (i.e., was he turning passive into active)? After a moment's reflection, the young man gave a brief snort, a smile, and reddened slightly; he realized that for years his family had accused him in precisely that way. That is, he was accusing the therapist as his parents had accused him, a turning passive into active mechanism. This insight enabled him to turn his attention from the analyst as tormentor to exploring why this underlying concern about his relationship to his family had masqueraded in his presenting symptoms.

I will now relate what emerged during the course of several years of therapy as the reason why his development had become so stymied: He claimed to have always been considered the black sheep by his family and the source of disharmony at home. His own theory was that this view of him originated from his father who was treating him as his own father (the patient's grandfather) had treated him (the patient's father). The patient admired and loved his own father. But he felt painfully disappointed by his father's failure both to understand him and to be on his side, and by his mother's failure to consistently try to offset his father's rejecting attitudes. He thought that his parents wanted him out of the way. He had felt so self-depreciatory, lonely, and tormented by being unable to move forward in his life, that for several years he would have felt grateful if someone killed him. The therapist asked whether he felt that his parents truly wanted him out of the way, wished him dead. He had felt this. Thus, the curious combination of his paranoid ideas that others wanted to falsely accuse him, and his feeling that he deserved such treatment, expressed his view of unfair parental attitudes toward him and, paradoxically, an acceptance of their attitudes. This accommodation to what he perceived to be his parents' wishes, culminating in his willingness to be killed, conflicted with his own stated desire to move ahead with his life.

A reader might react with skepticism to this formulation of a patient with paranoid symptomatology. For example, how could the therapist know whether his parents were against the patient? And even if they were, could their attitudes have arisen in response to his own nastiness? The quickest way to address those appropriate questions is to say that working on the basis of the dynamics just outlined, the patient was relieved of his symptoms, returned to college, graduated, and moved on with a much-improved relationship with his parents. The therapeutic task was to reduce his guilt-driven, compulsive need to act in ways which afforded his parents (and others) justification for rejecting him, which was what he perceived basically pleased them.

What is pertinent for our consideration of adolescent development is that this young man's adolescent turmoil which had continued in his symptomatic presentation as a young adult, did not involve integrating mature sexuality into his psyche; he felt comfortable and confident as a heterosexual male. Rather, his turmoil and symptoms seemed to be the outcome of a conflict between his self-expressed wishes to move ahead, to complete his development as it were, and his need to comply with parental attitudes toward him. What may have appeared to be rebelliousness toward parents, was at base an effort to give them what he perceived they wanted—justification for rejecting him. This represents a different developmental conflict from that posited by other theories, and one which accords different significance to parental interactions.

PARENTAL SPONSORSHIP OF THEIR ADOLESCENT'S DEVELOPMENT

Psychoanalytic theory correctly points out that one role of parents is to appropriately frustrate any realization of the adolescent's regressive, incestuous wishes; parents should neither be seductive nor overly demeaning toward the adolescent because of the parents' needs to defend against any resurgence of their own incestuous urges that have been stimulated by their child's pubescence. In addition, I am suggesting another, central role for parents, namely, what this young man pined for, an ongoing sense of parental approval and sponsorship of his progress in development. This differs from my reading of Erikson's psychosociological view in which the parent is seen almost symbolically as representative of the adult generation in welcoming a new member into its midst (1956). This is also different from Blos' similar view of the reciprocal, intergenerational aspect in the father–son relationship, which is important in ego ideal formation, and culminates in the father giving his blessing to his son's emerged manhood (1985). The dynamic which I am suggesting does not stop with mature ego ideal formation. Rather, it is a very family-specific need to support one's adolescent in an ongoing way. The parent's service as representative of the adult generation is of more peripheral importance. Also, as I will point out in the next quotation, this view of sponsorship differs from the self psychology view, because the individual's underlying self-esteem is unimpaired. It is an active, ongoing process, which antedates adolescence. And the reports that mentor-type relationships are sought out by men into young middle age (Vaillant, 1977; Levinson et al., 1978), suggest that a more circumscribed version of this sponsorship phenomenon persists after adolescence and thus transcends developmental stages. I understand the intrapsychic meaning of this interpersonal dynamic to be a wish to retain a positive relationship with parents.

I would like to illustrate this phenomenon further with a passage from the autobiography, *Memoirs*, of Sherwood Anderson, the American author who died in 1941, best known for his book, *Winesburg, Ohio*:

> You hear it said that fathers want their sons to be what they feel they cannot themselves be, but I tell you it also works the other way. A boy wants something very special from his father. I know that as a small boy I wanted my father to be a certain thing he was not. I wanted him to be a proud, silent, dignified father. When I was with other boys and he passed along the street, I wanted to feel a flow of pride: "There he is. That is my father."
>
> But he wasn't such a one. He couldn't be. It seemed to me then that he was always showing off. Let's say someone in our town had got up a show. They were always doing it. The druggist would be in it, the shoe-store clerk, the horse doctor, and a lot of women and girls. My father would manage to get the chief comedy part. It was, let's say, a Civil War play and he was a comic Irish soldier. He had to do the most absurd things. They thought he was funny, but I didn't.
>
> I thought he was terrible. I didn't see how mother could stand it. She even laughed with the others. Maybe I would have laughed if it hadn't been my father.
>
> Or there was a parade, the Fourth of July or Decoration Day. He'd be in that, too, right at the front of it, as Grand Marshal or something, on a white horse hired from the livery stable.
>
> He couldn't ride for shucks. He fell off the horse and everyone hooted with laughter, but he didn't care. He seemed to like it. I remember once when he had done something ridiculous, and right out on Main Street, too. I was with some other boys and they were laughing and shouting at him and he was shouting back and having as good time as they were. I ran down an alley back of some stores and there in the Presbyterian Church sheds I had a good long cry.
>
> Or I would be in bed at night and father would come home a little lit up and bring some men with him. He was a man who was never alone. Before he went broke, running a harness shop, there were always a lot of men loafing in the shop. He went broke, of course, because he gave too much credit. He couldn't refuse it and I thought he was a fool. I had got to hating him.
>
> There'd be men I didn't think would want to be fooling around with him. There might even be the superintendent of our

schools and a quiet man who ran the hardware store. Once I remember there was a white-haired man who was a cashier of a bank. It was a wonder to me they'd want to be seen with such a windbag. That's what I thought he was. I know now what it was that attracted them. It was because life in our town, as in all small towns, was at times pretty dull and he livened it up. He made them laugh. He could tell stories. . . .

He was always telling stories about himself. He'd say this or that wonderful thing had happened to him. It might be something that made him look like a fool. He didn't care.

If an Irishman came to our house, right away father would say he was Irish. He'd tell what county in Ireland he was born in. He'd tell things that happened there when he was a boy. He'd make it seem so real that, if I hadn't known he was born in southern Ohio, I'd have believed him myself.

And there was mother. How could she stand it? I wanted to ask but never did. She was not the kind you asked such questions.

I'd be upstairs in my bed, in my room above the porch, and father would be telling some of his tales. A lot of father's stories were about the Civil War. To hear him tell it he'd been in about every battle. He'd known Grant, Sherman, Sheridan and I don't know how many others. He'd been particularly intimate with General Grant so that when Grant went East, to take charge of all the armies, he took father along.

That's just one of the kind of things he'd tell. Of course, the men knew he was lying, but they seemed to like it just the same . . . As a boy that was what I couldn't understand.

When we got broke, down and out, do you think he ever brought anything home? Not he. If there wasn't anything to eat in the house, he'd go off visiting at farmhouses. They all wanted him. Sometimes he'd stay away for weeks, mother working to keep us fed, and then home he'd come bringing, let's say, a ham. He'd got it from some farmer friend. He'd slap it on the table in the kitchen. "You bet I'm going to see that my kids have something to eat," he'd say, and mother would just stand smiling at him. She'd never say a word about all the weeks and months he'd been away, not leaving us a cent for food.

But often I was filled with bitterness and sometimes I wished he wasn't my father. I'd even invent another man as my father. To protect my mother I'd make up stories of a secret marriage that for some strange reason never got known. As though some man, say the president of a railroad company or maybe a Congressman, had married my mother, thinking his wife was dead and then it turned out she wasn't.

So they had to hush it up but I got born just the same. I wasn't really the son of my father. Somewhere in the world there was a very dignified, quite wonderful man who was really my father. I even made myself half believe these fancies.

And then there came a certain night. He'd been off somewhere for two or three weeks. He found me alone in the house, reading by the kitchen table.

It had been raining and he was very wet. He sat and looked at me for a long time, not saying a word. I was startled, for there was on his face the saddest look I had ever seen. He sat for a time, his clothes dripping. Then he got up.

"Come on with me," he said.

I got up and went with him out of the house. I was filled with wonder but I wasn't afraid. We went along a dirt road that led down into a valley, about a mile out of town, where there was a pond. We walked in silence. The man who was always talking had stopped his talking.

I didn't know what was up and had the queer feeling that I was with a stranger. I don't know whether my father intended it so. I don't think he did.

The pond was quite large. It was still raining hard and there were flashes of lightning followed by thunder. We were on a grassy bank at the pond's edge when my father spoke, and in the darkness and rain his voice sounded strange.

"Take off your clothes," he said. Still filled with wonder, I began to undress. There was a flash of lightning and I saw that he was already naked.

Naked, we went into the pond. Taking my hand he pulled me in. It may be that I was too frightened, too full of strangeness, to speak. Before that night my father had never seemed to pay any attention to me.

"And what is he up to now?" I kept asking myself. I did not swim very well, but he put my hand on his shoulder and struck out into the darkness.

He was a man with big shoulders, a powerful swimmer. In the darkness I could feel the movement of his muscles. We swam to the far edge of the pond and then back to where we had left our clothes. The rain continued and the wind blew. Sometimes my father swam on his back and when he did he took my hand in his large powerful one and moved it over so that it rested always on his shoulder. Sometimes there would be a flash of lightning and I could see his face quite clearly.

It was as it was earlier, in the kitchen, a face filled with sadness. There would be the momentary glimpse of his face and then again the darkness, the wind and the rain. In me there was a feeling I had never known before.

It was a feeling of closeness. It was something strange. It was as though there were only we two in the world. It was as though I had been jerked suddenly out of myself, out of my world of the schoolboy, out of a world in which I was ashamed of my father.

He had become blood of my blood; he the strong swimmer and I the boy clinging to him in the darkness. We swam in silence and in silence we dressed in our wet clothes and went home.

There was a lamp lighted in the kitchen and when we came in, the water dripping from us, there was my mother. She smiled at us. I remember that she called us "boys."

"What have you boys been up to?" she asked, but my father did not answer. As he had begun the evening's experience with me in silence, so he ended it. He turned and looked at me. Then he went, I thought, with a new and strange dignity out of the room.

I climbed the stairs to my own room, undressed in the darkness and got into bed. I couldn't sleep and did not want to sleep. For the first time I knew that I was the son of my father. He was a story teller as I was to be. It may be that I even laughed a little softly there in the darkness. If I did, I laughed knowing that I would never again be wanting another father [Anderson (1939, pp. 45–49); excerpted from quotation in Kiell (1964)].

This quotation could be used to illustrate several developmental issues, including positive and negative oedipal constellations and the myth of the family romance. But psychosexual issues seem subordinate to young Anderson's perception that his father had never paid attention to him and the lad was reacting to never having felt claimed by his father. Interestingly and importantly, this factor does not seem to have left young Sherwood with a deficit of narcissism as Kohut describes, for the lad seemed quite self-contained and competent. Rather, his father's lack of ongoing sponsorship created a different order of developmental conflict, with which young Anderson partly dealt by turning away. That is, Sherwood acted as he felt his father acted toward him; the youngster exhibited identification with the aggressor, devaluing his father as we presume he interpeted his father's disinterest in him. The lad could only realize and accept his positive identification, and capitalize upon it in confirming his own future professional identity, after he felt that his father wanted to lend his strength to help Sherwood face his fear of open water. In both of the latter examples, the young paranoid man and Sherwood Anderson sought sponsorship by the parent of the same sex. While such seems important, I am persuaded that a sponsoring relationship by either parent can reduce the inevitable conflicts engendered by the antagonism of either parent to an adolescent's development. I am not convinced that this is a sex-related matter.

If continuing support from a parental figure is necessary for development to progress, then Freud himself offered a basis for its existence. In his later writings (Freud, 1930, 1940), which were not clinically oriented and never influenced his clinical theory, he wrote what now seems like great common sense. He said that the child's greatest fear is losing his parents' love, because his sense of security depends on that. This fear is so great that a child will assume responsibility for bad things which befall him, in his effort to retain parental love. In fact, Freud suggested this tendency to blame oneself for misfortunes which befall one continues into later life. This would help explain, for example, that tendency in the young paranoid man described earlier in this chapter. I have posited this as one underlying principle of adolescent development. It may seem opposite from the need to emancipate. Yet, an underlying sense of parental sponsorship for the adolescent's progress to independence, based on feeling that one has a positive relationship with parents, is a requisite for successful emancipation.

A THEORY OF ADOLESCENT DEVELOPMENT

If we return now to the threshold of adolescence, we can find another principle of development. For, as I have pointed out, we observe children who are progressing in every way through maturational spurts. They are getting bigger, stronger, smarter, more sexually mature. If the adolescent's physical, physiological, and intellectual development are all advancing, it would seem more reasonable to assume that progress in his or her psychological development occurs on a similar basis. There are references in the psychoanalytic literature to a concept which would align psychological development with these other progressive features. Ernest Jones (1922) and Helene Deutsch (1944) both wrote about inborn urges to grow up and achieve something. Anna Freud (1965, 1968) and Edward Bibring (1937) wrote about the importance of such urges to complete development in the curative process of child and adult analysis respectively. Ives Hendrick's (1942) instinct for mastery has a similar implication. More recently attention has been called to the same phenomenon: Harley (Panel, 1980) makes the point that "Maturation and spontaneous development are often most strikingly visible as the patient moves from early to late adolescence" (p. 162). Parens (1986) writes in a review of a book about breakdown in adolescence that, "As a result of years of direct child observation and child analysis I have come to the view that *usually*, a child's (boy or girl) powerful thrust to autonomy and self differentiation has to be thwarted quite substantially by the mother, consciously or unconsciously, to obtain what we find in Alan [the patient whose case Parens was discussing]" (p. 525). And Sklansky and Rabichow (1980) advanced the idea that, "The adolescent's push for autonomous functioning has the quality of an intense drive" (quoted in Brockman, 1984, p. 112).

If we posit three principles to underlie the process of adolescent development, (1) an urge to complete development which corresponds to the observable direction of their physical, physiological, and intellectual growth, and (2) the ongoing need for parental sponsorship, which enables the adolescent to feel confident that (3) he or she is maintaining an important relationship with their parents and pleasing them, then we can see from the experience of the young paranoid man (pp. 200–202) that trouble develops when these motives are experienced as being in conflict.

I submit that the process of development during the adolescent years is most accurately understood as an evolving, reality oriented, progressive effort by boys and girls to adapt to their increasing capacities, and to utilize these to reconcile unresolved earlier developmental conflicts. Many of the latter have arisen because during earlier childhood they had experienced their need to maintain a sense of security in relation to their parents as being in conflict with their strivings to complete development. Integration of sexuality is important during this period, but primarily because it is the last biological function to mature and imparts adult sexual capacities, rather than because it necessarily initiates the emancipatory process by virtue of conveying incestuous urges.

As illustrated in chapter 6, adolescent turmoil can have many sources, including problems integrating sexuality, or aggression, or new cognitive abilities, as well as conflict between urges to develop and to gratify parental wishes. Among the most important sources is the adaptive effort to try on new identities for fit, to experiment with new capacities and sensations, and to attempt to reconcile prior problems in relatedness to parents.

The great variation in the age at which individuals are ready to function maturely as adults does not lend this transition to a stage theory model of development. Most individuals at the chronological threshold of adulthood are able to live away from their parents and negotiate the problems of everyday living. Issues like emotional readiness for marriage, the freedom to live comfortably with moral and ethical standards different from those of one's parents, and readiness for a career commitment are often not resolved. For these accomplishments occur by the gradual resolution of a developmental process in which one's past history, one's real experience, influences the pacing and timing of the accomplishment of such developmental objectives; this is because of the ongoing importance of one's dual motives to complete development and to maintain parental sponsorship throughout development. As noted earlier, the findings of Vaillant (1977) and Levinson et al. (1978) that men seek out mentor relationships well into midlife suggest to me that parental sponsorship remains a developmental issue well past the time when a man assumes complete financial, physical, and moral responsibility for himself and a family of his own.

I have not found comparable published studies of women, but am persuaded that equivalent mentor relationships characterize their development. Levinson et al. (1978) reported that Stewart (1976) found that all subjects in a small sample of women in their middle thirties went through the same developmental periods as men, though some of the specific issues were different. I infer from this that mentoring was sought by women as well as by men; it is not a gender specific issue. It has been written that women have not been successful in the business world because of a lack of role models in corporate organizations.[5] I am persuaded that it is not a lack of role models, but a lack of having experienced sponsorship from male or female role models in those settings. Josselson concludes from her study of identity formation that mentor relationships are vital in accomplishing and maintaining the goals of those women who have made careers an important feature of their identity (Josselson, 1987). I suspect that the mothers themselves or aunts or older sisters serve the mentoring function for many women who follow the career of their own homemaker mothers. Such a sponsorship relationship which continues uninterrupted from adolescence or is reinstated again in young adulthood is potentially fraught with more difficulty because lifelong, familial relationships are more complicated than those one would usually have with a nonfamilial mentor. Nevertheless, the sponsoring process is as important in the development of women as men, but not as obvious in the home as in out-of-home workplaces.

THE ULTIMATE OUTCOME OF THE SPONSORING AND SUBSEQUENT MENTORING RELATIONSHIP

The continuing pursuit of sponsorship well past the traditional time when adolescence is thought to end also supports the wisdom of rethinking the value of the stage theory concept compared to one in which progress is understood to occur in a more evolutionary manner which involves issues that are not stage specific. In other words, if we can move away from the stage theory model, then the issue of defining criteria for the end of adolescence loses its importance; for development has been gradually evolving and different issues are resolved at different times, depending to a significant degree on the individual's unique past

---

[5]Role models are not necessarily mentors, but mentoring is also currently used to refer to a more focused, career-advancing relationship, which has been advocated as an antidote for difficulties women (and minorities) experience in this area. For example, "mentors help women in medicine accelerate through the ranks by showing them the ropes and pulling them up and into the inner circle of the medical establishment" (Higgins, 1994, p. 4). By contrast, I am using this term to describe a more broadly based sponsorship which has as its desired outcome the achievement of greater independence (e.g., via enhanced competence) rather than a calculated, rapid ascent up the equivalent of the proverbial corporate ladder.

history with his or her family. Understood this way, the sponsorship and subsequent mentoring sequence carries the individual from dependence through independence to mature interdependence. Interdependence is probably the most accurate way of understanding the relationship of mature adults who are in a close relationship to one another. Recognizing and accepting a reciprocity in important relationships becomes an indicator of maturity and a continuing and necessary strength throughout adult life.

COMPATIBILITY OF THIS THESIS WITH RECENT RESEARCH

Data which support the importance of real experiences in their own right, rather than as factors which simply color instinctual conflicts during development favor the view I am advancing: As noted in the Offers' studies (Offer, 1969; Offer and Offer, 1975) of modal adolescent males (chapter 6), the degree of upheaval which the individual adolescent experienced correlated directly with the magnitude of objectively identifiable disruptive factors in the family home. The latter ranged from differences between parents in attitudes, to illness, mental illness, separation, and death. This research supports the idea that real experiences are of utmost importance in the developmental process of individual adolescents; but since all their subjects were deemed to develop normally, these environmental factors were not sufficient to derail their development, at least during the years of their study.

Recent infant research, summarized by Stern (1985), suggests that the infant's ego apparatus is much more sophisticated than traditional dynamic theories have presumed. Moreover, the infant is attentive to and motivated by reality above all other motives, and development progresses through the infant's adaptation to reality not fantasy. A concept of strivings to complete development seems implicit in Stern's findings, which suggest the existence of ego instincts rather than, or in addition to, libidinal and aggressive drives. This concept of strivings to complete development is also compatible with the conclusions of Lichtenberg (1989) and the research of Emde (1988a, 1991). Stern concludes that, if anything, the infant separates his environment from a wired-in sense of himself. This implies a degree of inner motivation toward separateness and autonomy. Emancipating from childhood attachments to greater independence is the crux of adolescent development. So, if Stern's model of an ego oriented, adapting-to-reality modus operandi during infancy continues as the paradigm for development in childhood and adolescence, then a revision of the idea that adolescent psychological development and emancipation are prompted by oedipal fantasies is warranted. To be sure, adolescents are capable of more fantasy than infants, but fantasies more likely complicate the emancipatory process rather than initiate it.

These findings from empirical infant research are very compatible with results from the Weiss, Sampson, and the Mount Zion Psychotherapy Research Group (1986) control mastery studies on the psychotherapeutic process in adults. Their finding that the patient has an unconscious plan to effect his own cure is consistent with a theory of strivings to complete development. Their conclusion of the traumatic basis for psychopathology, like the Offers' research on normal adolescents, suggests the importance of real experiences as opposed to inner-generated fantasies. And the degree to which Weiss and Sampson's patients' strivings for success were thwarted by a compulsive need to comply with the wishes of others, is consistent with the idea that a sponsoring relationship is important for healthy development. The control mastery research provides a strong basis for the thesis I am proposing.

Robert Langs' (1985) clinical research on the therapeutic process has pointed up that patients attempt to cure inappropriately functioning therapists. Patients do this by unconsciously perceiving and trying to gratify nontherapeutic wishes of their therapists. Langs reports that in most cases these patients are sacrificing their own best interests in favor of pleasing the therapist. Therapists are typically experienced by patients as embodying the attributes and attitudes of their parents during the patient's childhood or adulthood. Thus, it seems reasonable to infer that the patient–therapist interactions described by Langs involve the same dynamic that I have described in adolescents, for example, the young paranoid man (pp. 200–202) and Cyril (p. 4), who sacrificed their own forward movement by acting in ways which they thought, accurately or inaccurately, would please their parents. Thus, Langs' findings are consistent with the model of adolescent development I am advancing.

To clarify the distinctions I have been making between my thesis and traditional psychoanalytic theory and to demonstrate the utility of my view, I will describe a patient whose presentation was typical of this late adolescent/early adult group. His psychopathology appeared to conform to the traditional psychoanalytic formulation, namely someone whose unresolved oedipal attachments prevented him from moving into adult commitments in love and work. Other factors which are consistent with my thesis and neglected by the traditional view, proved to be even more important in the outcome. I will also illustrate vicissitudes of the transference in these individuals, as I did briefly with the young paranoid man.

> Nineteen-year-old Alan sought treatment for problems with motivation in school and pursing a career, and because he felt bedeviled after breaking up with his girl friend, Ginger. Apparently a truly gifted fine artist, he had exhausted the curriculum at a local junior college where he still languished; and he was unable to get himself to complete a portfolio as part of the application to some prestigious art institutes, where his professors were sure he would be accepted. With regard to his other problem, despite having instigated the split from Ginger, because he knew he was not ready for marriage, he found himself acting with her in such a way as to feel that she was leaving him. He would feel devastated, unable to do without her, and then make motions to perpetuate the very relationship he wished to terminate.
>
> During our second meeting, Alan claimed always to seek and follow the lead of others, be it parents or peers. Yet, he then reported having refused to return to the last therapist urged on him by his parents, after that therapist humiliated him by saying he was a con artist, not a fine artist. I called attention to the disparity between that independent action and his avowed submissiveness, and wondered if Alan acted less sure of himself than he truly felt. Alan brightened noticeably, and replied that his mind had been blank at the beginning of the session. He thought that he had lost his thoughts (become "blank") to see whether I would either humiliate him (i.e., repeat the trauma inflicted by his last therapist), or force him to work in his studio (an allusion

to pressure from his father). Alan then began to associate more freely.[6]

With the un-self-conscious candor and insightfulness which characterize many late adolescents, Alan plumbed a number of conflicts, emerging with valuable understanding. He recognized that as the youngest of three sons he had felt a strong urge to remain the last child of his parents and particularly the confidant of his mother. Alan recalled always having felt left out during the dinner table conversations between his father and older brothers. He tried slavishly both to be like his father and to feel like one of the men in the family. At the same time he seemed to cherish his role as his mother's best helper and friend, even if his turn toward that special relationship had been partly by default when he did not feel accepted by the other men of the family. Nor did Alan exhibit any of the adolescent's tendency to devalue or temper his idealized, childhood view of his parents. He remained impressed by his mother's beauty and charm. He acted awed by his father's intelligence, accomplishments, wit, and patrician manner—ever the admirer of this self-made, powerful corporate attorney, who clearly let it be known that he could only be emulated, never surpassed. His father's own first love had been painting, which he had been unable to pursue as a youth because he had to work.

His parents, despite being solid individuals, tended to be trendy, and had sent Alan to an avant-garde boarding school as he entered adolescence, in hopes of promoting his artistic abilities. It proved, if not a den of iniquity, more like a school for scoundrels than a crucible of creativity. For Alan was encouraged by staff and peers into delinquent activity, introduced to alcohol and drugs, and then to sex by a young woman teacher who remained his lover for the duration of his year there. The latter experience, shared with his family, was apparently a matter of avid interest to all, mixed with envy on the part of his brothers and father. Alan felt frightened living away from his family and the year was disastrous academically and artistically. So, he returned home for the next school year, where delinquent activity and truancy persisted for a while.

At the new school, Alan engaged in more typical dating behavior. Less typical was his tendency to regale his parents with

---

[6]I focus on this little early transference trial balloon to make the point that adolescents and young adults try to find out from the minute they meet the therapist whether he or she will repeat the attitudes of their parents. If the therapist does so, then the treatment will more likely either come a cropper or stalemate in a transference reenactment. It behooves therapists to be especially skeptical if late adolescents/young adults present themselves as submissive or stupid.

descriptions of his sexual experiences, purportedly to their delight. In relating this period of his life, he focused on one romance at age 15. When that girl broke up with him, Alan had acted so devastated that his schoolmates felt he was becoming nonfunctional. The significance of that recollection did not become evident until very late in treatment. Subsequently, Alan had many girl friends, imitating his father's gallant manner in his dealings with them, before finding some way for the girls to end the relationship. The breakup with Ginger, which had prompted him to enter treatment, was the first one which Alan had overtly initiated.

Preoccupation with girls had long been Alan's most frequent way of distracting himself from schoolwork, drawing, and sculpting. When asked about his difficulty preparing a portfolio, however, Alan shared a long-time fantasy about having one-man shows at prestigious art galleries. There would always be one man at the opening who knew a lot about art and could tell that Alan was a fraud. When I asked who that man was, Alan immediately replied, "My father—Oh, my...," and he became moist eyed.

Alan had moved from home into a studio loft apartment with Ginger during his nineteenth year. He described rushing back after classes to tell Ginger about them while they cleaned up the loft together. I asked if cleaning up the apartment brought anything to his mind. His mother's face popped immediately into mind, and he realized with a sense of surprise that he had transported more whole cloth of his close relationship with his mother and his idealized view of his parents' own relationship into his new apartment than he had ever consciously realized. The observation that he was trying to imitate his parents' life led to the question of who couldn't do without whom. Alan realized that the funks and depressions into which he would sink when feeling that he could not live without Ginger were defensive. For his underlying purpose in feeling this way was to ward off even greater concerns that it was really Ginger (and behind her his parents) who could not live without him. Thus, he felt both very influential over them and responsible for them.

Up to this point, except for this last finding of his concerns about influence over and responsibility for others, the case conforms to psychoanalytic dynamics. For Alan's movement from adolescence into mature love and work pursuits was experienced unconsciously as being too close to an incestuous, oedipal relationship, that is, cohabiting with his mother and displacing/dispatching his father. So, to avoid the anticipated punishment of castration by his father (suggested by his fantasy of the man at the gallery opening), Alan could not allow himself the career to which his father had aspired (painting). Furthermore, any girl friend was tainted by Alan's own incestuous yearnings; so, he must avoid serious involvements. In this formulation Alan's competitiveness toward his father is defended against by reaction formation, which intensified his normative negative oedipal love for father and emerged as his excessive admiration of his father. We would expect to uncover his hostile rivalry as treatment progressed.

The only factor which is harder to reconcile with traditional psychoanalytic theory is the constellation which Weiss, Sampson, and the Mt. Zion Psychotherapy Research Group (1986) have characterized as omnipotent responsibility—feeling great power to influence parents and feelings of responsibility for their welfare. But this, too, could prove to be a reversal of Alan's own dependency needs, either based on his unresolved oedipal conflict or on a strong preoedipal relationship. In this formulation, Alan's adolescent turmoil, drinking, delinquency, and premature sexual involvement, would be understood as efforts to deal with loneliness at the boarding school and acting out of his incestuous longings with the woman teacher.

On the other hand, if his fear of leaving Ginger and his parents were not primarily efforts to avoid awareness of his own dependence, then his difficulty in moving ahead in his life reflected some compelling need to satisfy what he perceived, accurately or not, to be the wishes of others at the expense of his own need to emancipate. The remainder of this presentation will be devoted to outlining what was ultimately revealed in this case. I will also elaborate on how these patients work with the transference.

> Because Alan's symptomatic improvement fluctuated, I thought that more intensive treatment would help to consolidate his gains. So, mindful of the problems potentially created by making such a recommendation to an adolescent after six months of therapy, at a moment when he was remarking about how much he had to say and how long it was between sessions, I asked Alan what he would think about meeting more often. He immediately responded that he "guessed" that would be a good idea. I remained casual, asking him only to think about it. At the following session he brought

up the matter, but wished to suggest an alternative. Rather than doing so, however, he produced a litany of associations about having been dragged by his family to treatment as a youngster, to dinners and art galleries and museums, and wanting to get away from these. He then described having recently stopped private lessons from the best art teacher he had ever had. He had done so because he felt too important to that teacher, who in fact had treated him very specially. She had offered to teach Alan without charge and invariably kept him longer than their contracted time. When I tried to draw this into the transference, Alan simply replied that he had always thought of himself as a fascinating patient and harbored similar thoughts that teachers and others admired him. He did not think that I felt that way toward him, and he gave no further consideration to that possibility.

He did report a dream at the next session which was something he had rarely done: In it he was interred in a concentration camp. He and his fellow prisoners attempt to escape during a battle at their compound. He feigned death, lying over a side horse, only to find himself soon being mounted from behind by a fellow prisoner. The latter was short, boyish-faced, and obviously homosexual. Alan had not been able to determine previously whether this fellow prisoner was friend or foe. Alan stopped the other's homosexual advance, and they feigned death together. Alan developed a fondness for his fellow prisoner as the two of them lay there. Then, when all the escaping prisoners were being rounded up by guards who had regained control, Alan decided to bolt. As he did so, he looked back to see that all the others, including the young man, had been machine-gunned to death. He escaped.

In reflecting on the dream, Alan made no reference to the matter of more frequent appointments or to me. Even after I raised a question about the short, youthful-faced man (an accurate description of myself at that time), Alan emphasized that the dream figure was a younger, boy prostitute type. But prior to the next session, he recalled having wondered when he first met me if I were gay. From here he began talking for the first time about his own concerns about homosexuality.

So, although at this juncture Alan resisted analyzing the transference, he nevertheless used it to introduce an important developmental conflict. In fact, as his treatment progressed, he frequently initiated exploration of the transference or of the extension to me of his current feelings about his parents, often by wondering the same thing about me that he was about one of them. The content of the dream contained elements which support both theories of adolescent development. The homosexual theme fits with the traditional analytic view, and the desire to escape, which leaves his friend dead, that is, emancipation or survivor guilt, fits better with the model I am advancing.

Now, one would think that I had learned my lesson about the readiness of these patients to feel trapped, but I had not. The first week that he was to begin more frequent sessions, Alan had to cancel an appointment. Contrary to my previous behavior on such occasions, and related to my eagerness to increase the frequency of sessions, I offered him an alternative time. This aroused his fears that he was becoming too important to me, as he had become to his art teacher, and he wanted to reduce the frequency of meetings. He associated to his father's wishes that Alan, his last son, stay and work together with him in the father's studio in their home. Ultimately Alan's associations revealed his fear that withdrawing from people over whom he had such influence would kill them. This was an emotional, spontaneous thought, accompanied by a reddened face but no other associations. He subsequently recalled fantasies, between ages 13 and 15, of being at the center of the universe and that everything occurred with specific reference to himself; it was as if "someone up there" was planning everything as a lesson for his own development. He felt embarrassed recalling those fantasies which now seemed too egocentric, but they brought together the developmental phenomenon of self-centeredness and his fantasy that his emancipation to psychological independence would kill others. Especially since death wishes toward his father had not been uncovered underneath this fear, Alan seemed to be struggling with emancipatory guilt rather than oedipal guilt.

Alan's improvement was now more sustained. After he had recognized (from his fantasy of the art critic who would identify him as a fraud) that it was his father's criticism of his artwork that he feared, Alan had prepared and sent off a portfolio to art schools. He had also experienced an instructive progression of girl friends by this time. It had begun with Ginger, who had been incestuously tainted in his mind and not someone with whom he shared ego interests. Starr was his next girl friend. Alan and Starr seemed enraptured by each other, and most of their interest seemed to be mutual admiration, idealization, and idolization. At times they literally sat and gazed upon each other's beauty. Alan observed that part of their mutual interest seemed to be seeing themselves in the other. By contrast, Alan and his current girl friend, Cindy, were intensely preoccupied with talking about their relationship, to such a degree that Alan realized he was really working on a relationship rather than truly involved in one. Thus, in these relationships, Alan had demonstrated the progression posited by psychoanalysis—the incestuously tainted relationship which motivates efforts to emancipate, the narcissistic relationship (though as noted [chapter 6], this has typically been described to occur with a member of one's own sex), and the heterosexual relationship characterized by a playing-at-love quality.

As treatment progressed, Alan began to perceive his parents' feet of clay. Idolizing his father had enabled him to avoid awareness that his father's rudeness disgusted him; and his own faddishness warded off awareness of his distaste for that tendency in his mother. He was becoming appropriately self-assertive with everyone.

Alan was elated when he went to his parents' home to share the news of his acceptance at the premier museum school in Paris. His father insisted that the three of them celebrate with a hot tub in the nude. Alan was very reluctant but acquiesced, and felt uncomfortable at what he experienced as his father's exhibitionistic display of his genitals and what he perceived as his mother's "narcissistic" excitement at the sight of Alan's body.

Such data, plus their voyeuristic interest in his sex life noted earlier, suggested that his parents' behaviors had reasonably led Alan to conclude that they had a real and competitive interest in his own sexuality, and this had influenced his early adolescent behaviors. This is consistent with psychoanalytic psychology which accepts the idea that real experiences tend to intensify normal developmental conflicts. But, as the material which follows will illustrate, there seemed to be more to Alan's difficulties than that.

As he anticipated terminating analysis to pursue his studies abroad, Alan's now frequent dreams stimulated memories of earlier traumatic experiences. These recollections linked together his early adolescent turmoil and his late adolescent impasse. Late in the treatment, on one such occasion, he recalled an experience from age 15. His parents, who had always been so devoted to one another, had separated for several months when Alan's father suspected his mother of having a brief affair with her yoga instructor. His father had reacted very dramatically, with teeth-gnashing upset and depression, to the point of having an older son take him to a Crisis Unit where he remained overnight. Alan now associated that experience directly to his own similar reaction when the high school girl friend forsook him for another boy.

Alan's own delinquent, school-cutting, self-defeating, tumultuous behaviors had reached their peak at that time. He recalled an evening (at age 15) when his overwrought father, feeling miserably cockolded, was enraged by Alan's depredations. In what was apparently at least in part a displacement of the source of his ire, he was furiously kicking Alan who cowered on the floor in the corner. During the beating, Alan was feeling badly that he himself was virile and his father was declining. During this period, Alan spent his days away from school at the home of a married woman who would mock the small size of his penis and condemn him for premature ejaculation. Alan now realized that he had been demonstrating to himself and the world that he represented no competitive threat to his father and was no better than his mother, if she had been involved extramaritally (which was never confirmed). Working through memories like this one was associated with a more definitive cure than our earlier focus on oedipal concerns had achieved. Thus, at base, Alan's trouble emancipating seemed more closely related to efforts to buoy up, support, and preserve his parents and his positive view of them by demeaning himself, rather than to integrating his own mature sexuality.

To recap, Alan appeared unable to move ahead because of an unresolved Oedipus complex which had been intensified by seductive behaviors on the part of his mother and overbearingness by an impressive and self-impressed father. Alan had brought up his attraction to mother and fear of father early and easily in treatment, however, suggesting that incestuous concerns were not the major source of disabling conflict. Furthermore, any competitive feelings toward his father seemed subordinate to his wishes that his father accept and make him feel like one of the men in the family. Alan's adolescent turmoil correlated more directly with a period of breakdown in family functioning than with incestuous conflicts.

In my experience then, psychoanalytic theory accurately describes a number of phenomena observed in adolescents. Moreover, there are some youngsters whose emancipatory efforts seem to be initiated by puberty and some youth for whom oedipal conflicts can create developmental problems; that is, there are some whose course may be accurately explained by psychoanalytic theory. A much greater number appear, like Alan, to be stumbling on incestuous conflicts but prove to be primarily struggling with different issues; and there are some for whom oedipal matters do not seem to be at issue during adolescence. Existing psychoanalytic theory is not sufficiently encompassing to explain either the degree of variations exhibited by adolescents or the most basic dynamics of much adolescent psychopathology.

The perspective on adolescent development I am advancing is directly opposed to an important tenet of the traditional psychoanalytic view. In the traditional theory regressive urges must be overridden by self-protective and progressive necessities. By contrast I am positing that development occurs through progressive urges which can be impeded by regressive reactions that are perceived by the adolescent as necessary to appease his or her parents.

The view I am espousing provides a framework for understanding both those whose course through adolescence seems to conform to the traditional view, and the much larger majority of adolescents whose course does not follow that model. The revision accomplishes this by integrating more accurately the role of real experiences in the developmental process. Emancipatory guilt, which is implicit in the conflict between preserving the parental relationship, needing sponsorship, and strivings to complete development, is more crucial in this process than oedipal guilt. These features of development transcend stage progression, so the paradigm for adolescent development I have presented is not a stage theory.

Part III

Deviations from the Normal Developmental Process: Their Evaluation and Treatment

CHAPTER 8

Developmental Psychopathology

THE DEVELOPMENTAL BASES OF PSYCHOPATHOLOGY IN ADOLESCENCE[1]

Although adolescents are moving away from their parents psychologically, they carry over from childhood the idea that their sense of security depends upon pleasing their parents. Thus, the relationship with their parents remains more psychologically important than their outward behaviors often suggest. In fact, this is the period when conflict is most likely to arise between the adolescent's normal urge to complete development and the wish to maintain ties to his or her parents. If the adolescent has an underlying sense that the relationship is stable, and that the parents are strong and sponsor his or her progress, then pathological reactions are less likely to occur when disputes arise.

Adolescents tend to blame themselves for problems with their parents (Freud, 1930, 1940; Beres, 1958). They also tend both to feel responsible for maintaining the relationship with their parents and to feel that they have great power to influence them. The latter ideas have been referred to as concerns about

---

[1]Conditions that do not begin during adolescence, such as learning disorders, Attention Deficit Hyperactivity Disorder, and certain anxiety disorders will not be discussed here.

225

omnipotence by Weiss, Sampson, and the Mt. Zion Psychotherapy Group (1986); they delineated this constellation in empirical research which demonstrates the centrality of pathogenic beliefs in the genesis of psychopathology in adults. Adolescents typically ward off conscious awareness of self-blame by acting blameless or by blaming their parents. This need to reduce their guilt by reversal and externalization is one major reason why adolescents so often have difficulty acknowledging their own contribution to conflicts with their parents.

Adolescents tend to resolve this prototypic developmental conflict in two paradigmatic ways: by complying with parents or by behaving like their parents (defensive identifications). Compliance amounts to adopting behaviors that they think will please their parents at the expense of their forward movement. Such compliance is much more prevalent in the lives of adolescents than we are accustomed to considering it. For example, the young paranoid man described in the last chapter tried to please his parents by behaving in ways that enabled them to righteously condemn him as the black sheep of their family.

ACTING BADLY TO PROTECT THE PARENTS' SENSE OF MORAL SUPERIORITY

In a frequent variation of this paradigm, behavior that appears bad, rebellious against parental wishes or aimed at hurting them, proves on closer examination to be a compliance with what the adolescent accurately or inaccurately has perceived will please the parent or parents:

> A 16-year-old girl's parents suspected their daughter of sexual involvements with her male friends. Their suspicions were unfounded. The girl was not sexually active, but her parents continued to accuse and criticize her rather than trust her assurances. The girl eventually concluded, albeit unconsciously, that what pleased her parents most was to be able to put her down and feel morally superior to her. Without being consciously aware of her motive for doing so, the girl became sexually active in circumstances that her parents were able to substantiate. Thus, they could feel smug in castigating their daughter for sexual activity. The adolescent herself experienced little pleasure from the sex.

So, her seeming defiance of her parents was more accurately understood as an accession to what she had concluded truly gratified them, namely being able to righteously condemn her.

BECOMING TROUBLED TO BE LIKE ONE'S PARENTS

The other paradigmatic way that adolescents resolve the conflict is by adopting behaviors equivalent to those of parents whom they perceive to be troubled. I refer to these as defensive identifications. Alan, whose case was discussed in the previous chapter, was devastated and overwhelmed after his high school sweetheart dropped him for another boy at a time when his father was feeling miserably cuckolded. During that same period Alan would skip school to visit a married woman who mocked his sexual performance. Engaging in that adulterous relationship also enabled Alan to avoid feeling disdainful of his mother whom he thought was having an affair. Alan's basic motivation in both these defensive identifications was to preserve his own sense of security by dispelling any sense that he was stronger than, superior to, or critical of his parents.

THE PROMINENCE OF DEFENSIVE IDENTIFICATIONS IN PSYCHOPATHOLOGY

Identifications are basically imitative phenomena. They contribute to progressive development (chapter 6); however, they can also contribute to symptom formation. Defensive identifications can look to all intents and purposes like healthy identifications based on love and admiration. In fact, defensive identifications are often more obvious to an observer. Because they are maladaptive and thus are labored efforts to deal with anxiety, defensive identifications may appear more like carbon copies of the parent than do identifications based on admiration or love of the parent. The latter are usually more subtle and often not as evident to either parents or adolescent until the latter returns as a young adult. The parents and their young adult child then find to their mutual satisfaction that they share more in common than either had thought possible during the progeny's adolescent years (Anthony, 1970).

While there are probably inherited contributants to some characteristics, these shared traits and attitudes represent carryovers from
childhood and adolescence of those features of the parents which
contributed to the child's sense of security.

In the development of psychopathology defensive identifications are adopted in order to avoid worrying about one's par-
ent(s). Worry is most often prompted by the adolescent's
perception of weakness or instability in the parent or parents.[2] In
identifying with the weak parent, it is as if the adolescent is feeling
"I am not stronger than my parent. I am as weak or weaker than
my parent." Defensive identifications are also used to deal with
parental hostility toward the adolescent. In such instances of identifying with the aggressor (which is also a defensive identification), it is as if the adolescent is feeling, "My parent is not
absurdly hostile toward me, I'm the same as my parent," or in
other situations, "I'm not afraid of my parent, I'm just like him
or her."

As I explained in chapter 1 (pp. 12–16), developmental conflicts in which the adolescent is more concerned about preserving a parent he or she fears will be destroyed rather than
escaping from a parent the adolescent fears will destroy him or
her, involve emancipatory guilt rather than oedipal guilt.[3] When

---

[2]Parental instability may not be manifested as overt weakness; it may be
exhibited in cruel, overbearing, or inequitable behavior toward the adolescent.
For example, a child who is beaten capriciously by a parent for minor infrac-
tions certainly becomes fearful *of* that parent. He may also become fearful *for*
that parent, however; for the child concludes that the parent is unstable when
he observes the profound influence his own behavior can have on the parent
(Bloch, 1989). In my experience this latter fear *for* the parent invariably proves
more important than the adolescent's fear *of* the parent in impeding development and precipitating the psychopathological reactions that evolve from such
situations. Thus, preserving the parent's equanimity becomes a primary motive
in the adolescent's psychological makeup, and typically he or she has great
difficulty moving toward normal emancipation when there are questions about
the parent's psychological stability.

[3]As explicated in chapters 1 and 3, my clinical observation is that development is more accurately depicted when the castration complex and the Oedipus complex are understood as unrelated phenomena which, while they
function independently for the most part, can be brought together in certain
cirumstances. The former is related to observations of genital differences; it is
associated in development with ideas of "having" and "not having" and reflected in castration anxiety and penis envy which are common issues in devel-

emancipatory guilt assumes pathological proportions in adolescents, it is experienced like survivor or separation guilt.

EMANCIPATORY AND SURVIVOR/SEPARATION GUILT COMPARED TO OEDIPAL GUILT

Survivor and separation guilt (Modell, 1965, 1971; Niederland, 1981) are experiences of unconscious guilt which arise when an individual believes that he has survived or succeeded at the expense of another, usually a family member. He feels that he has prevailed either because he wanted a life of his own or more than his fair share (separation guilt). Such individuals believe that separation from their parent will kill the parent (Modell, 1965). Or, in the absence of any desire to supersede or survive another person, fate has given the survivor some advantage over the loser/victim (survivor guilt). The college student who was unable to study experienced survivor guilt associated with the idea of progressing when his retarded sister could not (footnote, pp. 163–164). I consider separation guilt and survivor guilt to be basically the same phenomenon, namely, unconscious or conscious guilt experienced when one feels one's success harms or is at the expense of another.

COMPARISON OF THIS THESIS WITH TRADITIONAL PSYCHOANALYTIC THEORY

Oedipal guilt, the hallmark of classical psychoanalysis, arises from a desire to supersede a parent toward whom one feels rivalrous. As such I consider it a subspecies of the more encompassing concept of survivor–separation guilt. For the

---

opment and readily observed in children. The Oedipus complex by contrast is normally a weak theme in development. It comes to prominence and becomes associated with castration anxiety only when the parenting is problematic in certain ways. This disjunction of castration anxiety and the Oedipus complex turns the primary focus in development from vicissitudes of incestuous conflicts to the more basic forerunner of the love relationship. That is what Freud (1912) termed the "affectionate current" of love which he identified as older than the "sensual current" and based on the "self-preservative instinct" and "directed to the members of the family and those who look after the child" (p. 180).

survivor–separation guilt continuum covers the special case of a person who feels competitive toward the other person. Oedipal guilt does not, however, account for the experience of an individual who feels guilty about surpassing another toward whom he does not feel rivalrous/competitive. Survivor–separation guilt is much more common than oedipal guilt in the development of psychopathology. This is logical since the Oedipus complex includes love as well as murderous wishes toward the same-sexed parent. In other words, it is more common for an adolescent to feel guilty about a wish to surpass a parent he or she loves and needs than to feel compunction about wishes to surpass a parent who is primarily hated. I find that distinguishing between such conflicts (or emancipatory guilt in the case of adolescent development) and oedipal conflicts is essential for understanding psychopathology which develops in adolescents. In my view the adolescent's desire to emancipate is a natural, inborn one. If the adolescent feels secure in the relationship with his or her parents, instinctual conflicts will be managed adaptively, and development will progress normally. So, adaptation to the environment (parents) in order to maintain the relationship is more basic to the developmental process of adolescent emancipation than defending against drive derivatives as posited by classical psychoanalytic theory.

Psychoanalytic theory does not neglect adaptation. It is one of six metapsychological (theoretical) viewpoints utilized to understand psychological phenomena. But in psychoanalytic theory adolescent development centers on resolving the Oedipus complex. While acknowledging that drives certainly play a role in adolescent development, I find that psychoanalysis has overemphasized the role of incest conflicts in the emancipatory process. For as the case of Alan illustrated (see chapter 7), even when oedipal conflicts complicate an adolescent's development, the concerns I have described are invariably present and a more important source of abortive development.

The prototypic developmental conflict in my thesis involves ego-oriented motives which have become irreconcilable with one another. Thus, in psychoanalytic terms it is an *intra*systemic conflict. It is nevertheless an intrapsychic as opposed to an interpersonal problem because the basic conflict is between the adolescent's strivings to complete development and his perception of his parents' reaction to those urges. By contrast, the core developmental conflict of adolescence traditionally described by psychoanalysis is also intrapsychic but is an *inter*systemic conflict between id urges and ego/superego controls.

Freud emphasized, and most psychoanalysts have continued to assume, that hormonal changes during puberty cause a resurgence of oedipal yearnings. Castration anxiety generated by these desires motivates the adolescent to move psychologically away from his or her childhood dependency on the parents. Thus, defense against unconscious incestuous and parricidal urges is the primary impetus for psychological maturation. The adolescent's love for the parent toward whom he or she also feels rivalrous is a secondary motive for emancipating. An adolescent who cannot successfully repress his or her desire for incestuous gratification, that is, one who finds oedipal yearnings too compelling, cannot advance developmentally. In psychoanalytic theory the adolescent experiences more necessity to emancipate (for self-preservation) than desire to do so. In my view adolescents experience a strong wish to resolve their developmental conflicts in order to emancipate. The process becomes impeded when the adolescent perceives that becoming independent is either not acceptable to parents or will somehow harm them or the adolescent's relationship with them.

CLINICAL ILLUSTRATIONS

The cases in this chapter will be presented succinctly in order to portray as clearly as possible the differences between my formulations and those of other theorists. My purpose is to illustrate rather than to "prove" my thesis. The subsequent chapter on treatment includes more extensive case descriptions. Here I will emphasize the dynamics that seemed most important in symptom formation as judged by the adolescents' own acknowledgment or by their responses in treatment. Contrary to the view of many therapists, I find that there are single, primary issues on which many cases turn.

DEPRESSIVE REACTIONS IN ADOLESCENCE

JEFF: DEPRESSION

A highly functioning, 17-year-old scholar-athlete was referred when he found himself unable to concentrate at school or study. He felt bad—pessimistic, self-doubting, discouraged, tense, and functionally immobilized. He had lost interest in his active life and felt alienated from but more dependent on his girl friend. He had begun to develop trouble with his tennis game. He lost his appetite and had trouble falling asleep. He couldn't understand what was the matter with him.

He was the only child in what had always been a tightly knit, well-functioning family. His father was a brilliant trial attorney who was anticipating appointment to a high-level judgeship. Jeff's mother was a homemaker who, along with their son, admired and loved the boy's father. In addition she considered Jeff to be her best friend and confidant. The lad's development prior to the onset of these symptoms was remarkable for its freedom from disturbance; he had breezed through everything in his life.

Several weeks before the onset of Jeff's symptoms, his father, who had always been self-assured and confident, became unsettled, unsure of himself, unhappy, and he announced that he wished to separate from his wife. This surprised the father as well as his wife and son, because there had been no prior indication of disharmony in the family. Jeff's father had suddenly found himself fascinated by a fellow attorney in the office building where he worked, and although they had talked, he was not involved with her. His father was perplexed but neither depressed nor psychotic. For once in his adult life, Jeff's father did not know what he wanted to do. In this setting the lad's puzzled, heartsick, and then outraged mother began to confide even more in Jeff and act in a dependent fashion. Jeff empathized with each parent and was himself unhappy about the situation, though unaware of feeling undone by it. Within a matter of weeks, however, he developed increasingly incapacitating symptoms of indecision, immobilization in schoolwork and tennis, dependency, and depression.

After a couple of sessions, the therapist observed to Jeff the similarity between his own behaviors and his father's symptoms. Jeff was struck by the parallel and wondered why he hadn't perceived that connection himself. He then realized that he was also acting toward his girl friend in the same helpless, hapless manner that his mother was evincing toward him. The therapist asked Jeff how he would feel if he were to continue along in his life as he had been, unscathed and successful, when both of his parents were severely troubled. Jeff's response indicated that he would feel misery and guilt, though he didn't know why. At the same time, he was aware of a wish not to be bothered by their problems.

Thus, Jeff was exhibiting a defensive identification with each parent, both of whom he felt were foundering. The therapist interpreted Jeff's adoption of behavior patterns equivalent to those of each parent as his effort to make his parents seem stronger by appearing worse off than them. His primary motive was to relieve emancipatory guilt associated with wishes to move ahead in his life while his parents seemed to be failing in theirs. As the pervasiveness of this pattern of dealing with these concerns was demonstrated and understood by Jeff, he overcame his depression. He still felt dragged down, however, and a bit disgusted by his mother's continuing unhappiness and the unsettled state of his parents' lives. He concluded that he would be better off away from home. So, he decided to transfer the following academic year to a boarding school that was academically superior and had a better program for a ranked junior tennis player than did the local prep school he had been attending.

At first glance Jeff's solution to leave home might seem like an identification with the way his father had dealt with confusion and uncertainty; however, it was not. For in contrast to his father's departure, Jeff's action was an age-appropriate, carefully thought-out and executed plan, made after his symptoms had reversed; and it represented an alternative which enhanced his options for personal growth and advancement.

A year later Jeff was asymptomatic and relating well to his parents who had separated. Jeff observed spontaneously that he was still maintaining some emotional distance from both parents for self-protective reasons; however, he anticipated returning to a closer relationship with each of them a few years hence. He was enjoying the boarding school, where he had made friends, and his academic and athletic performance were again in top form.

From the standpoint of current approaches to diagnosis and treatment, Jeff's case would be considered a depressive reaction by psychoanalytically oriented therapists. The dynamics do not, however, conform to the psychoanalytic formulation of depression which emphasizes turning aggression against the self. Rather, Jeff's depression was based on a defensive identification with the maladaptive behaviors of both of his parents which he had adopted to buoy them up, not because of hostility toward them.

Biological psychiatrists and other clinicians who base diagnoses exclusively on symptoms would give Jeff an Axis I diagnosis of Major Depression, Single Episode, on the basis of DSM-III-R criteria (APA, 1987). Currently such a diagnosis can justify treatment with antidepressant medication. Based on the outcome of the psychotherapy, medication would be neither advisable nor necessary in such a case. Moreover, prescribing medication might have communicated to Jeff that cure must come from outside his control rather than through ego-strengthening insight. I am not suggesting that medication never be used in adolescents. Rather, as I will demonstrate later, the decision to utilize medication in adolescents should usually involve consideration of more factors than a symptom diagnosis.

Jeff's case also illustrates that a relatively healthy person, facing serious emotional conflicts which have been precipitated traumatically, can develop severe symptoms and reverse them with therapy more quickly than their severity might have suggested possible. This is because the severity of symptoms correlates more directly with the intensity of the developmental conflicts whenever they arise, rather than with the age of the sufferer when the symptoms commence.

LISA: DEPRESSION AND ALCOHOL USE

For a year prior to her menarche at $12^1/_2$, Lisa had been getting drunk impulsively. Psychiatric referral followed a suicidal gesture. Her parents had divorced when she was 3 and Lisa had always lived part of every week with each parent. Her mother, a recovered alcoholic who still found herself tempted to drink, had expressed to Lisa the difficulty she experienced in remaining abstinent. Her mother also let Lisa know how much she valued her daughter's company as an antidote for her loneliness. Lisa's father tended to be somewhat strict with her. Since becoming very involved with a girl friend during the prior year, however, Lisa had sensed that he experienced her as a burden from which he would prefer to be free. It seemed that whenever her father began to feel this way, he became overcontrolling and overinvolved with Lisa, as if to disabuse himself of any idea that he preferred to be with his girl friend. Despite their individual difficulties and interests, Lisa's parents were taking care of her.

Lisa candidly shared those perceptions of her parents with the psychiatrist. She worried about her mother's lack of the companionship she craved. Lisa wanted to remain close but felt guilty when she preferred to be with friends. She also felt guilty about being a burden to her father. She expressed keen interest in forming a relationship with a young uncle who had recently moved to the area and who had shown some interest in her. His interest waxed and waned, however, and he himself had problems with drug use. So, his suitability as an influence on Lisa's development was by no means clear.

Lisa continued to drink impulsively, usually in circumstances which evoked her parents' attention. Exploration of the meaning of her drinking revealed that she was attempting to buoy up her mother, about whose stability she worried, by appearing more "alcoholic" than her mother. At the same time, drinking, which had been her father's reason for seeking the divorce, would give him justification for withdrawing from Lisa, which she sensed he wished to do beneath his overconcern.

The therapist interpreted Lisa's intense wishes to ally herself with her uncle as a normal way that many adolescents use to become more independent from their parents while not having to feel alone without parental-type support in the process. The therapist added, however, that he wondered if the intensity of her wish to become closer to her uncle carried an additional meaning. Namely, Lisa did not want to appear more independent than her mother, so she was trying to appear very needful of a man. In other words Lisa felt guilty or otherwise uncomfortable if she considered herself stronger than her parents. In this case stronger meant more independent, neither desperately yearning like her mother nor dependent like the way her father was acting toward his new girl friend. Lisa seemed to grasp all this immediately and the pressure she had felt to involve herself with her uncle diminished. Lisa became more behaviorally settled, her school performance improved, her peer relationships became less conflictual, she seemed happier, and her impulsive drinking abated.

Although the problems Lisa experienced with each parent were chronic and preexisting, the obligatory need to emancipate in adolescence activated emancipatory guilt that predisposed her to maladaptive efforts to support her parents. Thus, the same mechanisms adopted in an acute situation by Jeff were used by Lisa in a setting of chronic, problematic family relationships. Lisa and Jeff also illustrate that adolescents can gain and use insight very readily; this self-righting tendency is consistent with the existence of underlying urges to complete one's development normally.

The other points I want to stress are that in each case the adolescent's real experiences, current and past, seemed to be the most significant determinant of the pathological reactions. The other theories of adolescent development would formulate these cases differently. For example, a more traditional psychoanalytic formulation would interpret Lisa's efforts to establish a relationship with her uncle as multiply determined. Those determinants would include an effort to defend against her fear of regression to dependency on her mother which Deutsch (1944) considered to be the primary concern in early pubertal girls. At the same time, choosing an uncle as her new love object afforded Lisa neurotic gratification of her oedipal desire while simultaneously avoiding awareness of it by recourse to the defense mechanism of displacement. Lisa's drinking would be understood as a regressive, oral incorporative means of dealing with unfulfilled nurturant wishes from childhood. At the adolescent level, the drinking would represent a compromise formation which allowed Lisa both to defend against the regressive pull to dependency on mother by identifying with mother, while simultaneously gratifying the oral urge. Furthermore, by arrogating an adult prerogative, drinking, she was attempting to establish her independence from parental control as an emancipating adolescent. She was stuck developmentally, however, and not really emancipating because the neurotic, regressive oedipal and preoedipal (drinking) gratifications were too great.

These regressive, incestuous conflicts may have played a role in Lisa's psychopathology. The problem with that formulation is that Lisa was consciously aware of her unfulfilled wishes for more nurturant attention from earlier in her life. Moreover, she was readily aware of anger associated with these unfulfilled longings. Lisa did not experience any pleasure from drinking; nor did she feel any urgent desire to emancipate. So, those insights were not helpful in reversing her symptoms.

With respect to the Piagetian and self psychology formulations of the adolescent process, while Lisa was both perceptive and forthright with her therapist, she presented little evidence at $12^1/2$ of thinking about her thoughts (i.e., abstract thinking). While she could express disillusionment with each parent, the new "ideal" (uncle) she had chosen seemed basically more like than different from her mother and father. He was a substance abuser and tended to be overbearing like her father and to disconnect from relating like her mother. Thus, the self psychology and Piagetian formulations do not seem apt in this case.

In current diagnostic terminology from outside the medical–psychiatric model, Lisa's case would be diagnosed as Child of an Alcoholic or a Codependent. To underscore the relevance of developmental thinking to this group, I will present other issues which arise in such cases:

STEVE: DEPRESSION WITH SCHOOL PROBLEMS

Sixteen-year-old Steve had become frustrated, frightened, and depressed as he found himself unable to concentrate and study for his midterm exams. He was unhappy, emotional, and immobilized. When his mother called to make the appointment, she noted that Steve was currently very contentious with his father. Although Steve had always achieved excellent grades, he reproached his father for not helping him more with his studies. He also felt alienated from his friends whom he considered immature and self-centered.

Steve claimed that his father always had to be right and that he discounted Steve's complaints. His mother was quiet and reserved. He felt his teachers were neither helpful nor truly interested; he had no other explanation for his inability to study or for his chronic feeling that he was not learning as much as he could or wished. After expressing these frustrations to the therapist for a few weeks his mood lightened, he was able to study better, and in fact performed well, as he always had, on his semester exams. The therapist thought that the improvement occurred because Steve had not been criticized for his complaints about others. That is, the therapist suspected that Steve felt guilty about criticizing his parents and teachers and was relieved to a degree when the therapist did not defend the objects of Steve's dissatisfaction; doing so would have made Steve feel more guilty.

Steve subsequently revealed that his father was a recovered alcoholic, adding balefully that he guessed he was one, too, even though he had never drunk. For he had read that it is a genetically transmitted, familial disease. He became tearful when describing what little he could recall of his father's irritability when drinking. He remembered his parents arguing and neither of them being available to his younger sister and himself during those years. Steve recalled that his father refused to find any fault with his own attitudes and behaviors or to acknowledge his lack of help and attention to Steve during that period.

In reflecting on what he had described, Steve realized that those experiences with his parents formed the basis of his present-day expectations that teachers did not want to help him and that people would become angry toward him. He also realized spontaneously that those earlier experiences with his parents had held him back from feeling as close to friends as he would like. For he tended to be suspicious and to expect that friends would prove to be self-absorbed rather than interested in him.

Steve wanted his father to talk to him about that period, but knew his father would only become defensive and ignore any such request. The therapist encouraged Steve to explore his motives for wanting such discussions with his father. Beneath his wish that his father acknowledge the difficulty his drinking had caused his children, Steve proved to be looking for reassurance that he had not been responsible for his father's condition. His own inability to get started and accomplish anything turned out to be what his father used to complain about when his effectiveness had been compromised by drinking. His father had stopped drinking a couple of years earlier and Steve's presenting problems had been gradually increasing since that time. Steve harbored a superstitious fantasy that if he continued to have difficulty, then his father would not revert to drinking.

This case illustrates several points:

1. The feeling of responsibility that children unconsciously assume for their parents' problems contributes directly to the development of behaviors or attitudes in the adolescents that either duplicate or are equivalent to the parents' maladaptive behaviors.
2. The expectations developed from experiences with their parent or parents, in this case of not being attended to by adults, become transferred to other adults and peers.
3. In addition to those direct transferences, defensive identification with the parent's maladaptive style occurs. In this case it was part of Steve's effort to relieve guilt associated with his feelings of responsibility for his father's drinking.
4. The adolescent's problems sometimes commence after the foundering parent begins to recover or has recovered, and at

a time when the adolescent is in a position to succeed. This occurs because it is safer to reexperience the trauma in an effort to master it when there is less objective reason to worry about the parent. The adolescent attempts to master the trauma by repeating it in reverse, that is, turning passive into active. He actively perpetrates an equivalent of the parent's prior maladaptive behavior toward the parent and others (Weiss, Sampson, and the Mt. Zion Psychotherapy Research Group, 1986).

VIVIENNE: SUICIDE

Completed suicides are difficult to study. Based on a posthumous study of the letters, diary entries, and other writings of an intellectually gifted, emotionally precocious, and sensitive girl of 14 years, 4 months, who hanged herself, Mack and Hickler (1981) have presented a multifactorial analysis of suicide which they term an architectural model (Mack, 1986). Passages from the girl's writings, reported by those authors, point toward the type of dynamics I have been describing. Mack and Hickler report that Vivienne's father was a liberal, Universalist minister in a conservative, Roman Catholic neighborhood. He was being "criticized" in the community, losing his ministry and the family was moving at the time when the youngest of their three children suicided. The authors concluded that there was a "poor fit" between this family and the community. Vivienne's mother dressed Vivienne in clothes such as handmade smocks which were ridiculed by her classmates. After several difficult years in public school, at age 11 Vivienne transferred to the sixth grade at a private school where a male teacher took great interest in her. In the author's view, this teacher "brought her a great deal of caring, warmth, and support" (p. 34). Mack emphasizes the devastating impact of that man's departure as a precipitant for her suicide. A number of Vivienne's letter and diary entries related to that teacher. For example, when she was 12 years, 3 months, she wrote: "I wish Mr. May wouldn't go next year. And I wish Dad and Mummy wouldn't keep reminding me that he is" (p. 34).

It appears that Vivienne perceived her parents to be "rubbing in" the fact of her teacher's departure. In my clinical experience children often do not perceive such parental admonitions as efforts to help them master a disappointment by anticipating it (i.e., "forewarned is forearmed"). Rather, children experience such persistent, repeated reminders as an indication that their parents either want or need their child to feel unhappy.

After Mr. May's departure Vivienne wrote to herself:

> I am worthless, I am of no use to anyone, and no one is of any use to me. What good to kill myself? How can you kill nothing? A person who has committed suicide has had at least something to end. He must know joy to know misery. I have known nothing. Why live? Why die? One is an equal choice to the other. What do I do? I wonder if love would change anything. I don't know anymore. To know that the future looks worse doesn't help me any. I need people and there aren't any who care. It takes tolerance not to give in to death [p. 63].

She wrote to the teacher ten days before her death describing suicide attempts, but he did not receive it in time to alert her family.

Mack and Hickler consider many factors in their architectural model of suicide. From the dynamic standpoint, they ultimately focus on the significance to Vivienne of losing the teacher. They conclude that the teacher served a selfobject function for a girl with a strong identity and sense of self but who had disturbances of self-esteem and could not tolerate disappointments. The formulation I am elaborating may help explicate this paradox—a person with strong identity and sense of self who experiences disturbances of self-esteem and inability to tolerate disappointments: Mack and Hickler note that Vivienne often wrote that she felt under great emotional pressure from her parents, especially her mother, who turned to Vivienne with her (mother's) problems. Several months before her death Vivienne wrote:

> Mommy came to me for help. And I really have helped her whenever I could. But it puts a certain pressure on me; I'm not even fourteen yet, and Mommy's forty-eight. All the pressure and tension mounted up and I snapped. I decided that I couldn't be as

perfect as I wanted and I had to have some outlet. I've been smoking grass since around January. I've gotten stoned often enough, but I never really enjoyed it. Usually I just get high enough to relax [p. 83].

With that quotation in mind, Mack writes: "The psychodynamics of depression and suicide need to be evaluated, especially conflicts relating to self-esteem, which are demonstrated when the teenager focuses upon injuries to self-regard and expresses feelings of low self-worth. We are learning to recognize a personality organization that may contribute to low self-regard . . . overly hard superego elements, unrealistically exalted idealization, or ego ideal expectations, and evidence of an unusual degree of sensitivity to hurt and disappointment" (p. 72).

In fact, in the last quotation when Vivienne talks about helping her mother, it seems to be the mother's self-esteem that Vivienne felt was problematic rather than her own. I often find in such cases that the adolescent experiences guilt about feeling superior to the parent, and invariably does something to take him- or herself down. In this instance, Vivienne condemned herself, rather than her mother, for not being perfect and acted as if she needed to use drugs to relax. It was as if Vivienne were saying that she like her mother was not able to handle the problems of her life without turning to someone or something else. So, the overly hard superego elements and unrealistic expectations of oneself are self-punishing attitudes. They reflected the adolescent's effort to deal with emancipatory or separation–survivor guilt which resulted from feeling stronger and better able to cope than her mother.

Mack goes on to observe that, "Family dynamics which would disturb the teenager's psychic balance need to be assessed, such as, in Vivienne's case, the burdening of the child with problems that the parents are facing. It is important to assess whether parents are living out psychological needs of their own in relation to the teenager and failing, thereby, to see the child's distress" (p. 72). Mack may be hinting at the kind of dynamic I am advancing. His focus seems to be, however, that the parent–child relationship is problematic because the parents' preoccupation with their own problems prevents them from noticing their child's distress.

Vivienne's words in the last quotation and in the following letter written to her teacher three weeks before she suicided are consistent with the dynamic I have presented:

> We are having counseling for the family. *I know that I am probably the most destructive factor, but it's a little late for me to say that.* Once you said you were glad I was born. Now I have my doubts about the whole thing. *If I didn't have to worry about Mommy and Daddy, I wouldn't bother finishing this letter before I hung myself. But I have to stick with them. Sort of one burden holding up another, which isn't too stable a thing to begin with.* For one thing, I haven't got a single friend nearby. As a matter of fact, I have only one friend to speak of at all, and she lives in Belmont. With the gas shortage I see her solely at school [p. 111; emphasis added].

If one had had the opportunity to explore Vivienne's inner life with her from the vantage point presented in this book, as the last two quotations suggest, Vivienne would have acknowledged extraordinary feelings of responsibility for the welfare of her family. She felt stronger than her parents. It was they, not Vivienne, who had apparently become friendless in their community and whose situation was objectively dire. We would have found Vivienne held back from progressing in her life by survivor guilt concerns about being stronger than the parents. And the basis of her suicidal urges would have emerged in the conflict between needing to find a way to shore up her parents who were being ostracized and foundering on the one hand, and Vivienne's wishes to succeed in her life on the other. Vivienne made herself appear the friendless, ostracized, and despairing one to make her parents seem less troubled than she was herself.

PSYCHOPATHOLOGY RELATING TO CHOICE OF PARTNER (OBJECT CHOICE) AND SEXUALITY

In chapter 6 I described the normal practice of experimenting with different partners for fit in adolescents' object choices. But whenever an adolescent becomes involved in a relationship in which his or her strivings to complete development are thwarted, or in which he or she is psychologically hurt in other ways, almost invariably one finds two related factors involved. These factors are the appeal of the familiar and efforts to master earlier traumata involving parents. In my experience these are much more prevalent sources of aberrant choices of partner than are attempts to gratify or avoid awareness of oedipal yearnings.

THE APPEAL OF THE FAMILIAR

Adolescents who have had problematic parenting often tend to migrate to partners whose behaviors/attitudes resemble those of their parents. They do not do so because the parents' traits were appealing; rather, they do so because such individuals represent "known" entities to the adolescents. They know what to expect and how to respond to maintain a relationship with such individuals even if that relationship is not satisfying or desirable. For relating to such individuals is less anxiety engendering to the adolescent than are relationships with individuals who may be more suitable but whose modus operandi is unfamiliar. For the adolescent cannot sufficiently trust that the suitable partner is truly the way he or she appears to be. The adolescent always fears and expects that ultimately the more suitable partner will turn out to be like the trauma-engendering parent. This distrust is bred from the adolescent's earlier experiences with the trauma-inducing parent and by his or her feeling of responsibility for the maladaptive relationship with the parents which makes the adolescent undeserving of better treatment (Bloch, 1989). So, bad as it is to be involved with people similar to problematic parents, involvements with suitable individuals who hold out the hope of treating the adolescent in the proper way he or she truly prefers, can be experienced as even more anxiety engendering. The tenacity of these attitudes in adolescents who make inappropriate object choices is related to the second factor:

EFFORTS TO MASTER PRIOR TRAUMATIC EXPERIENCES DURING DEVELOPMENT

The other reason that adolescents choose problematic new partners involves the fact that people are driven to master traumatic aspects of their earlier relationships with parents. They attempt to do so by repeating prior, traumatic relationships with parent(s). The traumatizing relationship with a parent can be reenacted directly in the form of a conventional transference-type reaction to the new individual. Or, it can be reenacted in reverse, using defensive identifications in the mechanism known as turning passive into active. In the latter paradigm the adolescent exhibits the troublesome behavior of the parent toward the new partner. The importance of the latter mechanism in the process of therapy has been identified and explicated by Weiss, Sampson, et al. (1986).

The following examples illustrate the choice of unsuitable partners and friends by the adolescent on the bases just described:

An 18-year-old college freshman was in psychotherapy because of a tendency to blush, become panicky, and develop urinary urgency in social situations. She came to a session one day and announced that she hated all males. She had broken off with her boyfriend of two months because he was so passive. Now that her original symptoms were resolving and she was able to assert herself with greater equanimity, she didn't think it was fair that she always had to take the initiative in their relationship, especially since even when she did, he remained relatively unresponsive. The therapist asked her if there was anything familiar about what she was describing. She thought about other boys she had known toward whom she had harbored similar feelings.

The therapist then asked if this quality of being passive and unresponsive that she found so frustrating in boys bore any similarity to her father's style. She uttered, "Oh! . . . ," and became redfaced as she added, "I hadn't thought of that. I guess it's so." She proceeded to talk about her tendency to migrate toward such males, just as she does to girls with drug problems. (Her mother had struggled with a severe prescription drug addiction during the patient's preteen and early adolescent years.) She added that these are the only kind of people to whom she is attracted. She had tried without success to change her recent boyfriend and others before him. She claimed not to feel deserving or worthy of other types. More suitable young men would not like her if they knew what she thought or what she was like or about her background. The latter reference was to her mother's earlier addiction. Or else, if that knowledge didn't drive them away, she would have some ill-defined, bad, contaminating effect on decent young men.

The last association prompted the therapist to wonder if she struggled against believing that she had caused her family's problems, specifically her mother's addiction and her father's non-communicativeness and passivity. The young woman responded affirmatively. She had not caused her mother's addiction, but felt she had somehow contributed to its development. She went on to reflect that her parents had not been very affectionate during her growing years, though she had yearned for more expressions of their love. She had done everything she thought pleased them, but none of her efforts made them more physically demonstrative toward her. So, she had concluded that she must really be bad or undeserving. On further reflection she realized in retrospect that when she began high school she had found herself seeking out boys who were like her mother, that is, self-absorbed drug users. She no longer sought out such people; however, she found that such people were attracted to her and she has to be careful not to encourage such individuals.

She didn't know why, but sometimes she felt that she should just take the drugs offered by friends and acquaintances. After all, if alcoholism is genetic then drug addiction is probably also. So, abstaining completely as she did was ultimately futile—she was fated to become addicted. The therapist responded that this attitude appeared to mask guilt she felt about being responsible for her mother's drug problem and for feeling superior to her mother as well. The young woman again became red-faced and replied that that was probably so.

It is difficult to find evidence in material like this that the adolescent's choice of unsuitable partners is based on defending against a libidinal attraction to either parent. This young woman still sought love, approval, and responsiveness from her parents. Also, she wished exculpation from the guilt she harbored for her mother's illness and her father's personality deficits. There is little to suggest any effort to ward-off genital hetero- or homosexual desires toward either parent in her choices of friends and partners. I have found that the vicissitudes of object choice amongst adolescents are more frequently influenced by efforts like those of this young woman to complete unfulfilled developmental requirements from earlier life. But because of the central importance of drives in psychoanalytic theory, I believe that there has been a tendency in psychoanalytic thinking to mistake these tendencies for a libidinal attraction to perverse gratification. The following example illustrates this point in a case where sexual implications are more obvious:

A 20-year-old woman was being treated for recurrent anorexia nervosa with bulimia plus difficulties in establishing relationships with appropriate men and problems sustaining adequate performance in college. She had been raised on a hippie commune until her parents were killed in an auto accident when the girl was 9 years old. She then lived with a grandmother who was extremely compulsive, controlling, and fastidious, but otherwise self-absorbed and unemotional except for a preoccupation with weight and proper food intake.

In associating to the nausea she experienced prior to any date, the young woman revealed her fear of being raped. She associated this to a more basic fear of "a big man doing what he wants to me." This in turn brought recollections of her life on the commune during the 1960s as a preschool and school-aged child. She had witnessed a lot of wild people around her and recalled many people naked and having sex. She recalled her parents getting high on LSD and her father breathing marijuana smoke into her mouth with kisses, which made her feel nauseous.

As a young teenager she recalled not being able to say no to the requests of boys for sex. But during such experiences she would lie there crying, limp, and without experiencing any enjoyment.

Psychoanalysts have written that the symptoms of anorexia nervosa and bulimia represent a libidinization of food (Waller, Kaufman, and Deutsch, 1940). The anorexic and bulimic symptoms arise to ward off (anorexia) and gratify (bulimia) the girl's oedipal wish to have her father's baby, a wish that first arose during a time in her development when she thought that impregnation occurred through the mouth. One can understand how such a connection could be made from this patient's associations. When her history is considered in its entirety, however, it becomes more difficult to conclude that the repudiation of regressive oedipal desire is the basic motive for her anorexic and bulimic periods and her acquiescence to the sexual overtures of adolescent boys. The more crucial motives seem to be the girl's efforts to feel accepted and to reverse the apprehension and confusion she had experienced in this quest from capricious, uncontrolled parents and an overcontrolling grandmother. In this effort she turned to boys whose attitudes were familiar to her by virtue of their similarity to those of her parents.

PROBLEMATIC SEXUAL BEHAVIOR IN ADOLESCENTS

The previous two cases illustrate that the choice of romantic or sexual partners made by adolescents do not necessarily involve sexual interest. I will now turn to cases which involve specific sexual behavior but turn out to have a different basis than sexual curiosity or desire on the part of the adolescent.

SALLY: PROMISCUITY

Sixteen-year-old Sally sought treatment when she lost interest in schoolwork and became unable to perform academically. The youngest of four children, her parents had separated for several years when she was in grade school and had then reunited when Sally was a young teenager. Both parents tended to undercut their children's accomplishments, to take credit for them, and to sabotage their children's efforts toward successful independence. For example, after promising to support the older children through college, her parents had withdrawn their support at the last minute, so none of Sally's older siblings had matriculated. Although aware of being their favorite, Sally remained uncertain about whether they wanted her to succeed. This was reflected in the immobilization at school she developed at the time when she and her classmates began thinking seriously about college.

Sally had always been a shy, quiet child, who had harbored concerns that she had somehow caused her parents' separation. During the course of therapy the degree to which she felt obligated to accede to the wishes of others (friends, family, and strangers alike) emerged. This compulsion to comply proved to be based on her idea that to assert herself in the face of possible contrary wishes of other people would hurt them (emancipatory or separation guilt). Her parents' divorce had greatly reinforced Sally's feelings of responsibility for the welfare of other family members. This was particularly so with respect to her father's temperamental and volatile behavior. It was he who had initiated the separation and reconciliation. He acted readily offended and would literally walk away from interactions in which he was not getting his way. At the same time he was very aggressive in business to the point of rapacity.

During the second year of therapy Sally raised concerns about her very self-abasing and self-denigrating sexual interactions with boys. She would comply with their wishes for sexual intercourse, even though as she herself reflected, it was invariably the wrong person, the wrong place, and the wrong time. Guilt associated with the idea that boys' "egos" were fragile and easily hurt if they did not get their way seemed to be the most important psychodynamic factor in her compliance with their requests. It mirrored her apprehension about her father's inability to tolerate refusal of his wishes. As noted, this dynamic was operative in other aspects of her life as well.

Engagement in heterosexual activity with several different partners is not unusual amongst some teenagers. Sally's case is included with cases of sexual aberration because of the common psychodynamic factor in the genesis of these conditions. I refer to problems arising in the sexual development of adolescents based on conflicts regarding self-assertion and autonomy on the one hand, and on the other hand a need to maintain a relationship with others through compliant behaviors which have their basis in fantasies developed in the adolescent's real experiences with parents during childhood. Sally had experienced survivor guilt regarding her older siblings because she was acknowledged to be their parents' favorite and had not suffered at her parents' hands as they had. Sally also felt vaguely responsible for her parents' separation and experienced emancipatory guilt in separating from them. She nevertheless felt compelled to accede to the wishes of others, to atone for the hurt she feared she had caused her siblings (by being favored), and parents (by having caused their separation).

ALISHA: BROTHER–SISTER SEXUAL INVOLVEMENT

Alisha, a stunning, shapely, and talented 16-year-old was in therapy for depressive symptoms, shame, and guilt that were preventing her from studying. She was the younger child of a successful, ambitious, but arrogant and domineering research physician. Her mother suffered her husband's overbearingness in silence and basically pandered to his vanity while assuming much responsibility for the day-to-day administration of his grants and running his laboratory. In doing so she sustained herself with an underlying and perhaps accurate conviction that her husband could not function without her and she was the power behind his throne.

Alisha's father was particularly belittling and overbearing toward her brother, three years her senior, who strove mightily without success to gain the approval of his implacable and competitive father. The brother smarted also with unrequited competitive feelings toward Alisha, who was everything he wished to be—popular, socially poised, accomplished, attractive, and an outstanding student. His mother, with her attitude that males were fragile, tended to assuage her son's humiliation by infantilizing him. Alisha was not an object of her father's depreciation because in their family males were considered superior and achievement was not expected of females. Alisha felt both embarrassed and bad about her father's treatment of her brother, especially since she was spared her father's belittling. The ease with which she accomplished everything she attempted and the recognition she received for her accomplishments at school served to heighten her guilt about her brother's circumstances.

When Alisha was 13 her brother had begun to complain to her about his strong sexual yearnings and complete lack of success with girls. He subsequently began masturbating in her presence; this progressed to fondling Alisha and masturbating against her body. Initially Alisha tried to rebuff his advances; her brother would respond by acting so pathetically needy that she felt that depriving him would be very harmful. She feared that her brother was so defeated by his father's treatment and so painfully frustrated in his efforts with girls, that it would be very detrimental to him if she did not comply with his wishes. So, she pretended to be asleep and thus unaware of what he was doing. She would lie there, waiting for him to ejaculate so the event would be over. She experienced no sexual pleasure. Finally, after the single occasion when she started to allow him to enter her but stopped, her sense of shame and guilt became overwhelming and her presenting symptoms incapacitated her.

The therapist initially emphasized that Alisha's best interests were their most important consideration, and that she and he needed to determine how she could have let herself participate in experiences which were so mortifying to her. This approach helped reduce Alisha's guilt about the sexual involvement with her brother. Alisha also readily grasped the therapist's interpretation of the survivor guilt she felt with respect to her brother; this stemmed both from having been spared her father's cruelty and from being more successful than her brother. The latter feelings had been reinforced by her mother's intimations that males are basically weak. Alisha also readily understood how her mother's attitudes contributed to the development of Alisha's concerns about feeling responsible for her brother's welfare and having great power to influence him. This line of interpretation, namely that she had complied with her brother's wishes because of her survivor guilt, enabled Alisha to discontinue the sexual experiences with her brother and reverse her depressive symptoms.

TRISHA: STEPFATHER–STEPDAUGHTER INCEST

Sixteen-year-old Trisha was referred for symptoms of depression. While her mother was hospitalized for a complicated surgical procedure, Trisha's usually arrogant, tyrannical stepfather had prevailed upon Trisha to engage in sexual acts, including some of a perverted nature. When her mother discovered this upon returning home, she separated from and divorced Trisha's stepfather. Following her parents' separation Trisha became preoccupied with her stepfather's long-standing cruelty and she wished for revenge, but these thoughts alternated with feeling sorry for him.

The therapist soon observed that Trisha presented herself in such a manner as to elicit sympathy from others—how much she had suffered, how hard her lot had been. After acknowledging that the incestuous experiences certainly justified those feelings, he nevertheless wondered if Trisha recognized anything familiar in that particular manner of presenting herself. Trisha responded that that had been precisely the manner her stepfather adopted on those occasions when she had acceded to his sexual advances. He would present himself as very forlorn, needing her, and the victim of great adversity in his own early life. It then became evident that Trisha's prime motivation for acquiescing to his advances had been a fear of hurting him if she did not comply. So, she sacrificed herself in an effort to shore up her stepfather.

Adopting his manner after the parental separation, a defensive identification, amounted to a self-imposed punishment. She was making herself feel what she thought he had felt after being thrown out of their home. She felt responsible for that, and tried to relieve her survivor guilt by feeling what she feared she had caused her stepfather to feel. When these issues were interpreted, her depression lifted. The therapist was unable to ferret out any evidence that Trisha's most atypical, sympathy-seeking demeanor represented a resistance or defense against revealing any underlying incestuous longings to herself or others.

LISBETH: HOMOSEXUAL PREOCCUPATIONS

An 18-year-old high school senior became functionally immobilized in her studies and then in all other areas of her life as she began finalizing college plans. She described the indecisiveness, perplexity, and lack of confidence which had burgeoned of late and added that she no longer knew if she liked boys or preferred girls. She thought she might be homosexual.

She was the youngest of three and the only daughter of a competitive, controlling investment banker who took great pleasure in instructing his children in all areas of their lives. Her mother, who was independently wealthy, from a prominent family, and an astute businesswoman, had been instrumental in the rise to success of Lisbeth's father; however, Lisbeth's mother always remained in the background. This was a source of conflict for her mother who desperately wished to succeed in her own right but struggled with inhibitions against doing so. Thus, Lisbeth's mother presented a paradoxical stance of acting submissive toward her husband and sons, but considering males to be vulnerable and always in need of support. Lisbeth's mother also made it clear that she confided in and depended upon Lisbeth in a way she did with no one else.

Lisbeth was readily able to identify the degree to which she also kept herself back and inhibited her progress because of guilt and fear of hurting others if she succeeded. Initially she thought this represented an accommodation to her father's wish to always be the top man. After recalling regressive wishes to be cuddled by her mother, however, Lisbeth realized that she wanted to make her mother feel important and needed. Lisbeth recognized that she felt emancipatory guilt. She feared hurting her mother by leaving to pursue a goal to which her mother had aspired but failed to achieve; and Lisbeth was attempting to preserve the relationship she felt her mother needed. Her ideas that she was homosexual disappeared. Lisbeth's thoughts of being or becoming homosexual were understood as an effort to accommodate her emancipatory guilt as she prepared to venture forth independently from a mother who had used Lisbeth as her confidante and envied Lisbeth's opportunities to do what she herself had been unable to do.

MR. J: TRANSVESTITISM

Mr. J, a 22-year-old recent college graduate, sought treatment because he was preoccupied with transvestitism and had become depressed. His transvestite preoccupations were manifested in masturbatory fantasies involving transvestites and occasional cross-dressing in his bedroom.

He was the younger child of a socially isolated, working class couple. A much older half-brother from his mother's first marriage had not lived with the family for years. Mr. J's mother completely dominated his father who complied fully with all her dictates. Mr. J's futile complaints during childhood about the way in which his parents related, gave way to a sense of dismay, disgust, and frustration as a young adolescent. He tried not to feel contempt for his father's passivity with women and his mother's need to control men.

Throughout Mr. J's life his mother had often spoken of her wish that they remain close and that he not drift away from them as other children did from their parents. At the same time his parents frequently had talked about how their son was going to make everything right for them and elevate their social status. Mr. J was the first member of his family to attend college. Having completed his baccalaureate degree with honors at a local university, he was offered an excellent job in another city, where he wished to move. As he anticipated doing so, however, he became depressed, more socially isolated to the point of staying home, and his preoccupation with transvestites burgeoned.

He readily acknowledged to the therapist that he felt tied to home by his guilt over surpassing his father and escaping the environment in which his father was still trapped (emancipation or survivor guilt). He was also held back by guilt related to leaving his mother's domain because he felt she needed to control him and could not manage without him there (emancipation or separation guilt).

With respect to the development of his preoccupation with transvestites, both Mr. J's parents had openly bespoken their preference for a daughter for as long as Mr. J could recall. Also, Mr. J had found some transvestite magazines hidden amongst his father's belongings when he was rummaging around during preadolescence. This had led Mr. J to suspect that his father was interested in transvestites. His own preoccupation with transvestites began when Mr. J was 13 years old. He was convinced that he was heterosexual, however, though puzzled by the intensely sadistic nature of his masturbatory fantasies.

Mr. J presented himself to the world as mild and accommodating. These traits proved to be a defensive identification with his father's personality and a compliance with his mother's wishes to dominate. The defensive identification with his father kept Mr. J from experiencing the full measure of disdain he felt for his father's submissiveness (i.e., it was as if Mr. J were thinking "I'm like my father, not contemptuous of him"). Witnessing, as he grew up, his father's abject submissiveness to his mother's uncompromising domination, contributed to Mr. J developing the conviction that any self-assertion constituted defiance and aggression against another person. This was guilt-engendering and he dealt with it by acting compliant, yet this made him feel submissive, which aroused intense frustration. So, he alternated between feeling guiltily defiant and helplessly submissive. The intensity of his guilt that immobilized him in this obsessional way bespoke feelings of having inordinate influence over and responsibility for other people (omnipotence complex).

As these dynamics were elucidated in analysis, Mr. J began to demonstrate undoing. Any assertiveness on his part, in fantasy or action, was followed by feelings and expressions of weakness and passivity, and also frequently by intense transvestite masturbatory fantasies. In these fantasies he became the womanized man who was humiliated. His disgust for his mother and father and his degraded view of women emerged as he explored fantasies in which he was a "macho man" pushing women around. Whenever he entertained such heady, exciting fantasies he would immediately feel overwhelmed with guilt and reverse them into opposite fantasies in which he was a degraded woman (transvestite). So, he frightened himself by experiencing self-assertion (which he viewed as forbidden to males in his family) as sadism. He then punished himself for any self-assertive wishes by meting out to himself the very condition he feared his self-assertion had caused the other person to suffer, namely degradation and humiliation. Thus, his transvestite preoccupations were a self-imposed punishment for his wishes to get away from his mother, his disgust and disdain for her, and his contempt and feelings of superiority toward his extremely passive father who, as noted, had apparently been titillated by transvestites.

Mr. J's transvestite fantasies arose: (1) as part of a defensive identification with a weak father whom Mr. J had tried to build up in an effort to relieve emancipatory guilt; (2) to deal with emancipatory guilt associated with his self-assertive wishes to complete his development by compliance with a controlling mother who did not want him to emancipate and parents who had wanted a girl.

DELINQUENCY

In contrast to the last group of adolescents whose symptoms or behaviors related to their sexual development or behaviors, the cases which follow involve adolescents whose behavior brought them directly to the attention of the juvenile justice system. The term *delinquency* in this context refers to whatever behaviors a society chooses to stipulate as socially unacceptable for minors.

LUZ: HABITUAL TRUANCY

An intelligent, articulate, and ambitious 16-year-old girl was a chronic truant. Truancy had begun during her early grade school years and had proven unresponsive to all efforts by school and juvenile authorities. Luz was the middle of five children being raised by her mother. Luz's mother was an untypical, liberated, second-generation Hispanic woman who had become an outspoken, maverick community activist in their ethnic neighborhood. Her mother was truculent, opinionated, and exhibited a paranoid quality of suspiciousness toward anyone else's views. Also, though only modestly educated herself, her attitude toward Luz's early truancies, including her refusal to cooperate with efforts to help Luz stay at school, had led Luz to conclude that deep down, and perhaps unconsciously, her mother wanted to be Luz's only teacher. So, Luz's truancy, when considered alongside her ambition to get ahead, reflected a compliance with what she perceived pleased her mother.

Although a bit embarrassed in acknowledging it to the interviewer, Luz felt that she was more attractive, appealing, intelligent, and motivated than her siblings. And she was unique amongst her siblings and friends in neither having used nor sold drugs, drunk alcohol, nor become pregnant. Moreover, she did want to go to school. She had tried to overcome her difficulties by using self-help tapes and books. Thus, she exhibited significant personal integrity and motivation, but was unable to overcome her tendency to truant. She always returned home when she left school.

During a diagnostic interview Luz readily identified guilt at the thought of surpassing her siblings and her mother. And she recognized that truanting to return home was a compliance with what she felt her mother wanted. Thus, Luz was sacrificing her obvious wishes to move ahead in her development in an effort both to please her mother and to avoid emancipatory guilt associated with the idea of becoming independent of her mother's influence and more successful than her siblings.

STACEY: CHRONIC RUNAWAY AND INVOLVEMENT WITH GANGS

Stacey's maternal grandmother and mother had suffered abusive relationships with men. Stacey's mother had a long history of drinking and had herself run away from her own mother's care. Stacey's earliest memories were of being removed to a receiving home because her drug-using father violently threatened her mother and because her mother frequently left the children unattended to go drinking. From the age of 4 years Stacey recalled having felt responsible for watching over her mother and her younger twin brothers.

She and her siblings shuttled between her mother's and grandmother's care, and Stacey began running away at 5 years of age to avoid witnessing and experiencing brutality at her grand-mother's home. She ran to her father's home where he and his friends touched her genitals. By the time she was 14 years old Stacey had been in many foster homes and group homes.

When Stacey entered junior high school she had been placed again with her mother who had moved to a different area. Stacey entered the new school poor and unpopular. She then became the girl friend of a gang leader who was a few years older. Stacey observed that this involvement provided her with material goods she could not have had otherwise. It also gave her respectability and popularity at her school. Remaining true to her boyfriend was all that was required of her. She was not required to drink or to use or sell drugs, nor was she coerced into sexual involvements against her will.

By the time she was an early adolescent Stacey had run away from placements far from where her mother lived. She had trav-eled alone or with fellow runaways hundreds if not thousands of miles, without having been physically abused, seriously injured, or harmed, and without having been raped nor having contracted venereal disease, become pregnant, or involved in prostitution or drug selling. So, she had proven herself highly adaptable in very adverse circumstances. She even eloped from treament centers she liked, and always ran home to her mother or to her boyfriend and then back to her mother's domicile.

Stacey was a highly intelligent and remarkably insightful ado-lescent. She identified her problem as one of always looking for love and attention. She had never found the attention she sought from her mother and so turned to others and found it in the gang. In other words, she experienced more evidence of continu-ing interest, protection, and recognition from gang members than she had from her family. She observed that adults had proven so untrustworthy that peers rather than adults had become the objects of her admiration and the source of her standards. As noted above, the price of these benefits from the gang was only accepting the possessiveness of her boyfriend and the sometimes overbearing protectiveness of his gang. For someone who had been prematurely exposed to life's dangers, this hardly seemed bad or too constraining. By the time Stacey was 15 years old, her mother had been sober and stable for a couple of years but very rarely took the initiative to contact her daughter.

So why did Stacey compulsively return home? As noted, from the age of 4 years Stacey could recall worrying about and feeling responsible for her mother and her brothers. Her worry in part reflected her earlier experience with an obviously foun-dering and abandoning parent on whom Stacey nevertheless needed to be able to rely in order to feel secure. In an effort to obtain this sense of security she assumed responsibility for the cruel and rejecting behavior of her parents. So, she always returned to seek absolution from her mother for her fantasy of having caused the family's problems. Furthermore, by acting with motherly concern and worry toward her mother and the twins, she achieved a little inner comfort by feeling the way she wished her rejecting parent would feel toward her. It is as if she loved her mother as she wished to be loved by her mother. So, Stacey was compelled to run home to relieve her guilt and feelings of responsibility for her mother's welfare by assuring herself that her mother was all right, to feel cared for by reversing the role of caretaker, and at base to seek her mother's love.

Stacey always thwarted the sincere efforts of well-intentioned adults to help her. In addressing this puzzling matter Stacey herself said that she did not trust adults. She had unconsciously concluded from her parents' behaviors toward her that they did not want her to succeed; and she came to sense that what truly gratified her parents, and therefore by extension other adults as well, was to reject and punish her. So, in any therapeutic setting, Stacey did one of two things. She either tested caretaking adults past their limits of toleration, which then confirmed her view of their basic wish to punish her; or she ran away. She ran away both to reject before being rejected and to present herself as someone who deserved to be punished or rejected by adults after being apprehended. Thus, Stacey's runaway behavior, which seemed on the surface like defiance of adult authority, proved at base to be an effort to please adults. By pleasing them in this way, Stacey hoped in turn that they would provide her with the security she needed from parents. For at base she did not want to be let go of; she wanted to be held onto. She made it appear so much the opposite, however, that she ended up repeating, in her multiple out of home placements, the pattern of being rejected and abandoned and punished that she wanted to reverse.

SUMMARY

In this chapter I have described and illustrated how psychopathology arises in adolescents based on the model of adolescent development I have presented. When adolescents experience conflict between their strivings to complete development and their wishes to retain a positive relationship with their parents, they typically experience emancipatory guilt. This is the term I use to characterize separation and survivor-type guilt which arises in the development of adolescents. Adolescents often react to emancipatory guilt by: (1) blaming themselves for the problematic relationship, though they often ward off the guilt by acting blameless or by blaming parents; (2) feeling great responsibility for their parents' welfare, again often avoiding awareness of this by recourse to an opposite attitude; and (3) feeling a burdensome sense of great power to influence their parents, termed omnipotence feelings by Weiss, Sampson, et al. (1986).

These internal conflicts are often resolved by behaviors which represent either: (1) a compliance with what the adolescents think pleases their parents; (2) defensive identifications which amount to imitations of or equivalents of the maladaptive behaviors being exhibited by their parents.

As noted, these responses frequently reflect emancipatory guilt, associated with the wish to surpass parents, to be healthier and more successful than them. In cases where the adolescent experiences significant psychopathology, this emancipatory guilt can be more clearly characterized as guilt in the survivor–separation continuum. This view of the development of psychopathology in adolescents is contrasted with the more traditional, psychoanalytically oriented psychodynamic view.

Then a spectrum of problems and symptoms is presented to illustrate how the psychopathological reactions can be understood to arise from the prototypic adolescent developmental conflict I have presented. Case examples encompass: (1) depressive reactions, including those with substance abuse and school failure; (2) suicide (using a case published by other authors); (3) anxiety states; (4) sexually aberrant behavior, including promiscuity, brother–sister sexual involvement, stepfather–stepdaughter incest, homosexual preoccupation, transvestitism; (5) delinquency involving habitual truancy and chronic runaway behavior with involvement in gangs.

CHAPTER 9

Assessment and Therapy

Several factors conspire to render difficult the task of determining whether an adolescent warrants treatment or can be left alone:

There is a continuum between healthy and pathological adjustment. Thus, quantitative as well as qualitative factors must be considered and that moves the decision making into the realm of clinical judgment.

The same signs and symptoms can reflect normality or pathology. For example, failure to attend school can represent a reasonable adaptation or be the symptom of severe psychopathology (Mogul, 1969).

Many adolescents, particularly younger ones, are reluctant to reveal much to therapists. A lack of data always compromises clinical judgment.

Although the basic developmental tasks of youth have not changed for centuries, in our lifetime more avenues have become available to adolescents for working out developmental conflicts with narrower margins of safety before pathology or tragedy prevails. For example, one can experiment much longer with the traditionally used beer than with crack cocaine before serious addiction ensues. Or, as another example, reduced social prohibition has predisposed to more sexual experimentation amongst adolescents which, despite the availability of contraception, has increased the risk of tragic pregnancies and more recently of an incurable illness as well. This makes the job of assessing adolescents more anxiety provoking.

Therapists often have trouble using their intuitive and empathic senses with confidence in evaluating adolescents. It is difficult enough to know what another person is experiencing under any circumstances; and it becomes more so when one's feelings are changing rapidly, which is often the case with adolescents. Uncertainty about the "norms" of expected adolescent behaviors which, as implied in the previous paragraph, seem to have changed even if developmental goals have not, confound the use of the therapist's intuition and personal experience.

The attitudes of adolescents and the adult generation's reservations about them have been the same for millennia (chapter 2). Nevertheless, we must keep our assessment as uncontaminated as possible by preconceived notions of how things must still be because of the way they were, or how dramatically they must have changed given recent sociological reports about adolescents' manifest behaviors and attitudes. The best way I know of doing this is to use the individual as his or her own control subject.

I will outline an approach which has helped me arrive with more confidence at a clinical impression of the significance of an adolescent's presentation.

ASSESSMENT OF THE ADOLESCENT'S ADAPTIVE STYLE, STRENGTHS, AND RELATIVE VULNERABILITIES PRIOR TO ADOLESCENCE

Development during adolescence is a gradually unfolding process which can be complicated, prevented, or fostered by the environment. Thus, determining how essentially different the current behaviors/symptoms are from the adolescent's preexisting style of adapting becomes vital for understanding the significance of his or her clinical presentation. Many of the ways in which adolescents deal with stress are at base variations of previously used mechanisms. The surfer (p. 18) and the nerd turned rock musician (p. 96) illustrated this phenomenon. The conclusions one reaches can be much different if the therapist does not carefully differentiate between those features of an adolescent's presentation which are essentially continuous with his or her prior adaptive style and those which are new.

Therapists must obtain information about ego and personality assets that may be capitalized upon during adolescence by considering his or her earlier academic and interpersonal development during grade school with respect to the following: [1]

EGO STRENGTHENING

One aspect of ego strengthening involves control of impulses, particularly aggressive impulses. Determining whether obsessional defenses, and particularly reaction formation, have been integrated is helpful in this regard.

The child's capacity for sublimation is a second aspect: (1) This is most commonly estimated from how well the adolescent has developed the tools of precision learning and his or her ability to persist at learning tasks. The former does not necessarily equate with school grades, but if grades have been mediocre, the latter factor of frustration tolerance becomes relatively more important. (2) The acquisition of skills and the development of talents are similar phenomena. They represent ego assets upon which the adolescent may be able to capitalize in his or her movement toward greater psychological independence.

Evidence of the degree to which the child during the grade school years was able to control, order, and array fantasy is important. This is somewhat more difficult to determine.

AGE-APPROPRIATE CONSCIENCE FUNCTIONING

We can assess age-appropriate conscience functioning from the ease with which the child was able to differentiate, live with, and live by a sense of right and wrong; his or her ability to play by the rules without much auxiliary ego support; and a history of delinquent behavior.

---

[1]Writing from a libido theory perspective, Blos (1962) observed that "a prerequisite for entering the adolescent phase of drive organization is the consolidation of the latency period" (p. 56). He implies the kind of assessment I am suggesting, but he emphasizes the individual's ego resources for dealing with the upsurge of drive at puberty. I am focusing on the individual's adaptive capacities since I have found dealing with drives to be less critical in most cases.

PEER RELATEDNESS

Borrowing a metaphor from Harry Stack Sullivan, the term *peer relatedness* refers to the "silent miracle" of friendship, by which I mean aim-inhibited or ego-filtered altruism. A strong peer relationship during the grade school years represents the first movement away from the nuclear family. Evidence that this occurred augurs well for the adolescent's ability to use peer relationships to facilitate emancipation.

IS THE CURRENT THRUST OF THE ADOLESCENT'S DEVELOPMENT FORWARD MOVING? (THE PRESENT STATE OF THE ADOLESCENT'S STRIVINGS TO COMPLETE DEVELOPMENT)

Having developed some sense of what adolescents have brought from childhood into adolescence, I then try to determine whether their presentations are basically forward moving or stalled. To do so I consider how problematic behaviors or symptoms relate to what adolescents are trying to accomplish during this period. (1) They are attempting to feel increasingly independent of their need for parental guidance and influence with respect to managing impulses appropriately. This includes moving toward adopting a moral code of guiding principles for living which is not exclusively dependent upon their parents' standards. (2) They are attempting to maintain forward momentum of their capacity to learn and (3) to formulate an increasingly appropriate course for the next period of their lives based on reality considerations (i.e., probabilities rather than possibilities), and taking increasing responsibility for achieving that goal. (4) They are attempting to be able to move forward with pleasure and self-satisfaction, and anticipating the future with reasonable confidence and optimism, neither as the guilty man of Freud nor the tragic man of Kohut (1982).

If on balance the adolescent's development is not progressive, what is impeding it? Since the prototypic way in which adolescent development becomes problematic involves the relationship to the parents, this feature of his or her current life is evaluated.

THE ADOLESCENT'S RELATIONSHIP TO HIS OR HER PARENTS
(PRIMARY OBJECT RELATIONSHIPS)

Compulsively compliant behavior or defensive identifications suggest that the adolescent is experiencing emancipatory guilt. The presence of these behaviors are clues that the adolescent is avoiding awareness of some dissatisfaction with a parent or is protecting a parent and is inhibiting his or her own progress. Traumatic experiences involving parents or siblings which have precipitated survivor guilt are frequently the sources of these problems and are often relatively easy to identify.

Regarding technique for assessing problematic relationships with other family members, the most prominent complaints of many adolescents are often about other family members or friends. Rather than eschewing such complaints as resistance to dealing with inner conflict, I welcome such material as the best entree to the intrapsychic. For after listening to their dissatisfaction, *without contradicting or disputing their view,* I can then ask for their personal reactions to these interpersonal frustrations. Adolescents usually respond if I have not conveyed a sense of judgment or disapproval of their condemnation of family or friends. Thus, we have arrived where I hoped we would, at the threshold of the intrapsychic. This approach affords a more personal analysis than one that either concentrates on the interpersonal dynamics and thus risks accepting what may prove to be rationalizations on the patient's part, or one which focuses on traditional defense analysis, which risks distorting understanding of the case by forcing the patient's symptoms into line with psychoanalytic metapsychology.

An adolescent's relationship to his parents can often be clarified using a framework developed by Anna Freud (1958). She presented a series of prototypic responses of adolescents to their parents which she termed defenses against the libidinal object ties. They represent, in the libido theory model from which she writes, ways in which the adolescent attempts to avoid resurgent incestuous urges. Her description is very useful, even though I deemphasize the motive she ascribes to these behavior patterns. For these defenses can equally well be viewed as ways in which adolescents are attempting to deal with their wishes to become more independent from their parents. These defenses are:

1. Displacement of the childhood love for parents onto others. If the displacement of affection/admiration is to a laudable mentor, relative, or friend, then the reaction is adaptive. If the displacement is to an unscrupulous, charismatic leader, then this mechanism proves maladaptive or at least dangerous for the adolescent. The view of development and psychopathology I have presented offers a model for comprehending how this mechanism can become problematic. That is, to quote Blos (1967), my construct helps elucidate how the adolescent can find him- or herself "doing the wrong thing for the right reasons" (p. 167).

2. Reversal of affect in which the childhood love of parents is turned into anger and hatred. Anna Freud finds that guilt associated with this anger predisposes to depressive or paranoid reactions in adolescents who use this mechanism. Which reaction occurs depends on whether they turn their aggression against themselves or toward the outside world.

3. Withdrawal (of libido) into a schizoid-type state. Anna Freud finds that this potentially more dangerous reaction can lead to hypochondriasis or grandiosity. Which reaction occurs depends upon whether the adolescent cathects his or her body or psyche with the libido that has been withdrawn from parents (or more correctly in libido theory terms, from the adolescent's mental representations of his or her parents).

4. Regression to a potentially psychotic state of psychological organization.

While these four mechanisms form a continuum of increasing pathological potential, the use of any or all of these behavior patterns is not necessarily pathological. The intensity, degree, and exclusivity with which the adolescent uses them determines whether they constitute adaptive or pathological reactions. Pathology develops when these mechanisms are overused, overstressed, or when one is used exclusively.

SUMMARY

The evaluation is accomplished by:

1. Assessment of the adolescent's adaptive style, strengths, and relative vulnerabilities prior to adolescence. Subcategories include: (a) ego strengthening, (b) age-appropriate conscience functioning, (c) peer relatedness.
2. Determination of whether the current thrust of the adolescent's development is forward moving. Features of the adolescent's present life which serve to indicate whether or not he or she is advancing are enumerated.
3. Consideration of the adolescent's relationship to his or her parents. The presence of compulsively compliant behavior or defensive identifications are clues that the relationship to parents is problematic. A schema developed by Anna Freud for assessing the adolescent's way of relating to his or her parents is incorporated into this part of the assessment.

Synthesis of these elements helps one make a clinical judgment about whether the adolescent's presenting difficulties represent on balance forward movement or foundering development. Recommendations for treatment, for watchful waiting, or reassurance of the adolescent and his or her parents are made on that basis.[2]

FAVORING THE LONG VIEW IN ASSESSING THE ADOLESCENT'S PRESENTATION

The importance of keeping the long view of the individual's presenting symptoms ever in mind is implicit in a developmental perspective. By virtue of its progressive nature, the developmental

---

[2]Mogul (1969) describes an approach to assessment of adolescents that incorporates A. Freud's defenses against the infantile object ties plus the adolescent's developmental tasks and an awareness of the adolescent's "immediate social context in an historical perspective" (p. 31). The latter refers to an understanding of those current and past factors in his or her development which have influenced the adolescent's development. Because Mogul uses a libido theory perspective, however, his consideration of the social context in historical perspective serves to delineate factors which prevent successful resolution of the resurgent Oedipus complex. Thus, while Mogul's model for assessment includes several features similar to those I have described, he arrives at different conclusions about adolescents whose development is foundering. For example, his model does not make provision for my finding that traumas in relation

perspective inclines one toward a stance of cautious optimism. Operationally, this translates into always considering adolescents' acute problems in light of their underlying strivings to complete their development successfully. This does not mean we adopt Pollyanna's attitude, but rather that this vantage influences our view. For example, some adolescents use an underlying sense of confidence in their parents' support as license to experiment more freely and problematically than their parents find acceptable. If, for example, these strident strivings of a seemingly well-structured adolescent to become more independent from a previously close and compliant attachment to parents have become punctuated by habituation to amphetamines, then we do whatever we can to eliminate the latter. We cannot simply trust that as development proceeds and the rejecting behaviors toward parents moderate, he or she will necessarily be able to bring serious drug use under control. The therapeutic effort in other cases may be directed toward trying to help adolescents and their parents get through this period of development with the youth emerging sufficiently unscathed from their experimentation (be it from sexual involvements, lack of attention to academics, other risk-taking activity, or contumacious behavior), so that their options are preserved in young adulthood. These are the adolescents who particularly benefit from the almost unlimited opportunities for second chances offered by the American political system. Again, it is not that we routinely presume that adolescents will get better if left alone. But we look carefully for evidences of strivings to complete development, and therapeutic goals and interventions are oriented toward supporting the latter with the earlier mentioned optimism, even as we attempt to identify significant impediments to the developmental process.

THERAPY WITH ADOLESCENTS

The following guidelines for treating adolescents follow naturally from the view of development I have presented. These precepts have stood me well in conducting psychotherapy and psychoanalysis. It is important, however, to always consider each case on its

---

to parents most often cause adolescents' development to become impeded by emancipatory guilt rather than by oedipal conflicts.

own merits; thus, these precepts might not apply to every patient. After discussing these guidelines with reference to typical situations that arise in the therapy of adolescents, I will illustrate this approach by describing the treatment of several patients.

Precepts for approaching the basic developmental conflicts in adolescents which often appear in therapy follow directly from the three issues of adolescent development:

Adolescents may fear that they will cause a breach in their relationship with their parents as they strive for greater psychological independence under the impetus of their urge to complete development. Since they want to retain an important tie to their families as they emancipate, aberrant behaviors and symptoms often arise from this fear. The fear is that achieving autonomy will somehow hurt the parents, will cause them to feel rejected, or will motivate them to reject the adolescent. In therapy, however, adolescent patients often present the opposites of these fears. They act anxious about separating and express dependency yearnings or act exaggeratedly unconcerned about the impact of their behaviors on their parents.

The need for parental sponsorship has a counterpart in the therapist's need to transmit his or her support for the adolescent's efforts to progress. In other words, the adolescent patient must sense from the therapist something equivalent to the sponsorship he requires from parents in his ongoing development.

Many symptomatic behaviors in adolescents will become comprehensible if one uses this frame of reference when listening to the patients' material. Moreover, if you attend to these issues from the very outset and show the adolescent that you understand his or her developmental conflicts by practicing what I have just preached, then a therapeutic alliance or therapeutic detente (Bloch, 1981) may be formed. In other words, optimal conditions for working with an adolescent will have been created with this approach, and the patient will work with you if he or she is able to do so.

INITIAL CONTACTS WITH THE FAMILY AND PATIENT

Since his or her greatest developmental imperative is to emancipate, I remain scrupulously attentive to the matter of the adolescent's autonomy from the moment when preparatory negotiations begin for evaluating a youth. This consideration bespeaks the wisdom, for example, if the youngster is willing, of meeting with the adolescent, from age 12 or 13, before seeing the parents. In having parents prepare their child for that initial meeting with me, I ask them to emphasize that I am interested in talking with the adolescent about whatever he or she wishes to discuss. This, of course, may not correspond to the parents' concerns. But I am attempting from the outset to reduce the prospective patient's anticipation of being forced to do what the adults want; to convey my awareness of the importance of privacy and independence to the adolescent; and to communicate my wish that this experience be for his or her benefit, not for that of parents or myself. Implicit in this approach is my effort to begin demonstrating that the therapist has a perspective different from that of parents and other adults. While the therapist basically always takes the stance of the "good" parent, approaching adolescents in the manner that one would an adult rather than a child helps set such a tone.

IN OFFERING EXPLANATIONS TO ADOLESCENT PATIENTS AT ANY POINT DURING TREATMENT

Therapists have a tendency to overexplain to both younger and older adolescents. With respect to the former group, this tendency probably parallels the general inclination of adults to instruct, correct, and educate children. In the particular case of adolescent patients, this tendency often relates to underlying wishes, on the part of the therapist, to have the young adolescent conform, because many of the behaviors which bring adolescents to treatment are unsettling to adults. In the case of older adolescents, a tendency of therapists to overexplain may relate in part to certain underlying wishes that these fine young specimens, who are on the way up in their lives, be admiring of the therapist who, developmentally speaking, may well be at a point of relative decline in his or her life. Parenthetically, late adolescents will often become curious about you or your work, and ask questions about it. They may make veiled or direct references to wanting to become like you. Be careful and don't fall for the flattery, at least until you have convinced yourself that they are not trying to ascertain whether you can accept them not wanting to become like you. They wish the opposite of what they are implying, because they are working to achieve psychological independence from the compulsion to be influenced by others (autonomy).

IN MAKING INTERPRETATIONS TO ADOLESCENTS

Generally, when conducting therapy if one does not know what to interpret, one is well advised not to say anything. A therapist cannot be a "Great Stone Face" with adolescents, however, that is, too silent or too emotionally unresponsive. I have found that as much as anything can be axiomatic regarding psychotherapeutic technique, when in doubt about what to interpret, a therapist is much less likely to err with adolescents if he or she takes a stand on the side of the patient's efforts to feel more comfortably independent from the pervasive influence of parents. That is, one rarely goes wrong interpreting the adolescent's conflict over autonomy. (The word *autonomy* here refers to freedom from the compulsive, inhibiting psychological influence of others upon exercising one's developmental prerogatives.) Even in cases where the basic and most important issue involves the adolescent having felt rejected by his or her parents, I find it is usually safer from a technical standpoint to interpret the wish to feel comfortably autonomous before interpreting the patient's unrequited dependency yearnings. That is because adolescents are better able to acknowledge and face their vulnerability when they realize that their wish to be independent is respected and supported. If adolescents sense that you are allowing and appreciating their wishes for closeness rather than "encouraging dependency," they will be better able to reveal, share and bear such feelings. Wishes to be appreciated by the therapist, the counterpart in treatment of the adolescent's wishes to have been cherished by his or her parents, are an inevitable component of rejection conflicts. When the latter become evident, the therapist must demonstrate by his manner toward the adolescent patient that he values their time together. The several issues described in this paragraph will be illustrated in the case of Sam who developed an acute psychotic reaction during therapy (pp. 290–293).

THE EFFECT OF INTERPRETATIONS ON THE ADOLESCENT'S SELF-ESTEEM

Interpretations can predispose an adolescent to feeling like a child at a time when there is a desperate wish to assure oneself and others that one is self-sufficient. For this reason, I often preface interpretations or observations with such phrases as, "You may have already noticed this, but...", or "Are you suggesting that...," when the point I am trying to make may take off from the patient's observation, but is in fact somewhat tangential to the patient's point.

Furthermore, as part of the tendency noted above to want to impress late adolescent patients, therapists can experience an urge to make dazzling interpretations. In this regard, it is wise to always give the patient the "right of first refusal" before making interpretations. In fact, when he or she defers to you, the therapist is well-advised to press a bit more for the patient's ideas before presenting an interpretation. The dumber is the therapist, the smarter the adolescent has to become, which is what we are working toward achieving.

Lastly, the kind of behaviors and symptoms that bring adolescents to treatment are often troubling or threatening in some way to adults. This can incline therapists to clarify to the adolescent patient what he or she is doing wrong. In this regard adolescents are no different from other patients, and people in general; they fare better and become less defensive when helped to understand what is right about what they have been doing. I have *not* found that pointing out the adaptive effort in their behavior supports patients' rationalizations and increases their resistances. Rather, I have found the opposite more likely to occur, namely, they become less defensive. You are also demonstrating a different perspective than the adolescent expects from his or her parents and thus, by extension, from other adults as well.

The treatment will follow relatively naturally, especially if the adolescent senses that you are doing your utmost to understand what is troubling him (Frankel, 1994). In this regard, a point made earlier in the section entitled "Assessment" warrants repeating (p. 263): since adolescents often begin with complaints about parents or other people, the best way to help them move from the interpersonal to the intrapsychic where they live, is to hear their complaints without contradicting them, and then begin to explore their personal, internal reactions to these interpersonal complaints. (Very often, for example, their anger at other people masks/defends against awareness of their guilt. This was illustrated by Trisha whose stepfather had sexually abused her [p. 250].)

In their efforts to be neutral, fair, and to help the patient keep things in proper perspective, some therapists tend to immediately respond to an adolescent's diatribes against others by wondering what his or her own role has been in creating the troublesome situation. In my experience this approach does not usually produce further exploration by the adolescent. The adolescent will instead experience the therapist as an agent of parents or the environment rather than as a potential ally truly interested in understanding and helping him or her. The adolescent responds either by becoming more defensive or by complying with the therapist's implications of his or her culpability. The result of the former is that treatment bogs down, while the result of the latter is a superficially salutary outcome about which the therapist may revel in an illusion of success while the adolescent patient's underlying conflicts go unaddressed and therefore untreated. The best way to create a therapeutic environment where the adolescent can acknowledge his or her own contribution is through interested exploration which keeps the focus on the patient's experience.

ISSUES IN THE MAINTENANCE OF TREATMENT

THE ON AND OFF AGAIN NATURE OF THERAPY FOR SOME ADOLESCENTS

Because of the readiness with which an adolescent can feel his independence/autonomy threatened, the transference can frequently get overheated. In such situations, therapy can become an on-again, off-again phenomenon. Accepting this, and apprising the adolescent's parents that this is part of their child's developmental and therefore therapeutic process, can make one's life in treating them easier and perhaps their lives as well. It can also make the situation less awkward with their parents who may have to pay for missed appointments. This feature supports the wisdom of being willing to accept working on the developmental problem of that moment and waiting for the rest to come in its own good time:

> An 11-year-old girl with a very traumatic history was brought to therapy because of a serious symptom. She experienced symptomatic improvement over four or five months without seeming to have developed insight. At that juncture she suddenly refused to return to "that man" because, in her words, she could talk to her father instead, and preferred to do so. The therapist urged that she attend a final appointment, so she could see that he was not offended or hurt by her decision. She was brought in and that closure was effected.
>
> Four years later the girl insisted that her mother call the same therapist to get help for the girl's best friend who was experiencing a symptom similar to that which had precipitated her own earlier treatment. The therapist agreed to meet with the girl's friend only to make a referral. He explained his reason for doing so to the girl's mother: he did not want to treat her daughter's friend in case her daughter ever needed therapy again. And he maintained his position despite the parents' assurances that their daughter was symptom-free and faring very well.
>
> Four months later the parent called again, because the former patient herself was experiencing a severe recurrence of symptoms. The girl was willing to see the therapist and resumed treatment on an intensive basis which ended successfully several years later.

This therapist had no way of knowing that his former patient's symptoms would recur. The fact that the issues for which she had been treated were not resolved during the earlier period of therapy did not necessarily mean that her symptoms would return. Nor did the fact that the girl had her mother contact the therapist on her friend's behalf represent incontrovertible evidence that she herself would again have difficulties. At most that act suggested that she remembered the therapist as potentially helpful and not malignant, despite her adamant, precipitous termination. Nor can I be sure that the therapist could not have treated both girls concomitantly, though I am persuaded that it is always best to attempt to serve no more than one master. Therapy is difficult enough to conduct in the best of circumstances, so that one needs no additional complications. Issues of sibling rivalry, competitiveness, and survivor guilt are too rife in our population to risk encumbering the treatment of both patients if it can be avoided.

On the other hand, the proclivity of adolescents to break off treatment should not incline therapists toward a cavalier approach to their therapy. When an adolescent is pushing to terminate prematurely I always acknowledge the impossibility and undesirability of forcing him or her to continue, and I emphasize my wish not to do so in any event. I almost always ask, though, what the adolescent would think of me if he or she wanted to stop and I thought it premature but did not say so. This approach addresses the possibility that the adolescent is testing to see if the therapist really wants him or her to fall flat on his or her face; that is, the therapist does not want to help him or her work through his or her difficulties to greater true autonomy. So, this type of intervention deals with both sides of the conflict, the wish for independence and the need for assurance that the therapist wants the patient to achieve it. I take this approach even when I do not expect it will soften the adolescent's steely resolve to stop. In this latter situation, or in another common one in which an adolescent undertakes an evaluation but is reluctant to continue, it can be very helpful at times to tell him or her things from the evaluation to watch for as indicators of a more urgent need to work with a therapist. The fact that you are rendering him or her your considered opinion, as you would an adult, helps to soften the narcissistic blow of suggesting that the adolescent might harbor vulnerabilities at a time when it is important for him or her to be feeling symptom-free if not invincible. This approach also lessens the likelihood that the adolescent will experience such gratuitous information as a veiled threat in the form of a dire prediction, or as a reflection of the therapist's nose having been bent by the patient's rebuff. I provide the same information to the adolescent's parents.

In the opposite circumstance, whenever adolescents are willing to attend, I never question their motive and continue to see them, even if doing so is as seemingly unproductive as it appeared in the case of Sam (pp. 290–293) who burst forth with a psychosis after a couple years of seemingly unproductive therapy. If adolescents stay in treatment it is because they are aware at some level that they need assistance and that this forum holds out the hope of addressing that need.

TESTING BEHAVIOR

Many adolescents will flirt with danger under the guise of asserting their autonomy. They are trying to see if the therapist wants to control and direct them, or hover over them as do some parents. If they can convince themselves that the therapist is this way, then they can feel freer to rebel and to experience their conflicts as interpersonal, between the therapist and patient, rather than intrapsychic. So, one must be careful about intervening too much or directing too much. But one should never feel cowed by their assertions of autonomy into refraining from pointing out truly self-defeating behavior. For not doing so will communicate to them that deep down the therapist wants them to fail. In doing so, the therapist would confirm their fear that he or she is uncomfortable with their true independence. This kind of issue can arise around premature efforts to terminate treatment. Guilty adolescents who feel uncomfortable about becoming successful through therapy will often try to terminate prematurely under the guise of asserting their autonomy. They will argue that if the therapist agrees that they should be the masters of their own destiny, then they should be able to terminate their treatment now. In such cases, in addition to pointing out what may be the specific underlying dynamic, it makes sense to observe that assertion of autonomy and premature termination are different issues.

TRANSFERENCE AND EXTERNALIZATION

Adolescents are very prone to transfer and particularly to externalize current attitudes toward parents onto therapists, though this process may be observed most prominently in their defenses against transference. (The case of the young paranoid man in chapter 7 [pp. 200–202] demonstrated how quickly this can arise and jeopardize the continuation of treatment.) It makes good sense for therapists to capitalize upon this fact to its fullest for enlightenment about the patient even if not for making interpretations. This can be especially valuable with younger adolescents who are not forthcoming. The therapist can often discern a reenactment within the therapy hours of some important, ongoing experiences.

> Within a few weeks after beginning treatment, a 12-year-old, longtime latchkey child would arrive at the office, call his mother at her work (purportedly at her insistence), and then sit in the therapist's chair, eating crackers from a canister there, and staring silently at the therapist. The therapist thought that the lad was replaying his experience upon returning home every day. Thus, rather than picking up on other issues suggested by this material (i.e., competition; identification with the aggressor therapist in usurping his "throne"; orality), the therapist asked the boy what he does each day after school.

If you ask yourself, with respect to everything an adolescent tells you, "What is he or she trying to find out about me?" frequently you will find that they are attempting to determine whether you share their parents' view of their attitudes and behavior. If they can demonstrate to their satisfaction that you do, and adolescents are masters at doing so, then they will be inclined to recapitulate the family situation in your office in nonproductive ways or else they will soon leave treatment. (The readiness with which the transference can become intensified by even subtle actions on the part of the therapist was demonstrated in the case of Alan, chapter 7 [pp. 217–219], when I was increasing the frequency of his sessions.)

SELF-REVELATION ON THE PART OF THE THERAPIST

> A 13-year-old, learning disabled lad, who had been acting as if he were unperturbed by his parents' separation, came into a session wanting to see "if people in your generation are as smart as this one." He then began to quiz the therapist about state capitals, which he was studying at school. Several sessions later, during which he had reported his family's impending move, he complained about having to come to therapy and he began asking where the therapist was born. The therapist tried to avoid answering that question directly and the patient then started naming the

home of origin of all members of his family. He was born in Los Angeles, Michigan; his father in Detroit, Arkansas; his mother in Little Rock, Michigan; etc.

The lad's wish to leave therapy and his question about the therapist's birthplace suggested to the therapist that the anticipated move was reactivating the lad's unresolved feelings about his parents' separation. Since the boy had not acknowledged his feelings about the parental separation, the therapist had little confidence that a transference interpretation about feelings associated with leaving the therapist would be productive. So, he simply observed that perhaps he was telling the therapist that everyone in his family was not where he felt they should be. The lad became thoughtful, less contentious, and stopped asking about the therapist's birthplace, though this particular theme was not further developed at that session.

Therapists can feel a strong pull to respond directly to requests like that in the last example (i.e., for the therapist's birthplace), but therapists differ in the value or dangers they ascribe to self-disclosure. I rarely have found that it facilitates the therapy but I am uncertain about whether it is invariably harmful. The essential problem is that the specific information revealed by the therapist can inhibit the adolescent from bringing up whatever he or she wishes. For the information disclosed by the therapist is often experienced, accurately or inaccurately, by the adolescent patient as something about which the therapist might be sensitive. Therefore, these become areas about which the patient must be careful and censor what he or she says directly to the therapist. This potential problem is probably greatest when the self-disclosure is about the therapist's personal involvements (i.e., spouse or children). Acknowledgment of having children of one's own will invariably set up a situation in which the patient finds it difficult to share his or her wishes for a special relationship with the therapist; he or she will feel that he or she has been preempted from that by the therapist's family. So, such self-revelation is basically unfair to the patient, by virtue of limiting his or her freedom in the therapy situation.

It is possible that there are exceptions to this conclusion, but I suspect they are few and far between. For example, a patient who fears that a parent is possessive and thus anticipates a similar attitude from the therapist as well, might experience relief upon learning that the therapist has a family. If the adolescent patient receives this information early in therapy before the existence of that dynamic of possessiveness has been established, then the opportunity to gain insight into that crucial issue has been compromised by the therapist's revelation. And in my experience, if this issue comes up late in therapy and somehow requires a direct answer from the therapist, then there is a countertransference problem, because the therapist has communicated possessiveness to the patient rather than enlightenment about this issue of fearing being trapped in dependency by a parent.

Notwithstanding what I have just described, one does get the impression that some therapists do not perceive self-revelation about many issues to be problematic. For example, case reports of Selma Fraiberg, who numbers amongst the most widely quoted child therapists, convey this impression. The theoretical justifications for self-disclosure involve the need to create optimal conditions in which the ego of a patient who is developmentally suspicious of the therapist can function; the hope that the therapist's openness will serve as a model for the young adolescent; the notion that the new/real object (as opposed to the transference) component of the therapeutic relationship is more important for adolescents than for adult patients; and that self-disclosure will make the therapist seem less rejecting to the patient, and thus, for example, not like a pompous or withholding parent. Even in such cases, I try to buy time by telling the adolescent that if it is truly important that he or she know thus or such about me, I will tell them when we finish our work together. I have only revealed my marital status on the extremely rare occasions when it was known to the child from another source, as in the example which follows. If one concludes that it is advantageous to reveal anything about one's self during ongoing treatment, the likelihood of therapeutic gain is maximized if the adolescent's motives for wanting the revelation are understood.

A 12-year-old girl was dragged into therapy because of school failure and predelinquent behavior. After several sessions she commandeered the therapist's chair and kept it from that day forward.

She then began wondering if the therapist were married. She brooked no manner of evasion of the "Let's see what you'd think if I were or weren't" variety. In fact, she readily revealed an important, immediate determinant of this wish to know the therapist's marital status: Her symptoms had begun in reaction to her parents' separation the previous year. Problems at school had prompted personnel there to urge her mother to seek treatment for her. Her father, who sorely wished for a reconciliation, and toward whom the girl was trying to remain loyal as her mother became involved with another man, did not want his daughter treated. Her father resented the mother's boyfriend who was a psychiatrist; and her father shared a repeated joke with his daughter that people become psychiatrists because they want or need to see a psychiatrist and that they are usually divorced.

Her interrogation continued at the next session. This time she also wondered whether other kids from her school were seen by the therapist. She then chanced to say, looking up from under her eyebrows, that she knew that the therapist was married. She asked if the therapist knew Tom Jackson, her teacher. The therapist allowed that he did, and then learned that Mr. Jackson had told her that the therapist's wife had previously taught at that school. The therapist acknowledged that, feeling that there was nothing therapeutic to be gained by deceit in such a circumstance and not wanting to place the teacher in an unfavorable light.

The girl then began to again ask if the therapist were divorced. She did not appear perturbed, but rather imperiously and disdainfully demanded to know. The therapist reminded her of her father's view of psychiatrists, and asked, "Look, if I said I were not divorced, that would cast your dad in a poor light, and what good would that do?" The girl answered, "My father said psychiatrists *usually* are divorced." The therapist responded, "Which kind do you want me to be?" The child said softly, "The other kind." The therapist allowed that he was married. The girl literally expelled a sigh of relief, became red-faced briefly, and the therapist thought he heard her utter sotto voce, "Oh good." She then went on to ask whether the therapist had children, as well as whether he treated other children from her school, all of which questions the therapist did not directly answer.

OTHER VIEWS OF THERAPY DURING ADOLESCENCE

Much of the literature on the psychological treatment of adolescents is psychoanalytically oriented. It offers widely differing views ranging from pessimism to optimism about the possibility of treating adolescents. The problems presented by the adolescents' sexual and aggressive drives have been given foremost consideration in addressing this question about undertaking their treatment. The pessimists emphasize problems arising from two interrelated factors. The intensity of those drives threatens to overload the adolescent patient's ability to keep them in check. And forming a relationship with a therapist becomes anathema to adolescents because it threatens to throw them right back into the kind of dependent relationship from which they are trying to escape with respect to their parents. In the words of Anna Freud (1958), "the analytic treatment of adolescents is a hazardous venture from beginning to end, a venture in which the analyst has to meet resistances of unusual strength and variety" (p. 261); "One cannot analyze in adolescence. It is like running next to an express train" (quoted by Geleerd, 1957). In addition to the overwhelming quality of resistances which was also noted by Geleerd (1957), a rapidly changing presentation which requires multiple techniques (Eissler, 1958), and the overriding need for synthesis of the personality rather than analysis (Gitelson, 1948) have been advanced as prime sources of difficulty in treating adolescents.

Some psychoanalytic theoreticians assume that the problem presented by adolescents' impulses is that of being caught between childhood and adulthood. Unlike children, adolescents can no longer allow themselves to rely upon a parent to serve as an auxiliary ego or conscience in their efforts to cope with instinct. Unlike adults, adolescents do not have the inner stability which allows them to please their own conscience by controlling impulses, because they are in the process of integrating their own standards of conduct. While there is merit to those points, more so in some cases than others, that position overstates the issues. For as I pointed out in the chapters on development, the maturation of drives is not invariably tied to the desire to emancipate in the manner described by psychoanalytic theory. Also, adolescents normally look to parents to prevent them from letting their impulses get out of control. While they do not want to form new relationships of a parent–child variety, they nevertheless expect adults to aid their own efforts to keep impulses from overwhelming them to their detriment.

With respect to the other issue, that of forming a therapeutic relationship, Gitelson (1948) considers the problem to be a difficulty finding the proper emotional distance in treating an adolescent. Their unwillingness to relate to therapists leaves the latter without the benefits of transference which both facilitate understanding of the adolescents' inner life and help hold patients in treatment during difficult periods. Clearly such a view does not apply to all adolescents. Some do simply reject therapists; others form intense transferences which, as illustrated earlier (p. 272), can motivate them to break off treatment; still others work well in therapy and psychoanalysis. Yet, the type of difficulties reported above have led to an idea that only very passive individuals who are chronologically adolescent but developmentally preadolescent will accept treatment, and they remain unchanged by it (Anthony, 1970). In my experience the ego dystonicity of patients' symptoms (the degree to which their symptoms are experienced as bothersome by them), is a greater factor in determining an adolescent's willingness to stay in treatment than his or her relative passivity. Some authors emphasize that dogged determination is required for the arduous task of keeping adolescents and their parents in treatment because of the intensity of their collective resistance to change (Masterson, 1969).

By contrast, other psychoanalytic therapists remain more sanguine about the possibilities of therapy for this group. They view the psychically unsettled nature of adolescents, whose egos are threatened by instinctual forces, as offering a ripe opportunity for defense analysis. The outcome of this is strengthening of the ego in order to master threatening unconscious mental contents (Settlage, 1974b). Therapists of the more optimistic persuasion take pains to assure the hegemony of ego over id, even to the point of advocating much preparatory advance work with parents of early adolescents (Fraiberg, 1955). This technical approach, which emphasizes strengthening the ego's efforts to master anxiety, is congruent with the ideas I am presenting from a more adaptive standpoint.

Most psychoanalytic writers report that adolescents are much more willing to engage in therapy after they have successfully disengaged themselves from the incestuous ties to their parents that have lingered or resurged since childhood. It is generally true that the average expectable older adolescent is more willing to engage in psychotherapy than the average expectable young adolescent. In my experience, as I noted, however, the willingness for therapeutic help is predicated more on the degree to which adolescents feel themselves to be suffering.

Adatto (1958) finds that after late adolescents in analysis have accomplished that goal of "object removal" (Katan, 1937),[3] they experience a latency period during which they capitalize upon these developmental gains in their outside life and lose interest in further analysis. Adatto's observation is consistent with my point that adolescents are trying to complete their development; and when they feel they have done so, they want to continue on their own. As I have taken pains to point out throughout this book, however, conflicts that traditional psychoanalysis has attributed to instinctual drives are often not the most important hindrances to completing one's development.

STRENGTHENING THE EGOS OF YOUNG ADOLESCENTS

It has been noted both that young adolescents, those in the fifth through ninth grade age range, are often more difficult to engage in treatment than older adolescents, but that they can gain from ego strengthening (Settlage, 1974b). They are too old to engage in play therapy but many do not yet feel ready to talk to a therapist. I have found that with this group a concerted effort must be made to find some area of their interest. Generally this involves what they are doing well or trying to do well. The therapeutic tack starts with reinforcing and supporting and encouraging their accomplishments in that area. Accentuation of the positive, underscoring the adaptive aspects of what they are willing to tell you of their behaviors (i.e., pointing out the sense in what they are doing rather than the lack of sense), and demonstrating the seriousness with which you take their views by incorporating these into all decisions about their therapy, is often responded to by improvement in young adolescents without

---

[3]"Object removal" refers to a definitive separation via the defense mechanism of displacement from the parent to a new love object.

much insight being shared or imparted. Always finding something positive to impart about patients and their work with you
to parents or other caretakers is an important auxiliary aspect of
working with these patients.

WORKING WITH PARENTS OF ADOLESCENT PATIENTS

Given the adolescent's developmental imperative to emancipate,
I look to limiting my contact with his or her parents to the least
necessary intervention that is required to maintain the patient in
therapy. This can vary greatly, of course, depending upon the
nature of the adolescent's symptoms. Although I do not encourage parental involvement in the therapy, I do not want the parents to feel isolated from me. So, when I explain to them at the
beginning of treatment my rationale for not meeting regularly
with them, I nevertheless emphasize that I want them to feel that
they can have access to me at any time, both to impart anything
they want me to know and to ask whatever questions they have
for me. I urge them to forewarn their adolescent, however, for
by doing so he or she will not feel that they are trying to collude
with me behind their son or daughter's back. Also, if he or she
has been apprised of the parent's wish to speak with me, I can
bring the matter up directly with the adolescent patient without
compromising the parent's credibility in the adolescent's eyes.
While this approach works best, parents often wish to share observations without their adolescent knowing, because, for example, they don't want to appear as if they are tattling on their
child. In situations where the parents and I cannot find a way of
enabling them to broach the matter with their adolescent, I
would still rather have the parent feel free to speak with me, and
I look for material from the patient to explore the issue of the
parent's concern. In other words, I would rather live with feeling
a little duplicitous than have the parents feel they do not have
recourse to sharing their concerns with me. In times past when
the child guidance approach was popular, this problem was mitigated by having the parents see another therapist, and by the
therapists then conferring. I have never been persuaded that this
aspect of the child guidance model was preferable to the parent

having access to the adolescent's therapist, unless the parents were working on specific problems of their own with the other therapist. Even if that is so, the meaning to adolescents of information about them coming from the parents' therapist can never be salutary; for the issue of therapist indiscretion will always be raised in the patient's mind, and the trustworthiness of the adolescent's therapist is tarred by the brush of the revelations of the parents' therapist.

In some cases it becomes necessary to intervene on the adolescent's behalf. An example is lobbying for an adolescent to get certain freedoms from parents who feel, with justification in some circumstances, that the adolescent's behavior does not warrant the privilege in question. Well-meaning and well-intentioned parents can be holding to the very reasonable, traditional dictum that one's privileges as an adolescent are contingent upon exhibiting an equivalent level of responsibility. While always a good standard, some adolescents and their parents get locked into a battle around this matter, and adolescents conclude that their parents simply do not want them to succeed or move ahead or have what their peers have. In such circumstances it sometimes makes most sense for the therapist to explain this situation to the parents in encouraging them "to give a little"; in demonstrating their flexibility, the impasse between them and their adolescent can be broken. The adolescent may then identify with their flexibility and become a bit more flexible in turn.

In other cases, as that of Julie (pp. 294–296), who presented as psychotic and initially difficult to engage, the therapist must maintain frequent contact with the parents both to execute the treatment and to allay their anxiety about their adolescent's illness and their ability to manage the patient at home.

Pressures are, at times, brought to bear on the adolescent's parents from other areas of the adolescent's life, such as school. In such cases, it may be necessary to see parents more often to help them deal with difficulties presented to them from the other institution, as well as trying to find ways of reducing tension between themselves and the adolescent at home. In general, the goal is always the same. It is to help the parents become better able to reinstitute the age-appropriate parenting function for their adolescent and to fulfill the sponsorship function appropriately. This is accomplished technically by framing for them the developmental issues their child is facing, and explaining the sense (adaptive purpose) of their adolescent's behaviors, preferably with the patient's permission. At times this work includes helping parents bear via sharing with them the level of anxiety engendered by an adolescent whose experimentation or withholding is more than can be borne with equanimity by the parents (and may well be worrisome to the therapist too).

Since the problem for adolescents is intrapsychic, they must deal with the exigencies of their lives irrespective of their parents' behavior toward them. Thus, in general terms, working with parents is not something which assumes a role of any significance in my treatment of adolescents. That caveat notwithstanding, there is a spectrum of involvement that therapists have with the parents of adolescents.

CASE EXAMPLES

I will now describe in more detail the treatment of some types of cases that were not discussed in the last chapter.

OBSESSIONAL DISORDER: MALCOLM

Malcolm, a 13-year-old black youth, developed frightening, intrusive, obsessional thoughts a couple of months after entering junior high school (seventh grade). His initial preoccupations, precipitated by newspaper accounts of local witchcraft activity, were that he and his mother were members of that coven and that she would go to Hell. Then, to his horror, he began thinking that he would kill his mother, the person he loved most. Within a month after their onset, Malcolm's tormenting obsessions were shifting and spreading to thoughts that he was going crazy, would murder or rape someone, and end up in prison. These ideas panicked and depressed him.

Malcolm had been an easy baby who developed into a nonaggressive, popular, good student in his racially mixed neighborhood. His mother had always doted upon him, and Malcolm had always felt un-self-consciously fond and proud of his young mother. In fact he joked that soon she might be mistaken for his date. Although their mutual admiration persisted, physical expressions of affection between them had faded away in a natural manner as Malcolm became adolescent. Malcolm was exhibiting evidence of emancipatory urges in his preference to be with friends and in occasional complaints to his parents that he felt embarrassed and bored when with them in public. Malcolm felt some compunction about these sentiments because he realized they pained his mother.

Malcolm's father was an autoworker whose severe drug problem had come to a head when Malcolm was 7 years old. At that time his mother left with Malcolm for a year. Malcolm had always been a bit standoffish with his father. Yet, he had been very frightened by the separation, fearful that he would never see his father again, worried about him, and eager for the reconciliation. His father subsequently stopped using drugs by turning to a fundamentalist religion which became the center of his life. Malcolm now approached adolescence with his father's frequent admonition that Malcolm would likely become a drug addict because he had been one.

Malcolm was referred to a therapist to whom he related the history of his illness. The therapist told him that his obsessional ideas seemed to be Malcolm's way of punishing himself, and added that their task was to determine why Malcolm felt he deserved to be punished. Malcolm responded that in a vague way he could sense the accuracy of the therapist's observation. He himself thought that his symptoms were "10 percent" due to his father's admonitions that Malcolm would become a drug user, and "90 percent" due to worries about peer pressures he anticipated at junior high school. He sensed that his symptoms were somehow related to his conflict between wanting to drop long-time friends who clung to him and join a more popular group at his new shool.

Following that session Malcolm's obsessions became temporarily supplanted by devastating thoughts that other kids would not like him and that he would have no friends. Exploration of his fear of losing friends brought to light the fact that although other kids could criticize him, Malcolm never responded in kind. That material prompted the therapist to interpret Malcolm's "omnipotence conflict": Since Malcolm didn't deserve their criticism but never "fought back," Malcolm must feel himself better able than his peers to take criticism. Thus, underneath his mild and accommodating exterior, Malcolm must experience himself as stronger than other kids, since he was better able to tolerate abuse. Malcolm also worried that he would say the "wrong thing" to peers whom he wanted to impress and they would reject him. The therapist pointed out that Malcolm must fear that even his casual utterances could have a devastating impact on other people. Such interpretations of his omnipotence conflicts brought forth new themes. Malcolm realized that any critical thoughts he harbored toward friends or others were immediately followed by self-critical thoughts. Analysis of this defense of undoing made Malcolm aware that under his mild, accommodating exterior he did feel angry toward a number of people.

Malcolm realized that all the other students laughed when one of his male teachers would yell at them for being noisy during class, but Malcolm became scared and wanted them to quiet down. He didn't know what the teacher would do when angered. This led Malcolm to recall that he had not known what his father would do when he became angry while on drugs. At those times Malcolm would feel confused and fearful and would do whatever his father asked, in an effort to quell his father's anger. Malcolm spontaneously linked those experiences to his own fears that he would lose control if he became angry. (Since Malcolm never lost control, that idea was a defensive identification with his father.) He recalled wondering if he had caused his mother and father to fight and his father to leave. He was able to relate those earlier fears of never seeing his father again to his subsequent fears of losing his friends if he said the wrong thing. Subsequent to his parents' separation, whenever he encountered a problem with anyone, Malcolm's first reaction was to ask himself what he had done to cause it. Such material helped clarify how the traumatic experiences associated with his father's drug use precipitated concerns in Malcolm about his influence over and responsibility for his parents' separation during his childhood. These conclusions had frightened him then and were now complicating his adolescent emancipation because those concerns had been transferred to friends. Furthermore, dating from the time when his father began to recover, five years earlier, Malcolm had lost his confidence with peers and had developed a vaguely formulated but compelling idea that symptoms in himself would somehow keep his father from backsliding into drug use. That superstitious fantasy suggested emancipatory or survivor guilt.

Following these recollections and insights about his irrational guilt and feelings of responsibility for the prior family problems, Malcolm recalled more about his parents' fighting, and his symptoms diminished. He now found himself acting more self-assertively with peers. Whenever he became angry toward friends, however, he became fearful that his anger would drive them away. Then, as he began to remain asymptomatic at such times and felt confident that he was overcoming his illness, he would immediately develop symptoms. This continuing recourse to the defense mechanism of undoing, albeit in his mind, suggested that Malcolm still did not feel that he deserved to be symptom-free.

Malcolm now found himself becoming untypically angry toward his mother who observed that Malcolm was acting in a very self-centered way and was inconsiderate of her. Malcolm dismissed the therapist's suggestion that he was turning his childhood love for his mother into an opposite attitude in an effort to feel more truly independent from her. Malcolm responded that he had always been close to his mother and would never want to hurt her. He was more receptive to the therapist's idea that he might be displacing anger from his more restrictive father onto his more lenient mother. Fears of becoming a homosexual then replaced those of going crazy, raping, and murdering, and his depression deepened. This sequence suggested that Malcolm's guilt about emancipating had an oedipal component. For after the therapist had emphasized Malcolm's positive feelings for his mother and negative attitudes toward his father, Malcolm developed the intrusive idea of becoming homosexual, which would reduce the threat he posed to either parent in an oedipal constellation. Such a position hardly afforded a young, heterosexual adolescent any comfort, and he became more depressed.

As Malcolm began to recognize the pervasiveness of this pattern of becoming anxious when symptom-free, he began to sit with his symptoms longer, rather than immediately attempting to forcefully dismiss them by telling himself that they were self-punishment. As he allowed himself to entertain unpleasant thoughts longer, he realized that since age 11 he had been growing away from his mother, whom he loved, and that separation anxiety and his mother were somehow related to his symptoms. He couldn't understand how his love for her could be changed in his mind to fear of her dying and to thoughts of killing her. The therapist pointed out that maybe the emancipation process was difficult for his mother as well; his mother confirmed this. Malcolm's thoughts of her death reflected his fear of the impact of his emancipation on her. Malcolm then related his current-day fears of making girls cry to his earlier reactions when observing his mother crying while his father was using drugs.

At this juncture, after $1^1/2$ years of weekly psychotherapy, Malcolm was becoming quite familiar with his omnipotence concerns and his use of undoing, and his symptoms were markedly diminished. After two years of therapy Malcolm was contending with his parents in ways typical of emancipating youth—arguing, devaluing them, at times being rude, exhibiting some sneaky behavior—but all well tempered. His emancipatory guilt, the feeling that his advancement would hurt his mother and harm his father, was less evident. By the time he entered high school (ninth grade), Malcolm had been asymptomatic for several months. He experienced no recurrence of symptoms there and was approaching and talking with new and old friends easily and enjoying peer relationships. Therapy was phased out at the rate he requested over a six-month period.

Three years later Malcolm was symptom-free and performing well in all areas of his life. This case illustrates several points I have been making about the relationship between development and psychopathology and therapy in adolescents:

1. The influence of earlier real experiences on the emancipatory process and the importance of developmental considerations in understanding psychopathology in adolescents. Without this perspective one would be inclined to understand Malcolm's illness as a typical obsessional neurosis based on an unresolved oedipal conflict.

2. The technical approach utilized was that of psychoanalysis, namely defense analysis and interpretation. This began with pointing out his resistance, namely the omnipotence concerns that he could bear hurt and criticism better than others and thus must feel stronger than others underneath his mild, compliant exterior. This interpretative line was followed by evidence that he was using the defense of undoing. The guilt which motivated the undoing defense in turn served to maintain repression of his anger/aggression. The latter was frightening to this lad because of the dual problems presented by his father's fearsome behaviors when using drugs and his mother's strong affinity for Malcolm. Both of these features (father's fearsomeness and mother's preference) would tend to intensify Malcolm's normative oedipal strivings; these would then have to be defended against more rigorously. This was accomplished by reversal of his aggression into mildness and compliance and ultimately by regression to an obsessional state.

3. The foregoing formulation, while accurate dynamically to a point, fails to explicate why the illness occurred when it did—in early adolescence. Here the importance of the developmental process of adolescence as precipitant becomes evident, and the material illustrates a different meaning to what would have been considered a resurgent or persistent oedipal conflict. Malcolm's

wishes for new friends and fears of hurting old ones represented a displacement from his conflict about growing away from his mother. She herself, while resigned to and supportive of it, at times communicated her own unhappiness about Malcolm's inevitable need to emancipate; this engendered emancipatory guilt. Furthermore, the traumatic effect of his father's previous behaviors when using drugs had been to create or heighten feelings of responsibility in Malcolm regarding any problems he encountered in his relationships with other people. These included fear that self-assertion would have a bad effect on others and fear of retaliation for noncompliant behavior. This factor intensified his emancipatory guilt, giving it the character of survivor guilt. Thus, Malcolm was inhibited, by both the quality of past relationships with his parents and by the effects of trauma, from being able to use his peer group as a successful displacement away from parents. Rather, the conflict itself became displaced onto peers, in the form of exaggerated fears that breaking away from old friends would hurt them. He punished himself for this by fearing that he would be left alone. This is what he feared he had caused his father to experience during Malcolm's childhood, and what he now feared he would cause his mother to experience. So, Malcolm's emancipatory guilt became augmented to pathological survivor guilt by omnipotence concerns derived from the psychically traumatic experiences around his father's addiction, losses of behavioral control, and separation from the family.

PSYCHOSES

The choice of treatment modality for any adolescent should rarely if ever be made solely on the basis of symptoms. The latter proviso applies even to the decision to utilize medication in cases of psychosis for which there is probably the most clear-cut justification for medicinal treatment of adolescents. This view is "contrarian" to currently popular approaches which, espousing a medical model, emphasize diagnostic labeling of symptom clusters as the basis for therapeutic intervention. Actually, the approach I am recommending seems closer to the model of internal medicine which considers pathophysiology, not simply symptoms as the basis for diagnosis and treatment. For with respect to psychopathology, it is imperative to understand the adolescent's symptoms in relation to what he or she is trying to accomplish developmentally. This is because the degree of inner pressure some adolescents experience to emancipate and the wider range of options they have (compared to those of younger children) for expressing conflicts and interim solutions, can give rise to symptoms that are skewed toward appearing more serious, entrenched, and bizarre than they may actually be. Thus, there is an equally apt counterpart to the medication-oriented psychiatrists' appropriate caveat that patients should neither be denied relief-bringing medication nor made to feel psychologically inadequate nor morally weak when faced with illness which is biochemical in nature and out of the patient's control. The counterpoint is that it is equally unacceptable for an individual in the throes of his psychological development to be deprived of the invaluable, developmentally maturing opportunity to strengthen his ego and his self-esteem through insight-oriented and therapeutically enhanced tension tolerance by being told that cure is out of his control and comes in the form of pills.

SAM: PSYCHOSIS OCCURRING IN A CONTEXT WHICH ALLOWED FOR PSYCHOTHERAPEUTIC TREATMENT

Sam,[4] an 18-year-old high school senior, was referred because of school failure. He was attending school but not classes, spending his days in the student center with newfound friends after having endured several years of a relatively friendless existence. He considered himself socially immature, never a self-starter, and a mediocre student despite high intelligence. Sam was the youngest of seven children. His father was a physician who tended to be hypercritical of his children. Sam's mother was a warm, candid former nurse who enjoyed her children, but may not have had enough time to devote to her youngest. She observed that they probably had not protected Sam sufficiently from the teasing and tormenting of his older sibs, particularly the two next older sisters. No other telling developmental history was elicited and there was no family history of serious mental illness.

---

[4]This case was described in more detail in an article illustrating that distrust, developing from the individual's real experiences in his family, is the common core of paranoia and depression (Bloch, 1989).

Two years of twice-weekly psychotherapy failed to reveal the source of Sam's difficulties. He talked only about his social activities; was dropped from school; and continued to do nothing more than spend time with his friends. The therapist could not understand why Sam continued to see him. During the second year, when his parents requested for financial reasons that Sam's sessions be reduced to every other week, the therapist was surprised that Sam felt he ought to see the therapist weekly, even if for shorter sessions. Under that new schedule of half-hour, weekly sessions there still seemed to be no movement.

Then, after two years, Sam suddenly burst forth with psychotic paranoia and depression. The depression was manifested in self-condemnation, despair, suicidal thoughts, severe sleep disturbance, and difficulty concentrating. The paranoia was evident in his conviction that people were reading his thoughts and that an expanding network of knowledge about him was developing in which people were trying to encourage him to go out with girls. Radio songs contained specific reference to him in this regard. He could not leave home unaccompanied because he feared people looking at him, knowing about him, and trying to influence him. He was seething at home, throwing knives into doors, frightening his parents.

At that juncture Sam claimed that the therapist was the only person he trusted, though he had some reservations about him as well. When describing his delusions to the therapist he said that the therapist did not have to agree with his view, but that the therapist had to be on his side. The therapist could be neutral but he did not want the therapist to be against him. All he could say about the onset of his illness was that he had begun to feel that his friends wanted him to start dating girls and, by innuendo, were trying to push him to do so. Their "pressure" had made him more aware of his own inner conflict in the matter. For he wanted to date, but was "scared to death of girls." Thus, he faced an insoluble conflict.

The therapist, unsure of the basis of this psychosis, interpreted primarily from the content of Sam's material and was guided by his responses: He told Sam that his best guess was that Sam was attempting to free himself from childhood attachments to his family (i.e., the issue of adolescent emancipation). Since he had rarely criticized other family members, negative feelings, rather than positive ones, might be the source of his difficulty in emancipating. Also, domination by his older sisters might have rendered him fearful of being trapped by girls. If these speculations were accurate, then Sam might have to feel more independent before he could comfortably date girls. The therapist also suggested that Sam might feel guilty about functioning more independently. In response, Sam recalled never having felt like a member of his family. He had felt accepted only as the family baby, and continued to see himself in that role. The therapist interpreted the persistence of that role in Sam's mind as his effort to gain the approval of his family by complying with what he perceived made him acceptable to them. Sam then recalled his own feelings of sibling rivalry, that is, his wishes to compete with and advance in relation to his sibs, and he felt less paranoid.

The existence of guilt beneath his paranoia and depression soon became apparent. He was feeling intensely pressured by cars honking outside his home at night. He felt the drivers were trying to get him to go out with girls. He said, "I feel like I either have to comply or kill one of them (drivers)." The therapist reflected that Sam could only feel so pressured if he felt guilty about not complying with their wishes, and why so guilty? "Because they're right," he replied. The therapist then interpreted the issue of autonomy again, by first asking in a doubtful tone, "They know you better than you know yourself?" The therapist added that since Sam shared his friends' wish that he date, but felt doomed to failure if he tried now, what would be wrong with waiting until he felt he could succeed? After that Sam felt better able to control his moods, and went for longer periods without feeling paranoid and depressed. And he recalled earlier life experiences—aggressive outbursts when frustrated by his siblings; sadistic, selfish wishes; violent fantasies. He also recognized his long-standing defense against such wishes, in remarking, "I'm almost phobic about offending people." He felt this attitude (i.e., omnipotence concerns) had significantly hindered his development and he associated it to similar parental behaviors—they could criticize their children but not other people.

Sam seemed better, so his family and friends began to extend social invitations to him. As he declined these, his paranoia and depression would recur. This sequence helped confirm that his symptoms defended against guilt that was aroused when he did not comply with the wishes of others.

He recognized this issue of discomfort over asserting himself in the transference; for he struggled against a compulsion to find historical data to confirm the therapist's interpretations. He had always consciously avoided looking at the therapist and thinking about the therapist's possible reactions to whatever he said, for fear of not being able to talk to him. He then recalled the first time he hit his next sister, when he was 4 years old, and she crumpled. He had subsequently wished for but feared the power associated with that aggressive self-assertion that had made her fold. So, he gained insight into the development of "omnipotence" fantasies in his early childhood that intruded upon his freedom to assert himself as an adolescent. His sibling rivalry, his anger, and his anxiety about the impact of aggressive behavior toward his sister had contributed to this constellation.

Two years after the outbreak of symptoms, Sam was procrastinating about returning to school. He claimed this was because he feared failure. The therapist interpreted that as a reversal: to the contrary, Sam basically felt guilty about the possibility of succeeding and becoming independent. (Recall that Sam felt acceptable only as the family baby; the price of security was immaturity.) Very shortly thereafter he took the high school equivalency test. During the following year Sam and his therapist explored his "omnipotent" concerns that his success would devastate others.

Three years after the outbreak of symptoms, Sam decided to enter college because, in his words, he felt "no pressure from inside or outside myself" to do so. During the next year, he reported experiencing his feelings more freely. He felt that his discomfort over succeeding stemmed from an equation in his mind between succeeding and sadistically dominating, that is, badly hurting, others. At this juncture, $3^1/2$ years after becoming symptomatic, his associations suggested more oedipal-type conflicts than the therapist's earlier interpretations of guilt over succeeding had brought to consciousness.

Sam also spoke meaningfully about his long-standing wish from childhood to be loved, but never having felt loved and therefore not lovable. He claimed that his fear of succeeding, that is, of completing his development, was the threat of losing love, and that the bedrock of his paranoia was a general sense of being disapproved of and not liked by his family. So he held himself back to gain their approval/acceptance by remaining immature. He was feeling progressively better "without any reason for it."

This case illustrates how the prototypic developmental conflict of adolescence I have posited emerges in the course of the therapeutic exploration with a psychotic patient. The psychotherapeutic approach involved encouraging Sam to think, make decisions involving himself, and act autonomously. This was accomplished technically by the therapist's questions about what was wrong with doing things when he felt ready, rather than at the behest of others. These interventions were aimed at relieving his guilt over functioning autonomously. That guilt, which kept him from moving forward, enabled him to avoid awareness of his conundrum, namely that he would lose the tenuously felt love of his parents if he were other than the family baby.

This case also illustrates the value of keeping an adolescent in treatment if he or she wishes this, even if you are not convinced that progress is being made. For in my experience such adolescents invariably have a very good reason for staying. And since the developmental imperative of adolescents is to emancipate, therapists need not worry that adolescent patients will become "too dependent" on them.

It also bears repeating, in this age of ready recourse to medicating adolescents, that if one has a therapeutic relationship with a youth and a stable home environment, it is possible to treat even some psychotic reactions psychotherapeutically. This approach is always advantageous because it affirms the youth's capacity for self-control through self-awareness and bearing painful affects—a vital developmental acquisition. I will contrast this with the next case in which the circumstances under which the treatment began were markedly different and dictated the treatment approach.

JULIE: PSYCHOSIS OCCURRING IN CIRCUMSTANCES WHICH DID NOT ALLOW FOR EXCLUSIVELY PSYCHOTHERAPEUTIC TREATMENT

Having been unable to secure help closer to home, in desperation a farmer from an outlying area called a psychiatrist in a relatively distant city. Speaking laconically, he characterized his 21-year-old daughter as being under stress and agitated. The psychiatrist agreed to see them that day.

Julie arrived with her parents and indicated by her hesitation that she wished her mother to accompany her into the psychiatrist's office where she remained mute save for occasional isolated words unrelated to the conversation between her mother and the psychiatrist. She was restless, wandering aimlessly in the office, looking around blankly. Occasionally she stared at something intently or stopped to look searchingly at the therapist's face, sometimes returning his smile and at other times smiling spontaneously. She waved her fingers in front of her eyes to create a strobe light effect. She picked at her face and took off her shoes and socks, rubbed her feet and smelled her fingers. She was briefly responsive to her mother's directives, and after removing her blouse she immediately put it on again when the therapist instructed her to do so.

Julie's parents were able to offer little history to explain the onset of this condition. An only child, she had always been viewed by them as psychologically tough and competent. Her development had been unremarkable. There was no family history of serious mental illness. Julie had not been a drug or alcohol user. She was living at home while working to earn money for college. She had become somewhat withdrawn during the prior few months and on occasion untypically snappish and perhaps a little depressed, which her parents related to fatigue from working and helping with the farmwork. During the week prior to developing symptoms she had been visiting friends at a college. It seemed that she had had a frightening experience during the return trip home, but she could or would tell them very little about it. She had managed to get herself home where the symptoms fluctuated for a couple of days during which she didn't sleep and became increasingly agitated to the point of bolting from the house. Her parents feared that they could not contain her and sought help. Julie's mother perceived her husband as hypercritical and Julie's father felt that his wife was overprotective of their daughter.

An emergency workup for an organic brain syndrome including drug screening and a pregnancy test all proved negative. The family could not afford private hospitalization and the public facility, which was near their farm, had such "snake pit" associations to it that they did not want her sent there. The psychiatrist concluded that Julie's parents could manage her at home, especially if she could sleep. So chlorpromazine was begun, with the dose being built up to 250 mg daily by the fifth day. The therapist urged her parents to call him with any questions or concerns, and he called them daily for the first six days to reinforce the parents' feelings of security about having her at home. As is usually the case when a therapist underscores and demonstrates his availability, the parents never called.

He saw the family again four days later. On that occasion, the mother talked of her frustrations with her husband in Julie's presence. Julie became very still during her mother's complaint. That behavior prompted the psychiatrist to ask Julie if she worried about people. Julie replied that she did, and so the psychiatrist told her she need not feel guilty. Julie also acknowledged in response to direct questions that she sometimes felt scared and sad and sometimes happy, but never angry. Little more could be elicited from her. By the ninth day after treatment began, Julie wanted to meet alone with the psychiatrist. From that point on her mother was brought in toward the end of sessions, to discuss with Julie and the psychiatrist her observations of Julie's behaviors, her own worries, changes in the dose of the medication, and to continue to talk about the alternative approaches for proceeding with her treatment, namely, medication and/or individual or family psychotherapy.

Julie's psychotic withdrawal continued to abate and become replaced by a pleasant reserve. At weekly sessions, she revealed some of what had happened during her vacation. Prior to the trip she had experienced some puzzling physical symptoms, which were probably prodromata of her psychotic episode. These had arisen at a time when she was experiencing conflict about matriculating at the distant college she was visiting rather than at the rural college near her home that her parents had expected she would attend. Julie's conflict involved feeling that her parents needed her nearby. During the drive home, she had stopped in a city to eat, and allowed herself to be picked up by two men and a woman, which was untypical behavior for her. They all went to a ground floor apartment of the men where the others began to drink. Julie refused to join them and they wouldn't let her leave. She became frightened, and either was already disorganized or became so at that point as she managed to get away by climbing out a bedroom window. She drove her car most of the way home, where she was picked up for erratic driving by a deputy sheriff who knew her family; seeing that she was either under the influence of some drug or was acutely distraught he brought her home, where her state of agitation persisted. Julie was reluctant to reveal more of what she recalled. Typical of her style, she wanted to forget about the experience. Nor did she want to explore other areas of her life. She wished only to return to her previous routine.

Tapering of chlorpromazine had been begun on the twelfth day because of drowsiness and was completed on the fiftieth day. By the time she was off medication, seven weeks after it had been begun, Julie and her parents were politely but clearly communicating their wish that treatment end because of financial constraints, the distance from their farm, and the fact that Julie had resumed her normal activities and was functioning without symptoms. Treatment ended at that time. Two years later she was asymptomatic and attending college full time.

A comparison of this case with that of Sam underscores the point that it is not only the symptoms of a patient which determine or dictate the mode of treatment. Julie's psychiatrist was faced with a psychotic patient about whom he knew nothing, who seemed on first meeting unable to form a therapeutic alliance, and who lived at such a distance that he could not attempt to develop one quickly by seeing her daily. Her parents could neither afford private hospitalization nor accept referral to their state hospital. Thus, working solely psychotherapeutically with Julie was not a reasonable alternative.

ANOREXIA NERVOSA

Anorexia nervosa, with or without bulimia, continues to defy understanding, despite much interest during the past two decades in this long-known condition. The similarities in the presentation of anorexia nervosa patients are usually more striking to the clinician than their differences. The symptoms incline one toward thinking that there is a unitary condition of anorexia nervosa, which should prove to have very similar dynamics amongst sufferers, even if it can occur in people with different subsequent or underlying personality structures. For example, there is a preponderance of adolescent females; a profound avoidance of eating and tremendous fear of gaining weight, coupled with indefatigable exercising, idiosyncratic ideas about their figures, proclivity for obsessional behaviors, disinclination to think psychologically about their illness, frequent imperviousness to insight, and cessation of menses often before this would be anticipated on the basis of inanition. For this reason, the developmental perspective I have identified in other adolescent disturbances may prove helpful in understanding and approaching this vexing condition.

Those anorexics I have seen for whom the dynamics elaborated in this book proved important exhibited one or more of the following features:

1. A parent or parent surrogate of the anorexic is preoccupied with his or her own or the future anorexic's eating or dietary control (e.g., case on pp. 246).
2. The anorexic is acting as if she could not control her appetites (Galdston, 1974) in order to protect a parent who the patient feels has a similar problem. Or, the anorexic is attempting to protect a parent(s) whom the patient perceives to have eating problems of their own, by having more serious difficulties than the parent.
3. The anorexic is trying to avoid contempt for a parent.
4. The anorexic is complying with the parent's reluctance that the patient grow up (i.e., experiencing emancipatory guilt).

5. The anorexic struggles with the omnipotence complex of feeling both great responsibility for and having great influence over one or both parents.

OTHER VIEWS OF ANOREXIA NERVOSA

Historically, conclusions about its basis have covered the full spectrum from it being an organic disorder to it being a psychological illness specific to adolescence. These evolving formulations have reflected popular psychological theories of the times and the disenchantment that ensues when treatments based on each of them provide inconsistent results. Thus, the psychological formulations have shifted from the psychoanalytic view in the 1940s that the anorexic symptoms defended against awareness of oral impregnation fantasies. With the development of ego psychology in the 1950s a more general renunciation of sexuality and of adolescent emancipation, that is, of growing up as it were, was posited as the source of anorexia nervosa. In the 1960s, it was seen as a dyadic problem involving separation-individuation based on object relations theory. In the 1970s and 1980s, it was viewed as having multiply determined causality based on the resurgence of descriptive psychiatry, the importance of preservation of the self based on self psychology, and renewed interest in identity formation in the 1980s. Moreover, some views of the illness seem to emanate more from convictions about treatment methods than from a persuasion about the underlying cause or causes. The latter include most notably the view of structural family therapy and to a lesser extent that of behavioral therapy. In the view of structural family therapy the difficulty lies in problematic relationships between family members rather than within the anorexic; in the behavioral therapy view, the anorexic symptoms are considered learned behaviors which can be unlearned.

Bruch (1977), a widely quoted student of anorexia nervosa, has described conditions which fit well into the model of developmental psychopathology I am advancing. In Bruch's experience the future anorexic has typically been a compliant, achieving, nonproblematic child. Her parents sought affection and confirmation of their own worth from that child, who in turn felt obligated to fulfill parental demands for support (Bruch [1977] cites Selvini [1974]). This long-standing pattern of having submissively fulfilled their parents' needs of them leaves these young people ill-prepared for the self-direction and self-regulation that are required for adolescent emancipation. Bruch considers that the symptoms of anorexia result from efforts of the anorexic to establish a "domain of selfhood" when faced with the adolescent tasks of independence and identity formation. In my experience such youth are not crippled by their own inadequacies nor by a lack of a sense of themselves as autonomous individuals. Rather, they are immobilized by the developmentally intensified conflict between acceding to their parents' need to retain their relationship as it is and their own wish to become more autonomous.

Mogul (1980) contrasted asceticism (see footnote, pp. 163–164) practiced by healthier adolescents and the anorexic's use of this same mechanism in markedly exaggerated form. In his view, healthy adolescents can adopt ascetic practices as a creative use of self-discipline to accomplish goals and enhance confidence in their self-control and thus move toward independence (e.g., athletics). By contrast, the anorexic's abstention from all pleasure becomes perverted into an end in itself, rather than a means toward an end. The anorexic sufferer's self-esteem becomes contingent upon abstention, rendering it easier to understand why weight gain can be experienced as a defeat rather than success. That formulation provides a way of understanding how treatments which employ coercive methods to achieve weight gain can push the patient in the opposite direction.

Treatment strategies have varied greatly. Despite efforts of some approaches to avoid preoccupation with the patient's weight gain, this effectively becomes the first consideration in all therapies; that is because the patient is in a life-threatening and thus anxiety-engendering situation. Rates of relapse and final outcome appear to be similar for all treatment modalities. This raises the possibility of underlying, self-limiting, or self-curative factors in these patients, though this hardly appears to be the case when faced with an anorexic patient.

The dynamics I have been elaborating were prominent in all of the cases presented thus far in this chapter. That background plus the earlier enumeration of features I have observed in patients with anorexia nervosa should provide a clear enough sense of those whose illness conforms to that model. So, rather than illustrating such a case, two cases in which these dynamics were not as prominent will be described. In addition to illustrating other conflicts in this condition, these cases illustrate that the onset is not necessarily in adolescence and can involve individuals from very different backgrounds. Issues in these cases which seemed as or more important than the dynamics I have been emphasizing include:

1. Rigid self-control and fixation on dieting were used by the anorexic to relieve intense anxiety associated with her idea that she could not trust or control her perceptions.
2. The anorexic did not feel secure in her relationship with her mother; this made the prospect of emancipating problematic.
3. The anorexic struggled with guilt and fear of retaliation for her angry and aggressive impulses; the latter is associated with sibling rivalry and feelings of having been betrayed by her mother.

Jean was hospitalized for four months on a milieu ward for children with chronic illnesses at the age of 14 following a 60-pound weight loss. She was the younger of two children in an upper-middle class, educated family.

Jean's mother was an engaging lady whose family remained apprehensive of her derisive sarcasm which could be unleashed against any of them, and about which she felt "too old to change." She functioned effectively in her housewife role though she may have tended to interact with Jean in a more siblinglike manner than one might expect of mother and teenaged daughter. Jean's father was a highly intelligent, obsessional professional, who tended to remain somewhat emotionally isolated and aloof from the family. Jean's 16-year-old sister was a brilliant underachiever who had recently embarked on minor delinquent behavior.

Jean possessed her father's intelligence and her mother's perceptiveness; she also exhibited her mother's penchant for decimating people with scornful looks and a withering tongue. She tended to act aloof with peers and adults. Obsessional features in her developing personality, including isolation of her emotions, became more pronounced with the development of her illness which took the form of an ascetic approach to all potentially pleasurable activities.

During her several months of hospitalization, Jean maintained that she was not ill, that there was nothing wrong with her, and consequently she had nothing to talk about. She visited less of her sneering hauteur on her therapist than she did on others. She tended to externalize responsibility for her own distress and frustrations. For example, she contended that the staff kept her from realizing her primary wish, namely to go home. She also attempted to determine what others wished of her and to comply. She began to gain weight relatively quickly, but this prompted her to feel discouraged that she could not control her eating and to fear that she would overeat. Jean realized spontaneously that she had to rely on others for permission to eat in order to avoid feeling guilty about doing so. This plus her lack of insight into her condition after two months of hospitalization frustrated her immensely. She condemned her therapist, the person on whom she counted to help her, for only frustrating her wishes to go home; and she began to look upon her illness as incurable, as she observed previously discharged anorexic patients being rehospitalized.

Jean then began to eat because she wanted to, but this created conflict in her because she wanted to remain at 90 pounds. On the one hand she would like the ward staff to allay her guilt by taking responsibility for her eating; on the other hand that much "taking over" of her autonomy was unacceptable to Jean. The ward staff's approach to her eating at that juncture changed from one in which they assumed responsibility for her intake, that is, considering food to be her medicine and prescribing the amount of caloric intake she needed, to a stance in which they underscored their confidence in Jean's ability to regulate herself. The staff did so by assigning Jean a section in the refrigerator which was always stocked with foods she liked. They advised her about how to handle mealtimes, but did not make her ward privileges contingent upon eating.

Jean began to interact with staff in a more relaxed and easy manner and her weight gain resumed, but she became petulant, frustrated, tearful and reproachful toward her therapist, as she voiced helplessness and pessimism. (This suggested that she felt uncomfortable about getting better.) At that time she was allowed to spend a weekend at home.

From that point, after three months of hospitalization, she began to reflect more concertedly on her mental state. She observed that prior to her illness her image of herself had been of someone "dumb, ugly, and fat." She had come to feel superior to others by not letting herself be "controlled by food," that is, by not succumbing to her appetite. By the fourth month of hospitalization, while continuing to exercise and remain preoccupied with being slender, she had regained 40 pounds, was eating regularly, and was in no physical danger. She was discharged from the hospital and followed in outpatient psychotherapy.

Subsequent to her discharge, Jean exhibited a sensitivity to the plight of other children on the ward whose circumstances were not as fortunate as her own that she had not evinced in the hospital. For example, she reflected, "Eleanor with no mother; well, she was given to her grandmother when she was 6 months old and didn't have a father, and no mother to visit. In the beginning when I came here I didn't care whether I lived or died. But at those times I could think, 'Well, my mother is coming tonight'—I don't know what would have happened if she wasn't there." She observed that previously she had liked people at a distance but now she could like them "close up."

Jean seemed to be implying that the vulnerability she felt which had precipitated her defensive aloofness was related to anxiety experienced in relationship to her mother. This in turn had complicated her adolescent emancipation.

Also, during that first month postdischarge, Jean reported what she had realized lay at the base of her difficulty: "It's funny to just come in and tell you this—but I was walking down the hall in school—and I suddenly became afraid. I don't know why, and then I recall that it was a fear, a fear of I don't know what, that brought about this whole business—all the activity and the stopping eating—to avoid thinking about it. I thought of three other times in my life when this happened. The first was a couple of times when I was really, really sick—like I was never going to feel like anybody else again. The second time was at camp my first year. I got very, very homesick. None of the other kids did except me. I don't know why, but I thought about dying and did for the rest of the summer. The third time was when I was real, real little—five or six years ago. I used to wake up in the middle of the night and look at something little and then look up and everything else would look very little; and I would get very scared. I'd go to my parents—they didn't understand. I'd go to their door and say, 'I'm lonely,' and my mother would say, 'Well, so am I, go to your bed.' I would go and dream about it, like I was walking on a brick sidewalk and looking at the bricks and they would look very small and I would look up and everything around me would look very small. Everything I did was because I was afraid of being afraid—not eating—if I could think about being thin all the time and keep busy doing things, then I wouldn't get scared."

Jean seemed to be saying that at times during childhood she had experienced intense anxiety. One aspect of this was separation anxiety associated with fears of annihilation; another aspect was a terrifying sense that she could not trust or control her basic perceptual faculties (see also p. 113). At those times her parents had not provided security-engendering responses that would have enabled Jean to feel more comfortably autonomous. So, in early adolescence when this anxiety resurged in the setting of her developmental need to emancipate, Jean resorted to an all-consuming concentration on self-control of her eating in order to avoid experiencing that anxiety and to instill a sense of autonomy and self-confidence. This material is consonant with my thesis about the importance of the security-rendering aspects of the parents which must be manifested in the sponsoring relationship during adolescence. The emphasis in Jean's case was on the lack of the security-providing element in her parents' relationship to her prior to adolescence. Also, it was not clear why eating and weight loss rather than other symptoms were "selected" by Jean, except for the fact that eating frequently becomes an anxiety-reducing mechanism for many people by substituting a function performed by the parent for a healthy identification with the parent.

> During the next several months Jean talked about feeling very different from peers at times, and that she had become disillusioned and dissatisfied with everything during her sixth-grade year when her illness began. She had been happy but "in my own small world," and observed that "when you're sick you don't have to think about things, including being unhappy." She talked about how unhappy she had felt being separated from her family, particularly her mother, when hospitalized. Currently she occasionally acted like a much younger child at home, to get her parents to treat her as such. She claimed to feel hesitant about growing up. At the same time, she reported that her mother at times seemed to provoke her or her sister "just to start something in the family." Jean expressed concerns about being unhappy and adopting that tendency of her mother when she grew up. She noted that she seemed to eat more when her mother was not around.

Jean's latter three associations suggested that her behaviors represented compliance with what her mother wanted, namely a peer with whom to contend. Such compliance on Jean's part would be based on emancipatory guilt related to progressing developmentally beyond the type of relationship that she thought her mother wished to have with her. Those same associations also suggested that Jean was at risk of adopting her mother's contumelious manner (i.e., a defensive identification) in a characterological way to protect her image of her mother.

> Jean told the therapist that she harbored secrets that she would never share with him or anyone else. Six months following her discharge from the hospital the friction she was describing with her mother involved typical adolescent concerns about having to report to her mother. She claimed to feel natural at school, enjoying social activities, and was no longer an outsider there. Her mood was buoyant as she chatted happily about her life, and she agitated to stop seeing her therapist. She brought a note for him to read after she departed from their last session. It read:

> Dearest Doctor—I couldn't think of any suitable way to say goodbye . . . so, henceforth is an original poem.
>   From the bottom of my heart
>   (Where all the bad things stay)
>   I must admit I wish you
>   The worst in every way.
> Au revoir, and good luck always . . .
>   Love,
>   Jean

The transference implications of the poem suggest that Jean had felt caught in an ambivalence conflict, unable to reconcile resentments and loving feelings. This condition stemmed from her inability to derive a sufficient sense of security from her relationship with her parents to be able to feel comfortably autonomous. Those parental traits which had hindered this aspect of Jean's development, her mother's sarcasm and inconsistent emotional availability and her father's aloofness, reflected their own intolerance for emotional closeness. Jean was at risk for developing those traits which would arise as defensive identifications, motivated by her need to deal with the discomfort engendered in her by those same traits exhibited by her parents.

Jill was hospitalized for the second time at age $11^1/_2$. The onset was very similar to that of a prior bout which had required hospitalization at age $8^1/_2$. Abstaining from sweets during Lent was followed by progressive dieting, by increasingly obsessional behavior, by undertaking more and more household chores, cleaning and cooking for the family, and doing for others at the expense of herself.

She was the third of eight children born at an inconvenient time to parents who struggled in an economically depressed area. Her mother went to work when Jill was 5 months old. Jill, never much of an eater, was considered by her parents to always have been the most controlled, compliant, excessively religious, and emotionally contained of their children. Jill never liked to feel angry; she considered it a "bad habit" which would turn others against her.

She remained reluctant to volunteer any information about herself during her two-month hospitalization. She did allow during the initial meeting with her therapist that she had been very surprised by her mother's most recent pregnancy ten months earlier. She also acknowledged lagging behind her girl friends in developing any interest in boys. And most strikingly, she allowed concern about her mother's health and welfare; she feared that her mother would get too tired from working so hard and have a "fatigue breakdown." Her mother had been hospitalized once in the past for depression. Wishes to protect her mother were Jill's ostensible reasons for beginning to do so much of the family cooking and gardening.

From a more traditional psychoanalytic/psychodynamic standpoint this behavior would be understood as a reaction formation defense against anger experienced toward her mother and rivalry toward her new sibling. But in acknowledging feelings of responsibility for and influence over her parents and sibs, Jill bespoke separation guilt conflicts, namely that getting what she wanted would be at the expense of her mother or sibs. Which of these conflicts, reaction formation against aggression or separation guilt, was more basic in Jill's psychopathology was not clarified.

During the initial weeks of hospitalization, Jill considered that she had no problems; nor did she seem to be developing insight into her condition. Rather, in a compliant manner she appeared to be making an ostensible effort to gain weight in order to return home. This burst of health was short-lived, and she was soon losing weight, exercising vigorously, and repeating the pattern she had embarked upon at home: She engaged in a flurry of activities to help the ward staff, for example, passing out food trays to other patients rather than eating herself and helping the ward clerk rather than meeting with her therapist.

Gradually Jill began to acknowledge that she had always felt herself to be the child in her family who loved and needed her mother most. In fact she felt betrayed, having given so much and gotten so little in return. When she experienced this abject loneliness and hurt she would cry uncontrollably. She accused the therapist of creating these emotions in her: "You make me cry," was her understanding of the source of her tears, and she would continue to insist that she had no problems and run out of sessions to avoid talking more about these painful thoughts. The intensity of her jealous angers toward certain other family members and her fears of being thought of as a bully if others knew of her wishes to bite, stomp, kick, and hit emerged gingerly. So, too, did the degree of her "hunger" for love from her parents and loneliness about which she cried a lot, while steadfastly disclaiming any connection between this and the genesis of her anorexia.

After six weeks of treatment she revealed having heard (sometime prior to the hospitalization) that babies were born in a very dirty and disgusting way. This had led to her decision not to grow up and have babies. She would not mature and this could be accomplished by not eating. By this point in treatment, however, she observed with some perplexity that she was neither running nor skipping as much and was eating more.

After two months of hospital treatment Jill had gained twenty-five pounds and was taking good care of herself, having fun with other people, expressing her feelings to others, acting in a more relaxed way, wearing more feminine outfits, and behaving a bit more like a growing girl. She was discharged and seen only in periodic follow-up because of the great distance from her home.

Both Jean and Jill exhibited the common behavioral features of anorexia nervosa. Between them they presented isolated pieces of data which would fit into most of the different formulations I referred to earlier. Specifically, Jill evinced disgust regarding heterosexuality and procreation. Both expressed fear of maturing, Jill because of sexuality and Jean because of the extremely frightening concern that she was losing her capacity to discriminate reality with respect to perceptions, and feared being unable to control her appetites (Galdston, 1974). Separation from their mothers was an important issue for both of them. Yet, they came from remarkably different psychosocial circumstances and one had the onset of her illness prior to adolescence.

Each girl indicated that the relationship with her mother was of greatest importance, ambivalently held, and associated with fears of rejection—for Jean from her mother's sarcasm and for Jill from her mother's lack of availability owing to being spread too thin amongst a large, struggling family and from her own depressive inclination. The intense wish to be reunited with her mother was the ostensible motivation for each to improve her nutritional state and regain weight. The most striking psychodynamic revelations of Jean were her awareness of dependency on others, the adoption of rigid self-control in a compensatory effort to substitute feelings of superiority for those of inferiority, and the use of rigid self-control to relieve intense anxiety associated with the idea of being unable to reality test and control her perceptions. Jill's most striking self-revelations were of feeling betrayed by, ambivalent toward, worried, and guilty about her mother, and fearful of experiencing and expressing anger because she anticipated retaliation for aggressive impulses.

Part IV

Further Consideration of Intensive Therapy for Severe Psychopathology

CHAPTER 10

Psychoanalysis of an Impulse-Ridden Adolescent

Almost all of the pathological conditions described to this point were first manifested during adolescence and derived from conflicts directly related to the process of development during adolescence. To be sure, harbingers of future problems could be identified in the earlier childhoods of several of the cases. Those future patients, however, had managed to adapt adequately until faced with the developmental imperative to emancipate. By contrast, most impulse-ridden youth have struggled unsuccessfully to achieve self-control during childhood and this pattern usually continues unabated during adolescence.

The increasing numbers of adolescents who exhibit such pathology represent the rationale for presenting such a case in detail. In this patient the development of impulse-ridden behavior correlates with the absence of a constant, positive, sponsoring parenting experience during childhood. The process by which this lad achieved self control in the treatment is also illustrated; he replicated with the analyst, in an almost caricaturish way, the type of interactions by which parents normally help very young children to consolidate impulse control.

It may impress readers as quaint even if not antiquated to present such a case in a day and age when we are primarily looking for ways of minimizing contact with therapeutic personnel. However, at the very least, insights gained from intensive therapy should prove helpful to those who are searching for less labor intensive approaches, because understanding behavior is one important step toward changing it. At worst we may have to accept that we are barking up the wrong tree if we expect Romes to be built in a day.

Recent retrospective investigations using a large source of data on psychoanalyses and psychotherapies of children support my contention that there may be no shortcuts to some cures. These researchers find that longer and more intensive therapies correlate positively with better outcomes; and beginning the therapy intensively (4 or 5 times a week) significantly reduces the likelihood that the patient will terminate prematurely (Fonagy and Target, 1994). Also, the more severely disturbed children are much more likely to show reliable improvement if treated intensively (4 or 5 times weekly) compared to those treated 1 to 3 times weekly (Target and Fonagy, 1994). The children in these studies began treatment when they were 2 to 3 years younger than the lad whose treatment will be described. Nevertheless, I suspect that the same conditions hold for older children with severe disorders, even though it is more complicated and difficult to bring adolescents into intensive treatment.

In describing Eddie's treatment I will illustrate several points:

Such individuals can be treated psychotherapeutically; as a corollary, when treating an impulse-ridden adolescent, in addition to anticipating an impulse-ridden therapy, we can expect impulse-ridden families and impulse-ridden external impediments to maintaining the treatment. Thus, factors outside the therapy conspire against the likelihood of success. One approach that has been advocated to deal with such cases involves concentrating therapeutic resources on the child's supporting environment. Without intending to dismiss that view, I will illustrate a different approach. Namely, if one can get the adolescent into the office several times a week, then the therapeutic effort can be focused almost exclusively on the patient's ego, and the chips of his or her outside life can be left to fall where they may. This approach is a natural outgrowth of the importance I have placed on adapting one's strivings to develop to one's environment. We have to presume the existence of underlying urges in people to correct their disabilities. Many of the environments from which impulse-ridden youngsters emerge are more difficult to change than are the young people themselves. It may ultimately be as cost effective to train a cadre of therapists who can treat these youngsters as to attempt the "preventive" approach of trying to educate, treat, and support the environmental crucibles in which these youngsters are formed. For it is these youths themselves who will determine the outcome of their own progeny in the next generation.

The individual strives throughout his or her development for a stable relationship with a parent in which he feels both claimed and sponsored so that development can be completed with a sense of inner security.

Prominent adaptive mechanisms developed by individuals who exhibit pathological impulsivity include turning passive into active and reversals into the opposite behavior, attitude, or feeling (counterphobia).

The therapeutic technique, dictated by this patient's presentation, involved almost exclusively working with the relationship the lad exhibited toward the analyst as opposed to exploring his past history and his present life outside the consulting room.

The kinds of feelings engendered in the therapist by this type of patient and the role of the therapist's emotional responses in facilitating rather than inhibiting the treatment will be described.

EDDIE

Eddie, a 12-year-old seventh grader in long-time foster care, was referred by his welfare department social worker: Eddie had a long history of presenting himself in a smiling and affable manner, while only allowing people to have the most superficial relationship with him. Always demanding and selfish, Eddie neither expressed nor conveyed any sense of gratitude nor attachment to those who cared for him. His case worker considered Eddie's lack of appreciation to be the major reason for the several changes in his foster home placements. He was immature with peers—overbearing, a know-it-all, and bossy. He fought frequently and had no lasting friendships. He had a long history of lying and petty thievery about which he exhibited no remorse. He always wanted things, stuffed himself with food (particularly sweets), and was oriented toward immediate gratification, exhibiting limited frustration tolerance and a short attention span. He was talkative and disruptive at school and clowned so much that he alienated classmates who by now tended to ignore him. His IQ had been assessed at 140, yet he was barely passing his courses. The immediate precipitants for his referral were his marginal school performance and stealing money from his foster father following a visit to his natural mother.

BACKGROUND

A paucity of history was available. Eddie was the youngest of three children. His seven-year older brother had been treated for bipolar disease and his five-year older sister had been hospitalized for psychosis, presumably schizophrenia. A sibling between the older two had died shortly after birth. The long-distance trucker whom Eddie considered to be his father had been killed in a big rig accident when Eddie was 18 months old. The family had stayed together with various relatives from then until Eddie was 5 years old. At that time his mother was hospitalized for a psychotic illness and the children were placed in foster care. Eddie's mother, variously diagnosed as schizophrenic and manic depressive, had been rehospitalized intermittently. At the time of Eddie's referral she was living alone in a nearby town and functioning marginally. Her long-time gentleman friend lived close by and was said to bear a striking resemblance to Eddie. The boy wished to live with her and tried to see her more often than his authorized monthly visits. Behaviors like stealing occurred more frequently after he had seen his mother.

The three siblings proved unmanageable when placed together, so they were separated. Between ages 5 and 7 Eddie had at least three foster home placements. At age 7 he was placed with the foster parents with whom he lived when he began treatment. They anticipated keeping him as long as they could. An older couple, grandparents in their own right, they liked Eddie and exhibited great tolerance for his aberrant behaviors. They were frequently exasperated and at a loss to know how to get him to behave. Yet, they treated him with an understanding that reflected wisdom about human relationships, acquired over long lifetimes. They were people who understood a lot of what they experienced, who knew their own feelings, and who were friendly, straightforward, and unpretentious. Their complaint about Eddie was that "he doesn't mind." He would not do the minimal chores expected of him and performed jobs properly only when watched. The minute he was unsupervised he reverted to doing tasks quickly, sloppily, and superficially. If he was sent on an errand and met other kids on the way, he would not return home. "You can tell him, but he'll do like he wants." He played with everything and preferred the toys of younger children. His foster parents reported that "all hell broke loose" when Eddie's brother or sister visited; they became rowdy and destructive.

Even when his foster parents withheld soccer, Eddie's passion, he did not behave or perform in school. He often walked in his sleep from his bedroom to the kitchen or to his foster mother's room. He frequently asked them when he could live with his mother, especially when he was "all wound up and day dreaming" after having visited her. But when his foster mother would then threaten to send him away, Eddie always looked worried and said that he wanted to stay with them.

Eddie had had weekly psychotherapy during fifth and sixth grades for stealing, lying, and trouble and fighting at school. His psychiatrist reported minimal movement and Eddie was allowed to terminate when he wanted to do so. Also, his foster parents had taken a course in behavior modification child management techniques, but these, too, had proven ineffective.

INITIAL EVALUATION OF EDDIE

Eddie was a good-sized, nice-looking lad with red, curly hair and sparkling blue eyes. He bulged at the seams of his clothes with a "baby-fat" look, and he wore an ever-present, wide grin. He talked in a rapid and animated manner, walked rapidly, and was always dressed neatly and well groomed.

Eddie remained bright and cheery during the two months of his evaluation. He offered little spontaneously, except about soccer games, and was decidedly uninterested in exploring anything. He described the series of foster homes in which he had lived, recalling problems within those families as the causes for leaving them. He never remembered or at least never reported any contribution of his own mischief to the failure of those placements. On occasion he would play un-self-consciously with toys typically used by much younger children, such as puppets and the doctor's kit. He told me he was in a special class for kids with high IQs. When I attempted to explore this in light of his marginal academic performance, however, Eddie began looking around, yawning, and we got no further. When I broached his stealing and lying, he could not correlate them with visits to his mother. He claimed to lie solely to avoid punishment. He did not have problems, or if he did, he was not interested in trying to understand them better in an effort to master them. They would go away by themselves. When I pursued his stealing, though, using defense analysis technique, Eddie acknowledged not wanting to talk about it because he felt ashamed.

When at our last session of evaluation I presented Eddie with my reasons for offering him intensive treatment, he didn't understand. But when I reflected on the problems we would face in trying to sustain this treatment (i.e., when I seemed perhaps to be withdrawing the opportunity), Eddie countered with ways of overcoming these obstacles. At hour's end Eddie described car crashes he had seen on the highway near his home, from "little rear-enders" to conflagrations, including a fire in the house next to theirs which could have destroyed Eddie's home as well. In this equivalent of free association and his earlier effort to counter my concerns about maintaining the treatment, I felt Eddie was conveying an awareness of underlying anxieties and his need for the treatment which he overtly disavowed. That awareness reflected among other things his underlying strivings to complete his development. His associations to car accidents and house fires suggested that, despite his seeming insouciance regarding his behaviors, he feared that things might go out of control in treatment with potentially devastating consequences.

Eddie's foster parents reported that he had been more settled during the two months of our evaluation. They attributed this calming effect to Eddie not having seen his mother. His case worker reported that Eddie frequently imitated me, always in good humor. So the importance of the tendency to identify, albeit seemingly in a mocking way, was apparent from the beginning of the therapeutic experience, and presumably reflected the strength of his wish for a stable (parental) relationship.

INITIAL ASSESSMENT

ADAPTIVE STYLE, STRENGTHS, AND VULNERABILITIES PRIOR TO ADOLESCENCE

Eddie's maladaptive behaviors and style capitalized upon the defense mechanisms of denial, rationalization, minimal reaction formation (his smiling and superficial friendliness), and isolation of affects. His counterphobic style, delinquent behaviors, and his markedly compromised ability to control his behavior all antedated his adolescent years.

His strengths which represented potential assets in treatment included: (1) his unabashed wish to be with his mother and seeming interest in forming a relationship with the therapist; (2) his intelligence, which was reflected in facile use of language and memory. It seemed that his academic problems related to a failure to produce assignments rather than a failure to have integrated basic rudiments of precision learning. (3) There was his brief acknowledgment of shame regarding his stealing.

Conscience functioning was not age appropriate. He appeared to be functioning with a sociopathic orientation. His acknowledgment of shame regarding stealing was the only suggestion that he was in conflict over wrongdoing, rather than exclusively concerned with avoiding punishment.

His avid interest and perhaps above-average ability in soccer seemed, in addition to his intelligence, to be the only skill or talent that he had developed which could aid him in the adolescent emancipation process.

He had formed no solid peer relationships, so did not have this important experience to aid his continuing advancement.

CURRENT THRUST OF DEVELOPMENT AND RELATIONSHIP TO PARENTS

Eddie did not exhibit evidence of efforts to emancipate. In fact, a major interest seemed to be reuniting with his biological mother. Little was known at that time about his relationship with his mother, though it appeared that he was always very compliant when with her in an effort to stay in her good graces. Thus, there seemed little evidence of adolescent development unfolding.

Several extraclinical features made the likelihood of sustained analysis problematic. Eddie's aging foster father would have to transport him a considerable distance in heavy commuter traffic for early morning appointments four times a week. The specter of his biological mother initiating a custody battle in the future hovered around the case. Also, fees (totaling 50% of customary charges) would be paid by two public agencies, either of which could withdraw financial support at anytime. Both agencies required frequent reports to authorize continuing the treatment and they would expect evidence of progress to justify these expenditures.

BEGINNING OF TREATMENT

Eddie's initial treatment hours were characterized by increasing interest in learning about my personal life, with his frustration mounting as I attempted to explore such questions as whether I had a family. I realized in retrospect that despite my explanations to him, Eddie began to experience my efforts to maintain therapeutic anonymity as evidence of hostility toward him.

Sessions were otherwise taken up with card and board games at which he was very quick and intensely competitive, though whenever I was close to winning, Eddie's skillful play deteriorated. This suggested that he became readily anxious and was in greater conflict about competing than his outward manner suggested. With a smile he could acknowledge feeling angry when he lost and he would become boisterous. He perfunctorily denied discomfort over winning or losing, but his behavioral reactions belied those disclaimers. For he became increasingly frustrated when I won games and eventually began to accuse me of enjoying beating him. Yet, after he would win he began to become solicitous of my comfort (e.g., wanting me to have a comfortable chair and to choose the color checkers). This pattern suggested that he felt in some conflict about both winning and losing. But rather than being willing to explore these reactions as they intensified, Eddie invoked magical thinking in the form of good luck rituals to reduce his anxiety and guilt as he became more intensely preoccupied with beating me in board games.

After playing all the age-appropriate games in my office during the first month Eddie became a little anxious, as if concerned about how he could avoid his conflicts. He asked more often how I wanted to spend our sessions. It seemed that he was keenly trying to figure out what I wanted of him. The posture of analytic neutrality was increasingly frustrating. Whenever I explained the rationale for my stance he would claim that he did not understand me and also state that he did not want to talk about himself. Yet his associations demonstrated that he had understood my explanations. And he carried material and themes over from one session to the next. This suggested to me that underneath his disclaimers, he was involving himself in the treatment process. I understand this to be a reflection of his underlying striving to complete his development. Fantasies began to slip out; for example, he would ask, "What happened to this toy soldier's leg? Someone bit it off? Someone must have been very hungry!" Eddie's level of motor activity escalated at such moments.

Also, his seemingly overweening, buoyant self-confidence began to appear less solid. For example, after I won board games his bravado would diminish and he would look to me for assistance with his moves. As his competitive wishes became even stronger, he would as noted exhibit undoing after winning. This took the form of feeling that I should then win some games. Or, after drawing something he would assert, "It's good!" but then ask me almost imploringly, "Isn't it good?" In line with the themes of this book, it was not clear to me at those times whether his self-esteem regulation was fragile or whether he was unsure if I wanted him to succeed and thus was acting more dependent because he could not be certain from my responses that my attitude was one that sponsored his advancement.

As his frustration with my therapeutic neutrality mounted, Eddie's undoing began to assume physical forms, accompanied by giggling, which reflected his anxiety. For example, after a marble he rolled brushed against me, he asked if it had hurt me and wanted to rub the spot on my arm. At the same time that his anxiety was mounting because he was unable to determine what I wanted of him or what would please me, he began to control our board game play. He would either decide what moves I could make or would convert games of skill to ones of chance by introducing dice, a pair of which he brought to the office and left with me. Leaving his possessions in my office suggested that Eddie was becoming more interested and involved in the treatment process and wanted to feel closer to me than his refusals to explore matters might have indicated. At the same time, dealing with his anxiety by invoking control over the other person amounted to the introduction of an immature obsessional mechanism; this mechanism is thought to function importantly in the process of integrating basic rudiments of self-control during early childhood development. Eddie's tendency to use undoing noted above was another rudimentary obsessional mechanism he adopted to deal with guilt or anxiety associated with winning.

As the first summer vacation approached, after a couple of months of analysis, Eddie's biological mother was becoming manic and gave her 13-year-old son sandbox toys to take to summer camp. Eddie never mentioned more about visits with his mother than where they had gone together. He expressed reluctance about continuing four times a week after vacation because of inconvenience to his foster father. Also, he threatened to remain silent and to "do something bad" if I did not tell him, during our last session before vacation, whether I had a family. I still did not comprehend the intensity of his interest in who had my attention.

DEVELOPMENT OF THE TRANSFERENCE RELATIONSHIP

Upon resuming after the three-week vacation, Eddie sat in my chair and complained about my "crummy" office. He reproached me for not asking him about his experience at camp (i.e., for not expressing interest in him). He disparaged me as committable (i.e., it was I not he who was sick). And he reflected his wish not to be here and characterized my patients as "victims." He dismissed my questions relating these attitudes to the recent interruption of our meetings and to concerns about having the type of "committable" illness suffered by his mother and siblings. Thus, while his associations suggested that he harbored a problem involving separations, he denied it and used reversal to disabuse himself of this problem; that is, he did not want to be with me rather than he had not wished to be separated from me. This concern about being separated from me would reflect the developing transference in which he experienced toward me what he had toward his parents during early childhood.

Eddie became increasingly upset by my failure to answer questions directly, interpreting this as hostility toward him. In turn this became his justification for provocative behavior. At the same time that he was disparaging me more, he also wanted to show me his good works and to obtain my approval of them. In retrospect I might have facilitated the treatment by acknowledging relatively innocuous questions. For example, he described having punctured his foot on a nail at camp and then wondered if the same thing had ever happened to me. I might have allowed that most people have had such experiences and they are worrisome. For if Eddie was trying to learn how to manage such situations, since his affects were isolated at that point, such a response from me would have given him permission to have feelings about troublesome experiences. Such a response from me would have also served a sponsoring function, letting him know unequivocally that I wanted him to be able to master anxiety-engendering circumstances.

Eddie bespoke his perplexity about my approach to his therapy more directly in a puppet show. He had a troll recoil upon seeing me because the troll "just didn't know what kind of being" I was. I reflected that because I did not answer his questions directly, that is, did not respond like other people, Eddie did not know how to relate to me. He became angry when I would not consistently reciprocate and perform puppet shows for him. He threatened to leave and did so, though he always returned immediately. He called me "stupid" because of my recent haircut. The evident association in his mind between not being able to control what someone else did and leaving suggested again that he harbored anxiety about separations from parental figures; and he typically tried to quell that anxiety by feeling he could control the behavior of others, in this case, the therapist. That is, he turned something anxiety provoking which he had experienced passively at the hands of someone else into an active experience by perpetrating it on another person, the analyst. The meaning of his accompanying criticism about my slightly altered appearance became more comprehensible shortly thereafter.

Eddie's intense frustration at my lack of directness and his inability to explore any of his productions became more understandable after another tendency was identified: this was his unusually keen perceptiveness. For many months at the beginning of treatment Eddie would walk into the office, casually glance at the cluttered toy shelf, and remark, "You've got a new roll of scotch tape." (The new roll would look exactly like the last one.) He was always accurate and this exquisite perceptiveness occurred so often as not to be by chance. Rather, this hypertrophied sensitivity to nuances in his environment appeared to be a capacity he had developed in his effort to adapt to an uncertain and changing environment. That is, the instability in his environment during his first seven years of his life, necessitated such hypervigilance to nuances of change in his environment. He had not had the luxury and opportunity during his early life to feel secure in relationship to a parent, and thus to be able to feel confident that others would look out for him. Rather, he had to remain hyperalert to his environment, to "read" people and their wishes, in order to adapt. Thus, his preoccupation with what I wanted and his frustration over my failure to respond were sources of real anxiety for the reason Eddie had indicated in the troll puppet show. (One and a half years later, when Eddie was much more confident of my constancy, he lost this capacity. For example, he would ask with obvious perplexity, "Is this gun new or has it been here?")

Moreover, his tendency to be made anxious by such minimal changes in my appearance as a haircut, and his criticism of me for this when he could not control my behavior, provided a clue as to why he responded with such intense frustration when I would not interact reciprocally with him. Some features of his earlier development, presumably related to the long absences and loss of his putative father, the separation from his mother, and multiple foster home placements had subtly compromised his capacity to confidently retain a security engendering sense of a parenting figure. It was as if he recognized me but with some residual anxiety which he tried to allay by feeling confident that he could control my behavior. (Almost two years later, following a two-week vacation, Eddie pleaded to look through my file containing his previous artwork. I asked if he were doing so to reacquaint himself with his treatment and me, to make sure that things were the same. He replied, "You're smart.")

INTENSIFICATION OF THE TRANSFERENCE AND OF TURNING PASSIVE INTO ACTIVE; EMERGENCE OF ONE MEANING OF EDDIE'S USE OF IDENTIFICATION

Eddie's provocative behavior when frustrated progressed quite quickly to destructiveness. He giddily cut and bit the heads and arms off plastic Indians, whilst allowing his wish to cut off my head. He broke cars and flirted with messing with glue. He tried to force me to eat clay and smeared it on me. He wanted me to get "mad" at him and kick him out so he would not have to see me. At the same time he wished to maintain physical contact with me. For example, in doctor play all of my body parts were broken in a car accident. Eddie took me to the hospital where I died. During the next session he traveled faster and faster between our homes, until he had a needle extending from his home to mine, and I was alternately dying and being revived by his injections. This play suggested that Eddie may have harbored some omnipotence fantasies about his father's death and feelings of responsibility for rectifying that situation. As with all other material, Eddie refused to explore his thoughts about that tragedy. In this paradoxical behavior (his ostensible efforts to get me to kick him out while trying to hold onto me), we could see the adaptive style he had developed to deal with his anxiety or guilt over separation, namely to reverse or turn what he felt into the opposite (i.e., that he wanted to get away, not stay close).

Another basis for his specific impulsion toward physical contact became apparent when I met for the first time with Eddie and his natural mother. Her condition had stabilized and she was not overtly psychotic for the duration of Eddie's treatment. During that meeting Eddie sat at her feet and his mother rubbed and stroked him almost continuously. Eddie in turn repeatedly traced the sole of her shoe with his finger. When Eddie and I met afterwards he repeatedly touched my face and everything in the office. He acknowledged that his mother frequently touched him. I suggested that his own tendency to touch me, especially occurring in heightened form after seeing his mother, represented his way of keeping her memory alive when he was separated from her, by identifying with (imitating) her behavior toward him.

VICISSITUDES OF CONSCIENCE FORMATION AND FUNCTIONING IN IMPULSE-RIDDEN YOUTH

For a long time Eddie also blamed me for any short-comings of his own. For example, when he could not build a card house to his satisfaction he accused me of causing it to fall down. Or, after inadvertently cheating at a game, with a giggle he would accuse me of cheating. Since he flew into rages when he failed to accomplish what he wished to, he could not bear the intensity of such frustration turned onto himself. For more than a year he vociferously blamed me for all his frustrations. Then he began to blame the object of his frustration (i.e., the task he was undertaking). Then he would literally alternate between blaming me and condemning himself. Eventually he began to call himself "dummy." Finally, he denounced stupid moves on his part. By that time the intensity of these tantrums had lessened significantly.

We can understand from this progression at least two important things about such youth. One is that although they may act as if they have no sense of conscience, some such youngsters are acting this way to avoid overweening self-condemnation. It is very difficult both to perceive this when engaging with them and to help them recognize it beneath their sociopathic-appearing attitudes, their use of projection and displacement. The other feature worth noting is the process by which this tendency is reversed in therapy. My best understanding is that the patient identifies with the therapist's capacity to tolerate being the object of such harsh and unfair condemnation with equanimity and without his/her own self-esteem and confidence being eroded. The patient then gradually adopts and integrates the therapist's tolerance of criticism by identifying with the therapist's attitude and becomes better able to accept responsibility for his/her own failings.

THE FUNCTION OF COUNTERPHOBIA IN SUCH YOUTH

Counterphobic behaviors were related to the type of punitive conscience function just described. Whenever I suggested that Eddie might be acting provocatively to prove to himself that I would not retaliate, his response was, "I'll do it more." When I suggested that he would be doing it more to further assure himself that he was not worried about me getting angry, he would stop that behavior at least for a short while.

A relationship between these phenomena, namely intense, underlying tendencies to blame himself for bad things which happened to him (which were massively defended against by opposite attitudes of being blameless), and the expectation of retaliation for his actions on the one hand, and an underlying sense of not having experienced the security-engendering features of a positive relationship with parents became evident at this time.

Following a two-week absence due to sickness, Eddie became a storekeeper and then a customer, stocking up on and eating food, while asking about my purported children. He discounted any possible connection between this play, his questions, and the recent interruption of our sessions. He then made a clay effigy of me which was thrown from a car, smashed, and killed (recall that his putative father had died in a truck crash). Eddie frequently described natural holocausts or movies with similar themes, and he usually did so around vacation times. The association between separations and the death of others, and between death and his own aggressive impulses or his fear of responsibility for such, seemed clear enough and consistent in his play and associations. He could not, however, acknowledge conscious awareness of these themes in his life. Eddie also elaborated play in which we took turns being a robber who was subdued and jailed, but then fed and solicitously cared for by the policeman-jailer. Thus, Eddie seemed to be trying to develop a more benign, tolerant attitude toward his underlying view of the responsibility he felt for bad things which had happened to him.

Despite such revealing material which suggested that Eddie was feeling more secure in the office, his provocativeness persisted at a more intense level than I would have anticipated solely in response to my consistent posture of anonymity and neutrality. I later learned at this time that the long-time boyfriend of Eddie's mother had told Eddie that he was his biological father. The ostensible reason for this revelation was to have Eddie's orthodonture covered by that man's insurance. Eddie never mentioned this to me, but rather, expressed wishes to stop his treatment. He always refused to discuss this matter, becoming hyperactive whenever I brought it up. Eddie only wanted to live with that man so he could be near his mother. His mother subsequently confirmed the story, though she considered the revelation to have been unnecessary. She claimed that Eddie's putative father had always felt Eddie to be his son and that Eddie and he had had a wonderful relationship. Eddie would run to the door whenever his father came home.

The paradoxical aspect of Eddie's presentation in therapy noted earlier was now even more strikingly evident. He was frustrated with me and ostensibly trying to provoke me to kick him out. At the same time, he was expressing wishes to hold onto and to preserve me (in elaborative play), to gain my approval, and to have physical contact. I again attempted to interpret this counterphobic behavior in the seventy-fifth session with an interesting result: Eddie began the hour claiming to be happy because his social worker had told him he would only have to continue seeing me for two more months. He refused to discuss this, so I wondered if perhaps he found what we did here more confusing than understandable and helpful, and perhaps it was very different from his prior experience in therapy. Eddie agreed and wanted to know why he had to come four times a week, asserting it was for the money (i.e., my avarice). I wondered why I'd be that kind of person. He didn't know, I just was. I wondered, from his view of me as someone who would exploit him for money, rather than someone who could help him, if he were experiencing me as he had other people in the past, specifically his multiple foster parents whom he thought might have done that. Eddie's response was to roll a toy car across the table toward me. It fell into my lap, and he reproached me, "You were supposed to stop it!" He demonstrated how difficult it would have been to stop it himself. Thus, he was saying that I rather than he should be responsible for assuring the safety and security of things between us. I addressed this approximately by suggesting he was telling me that if his feelings emerged here, he wondered if I'd be able to help him control them. Eddie put the car back on the shelf. I added that one thing that might lie ahead in his treatment were angry feelings about things that had happened in his life.[1] He soon asked what I would do if he left now. I replied that while I could not force him to stay, I hoped that we would be able to work together as long as it took for him to gain better self-control, and consequently to be able to use his energy and abilities in more constructive ways. Eddie asserted that my keeping him in treatment (not letting him go) was the source of his anger and hatred of me and the reason for his not liking to see my face anymore. He began to threaten and smudged my hand with a pen. I said that sounded like a reversal, and I thought maybe he was mad because people had not hung onto him but had let him go. He asked what I meant. I recalled the premature death of his putative father, the removal of his mother through illness, and his several foster home placements after that. All these experiences had occurred at ages when kids did not want to be let go by their parents, but rather they wanted to be hung onto, until they were old enough to be let go. Eddie had been drawing lines while listening, and he now told me that he was just 5 when his mother was hospitalized. I suggested that that

---

[1] I was at that time developing the ideas which form the basis for this book, and I interpeted his conflict as instinctual, that is, fear of his aggression. That was a more classical psychoanalytic understanding than I currently espouse. While that interpretation did elicit an enlightening response and may well have been accurate, I would now interpret his own underlying feelings of responsibility or his fear of being held responsible for the bad things which had happened in his life as the more basic conflict. His fantasy was probably that his anger or aggression were responsible for depriving himself of the kind of relationship he needed from his parents.

made kids angry.[2] He then asked me what he was drawing. It was a teddy bear. I asked if he had one, and he told me about the three-foot tall teddy bear his mother had given him when he was 5, perhaps when she left. He told me about his current teddy bear and the other stuffed animals he puts on his bed. Then he mumbled something about wanting me to be his teddy bear. I repeated this, but he said, "No," he couldn't stand me with him all night. Next, around the bear, he drew a car of the model and color that I drive, so that the bear was driving my car. He asked my license plate number and inscribed it on the car as the session ended. His doodling had belied his verbal disclaimer of wanting me, as object of a parental transference, with him.

During the next several sessions, Eddie talked anecdotally for the first time about his early childhood. He described the family home, burying toy soldiers and Indians in their backyard, wrestling with his brother, and dangers he had encountered. He played with toys which were appropriate for much younger children and crashed trucks in elaborate play. I questioned a relationship between the latter and his father's death. He reported that to have been a single truck crash (and thus by implication not what he had just been playing out). Then, for the first time, he asked for a graham cracker from the canister in the office which children are allowed to eat from at will. He adjudged the cracker to be "good." He mapped out an unfinished checkers game to continue the following day. He feigned injury to his arm and left the door open as he departed. These behaviors reflected a wish for ongoing contact, leaving the door open for further work, plus slightly lessened defensiveness against engaging in a relationship of therapeutic benefit.

Aspects of the way Eddie was now trying to feel more aligned or allied with me took on slightly grotesque qualities. In addition to asking more questions about me and frequently imitating my posture (to which he himself would call attention), Eddie was examining such things as my teeth at very close range in order to count and locate cavities, identify cracks, and so on. In the

---

[2]Now I would point out that it threatened his source and sense of security and made him scared; however, he disabused himself of such thoughts and feelings by acting angry, unconcerned, and not responsible for anything.

absence of other knowledge he seemed to want to know me in these ways. At the same time evidence persisted that he could not trust that I was benign. For example, after diffidently asking my permission for a second piece of Kleenex and a second graham cracker, he forced me to take some also. In so doing he was protecting himself from apprehension that he would arouse my envy or enmity for taking more than his fair share, a separation guilt-type dynamic. He bit my finger and thumb lightly. Following a ten-day Christmas vacation, Eddie exhibited a mixed reaction of wanting to shut me out of the office, which he literally did, wanting to compete with me in arm wrestling, but also wishing to keep me with him. The latter was evidenced by putting on my glasses and asking to take a toy home from the office. Yet, he still could not acknowledge any relationship between those wishes and the interruption of treatment for the vacation. Nevertheless, he took my professional card when he left. Thus, it appeared that the experiences which had bred out these attitudes had been so traumatic that he could not yet allow them into consciousness.

By this point in treatment (100 hours), Eddie no longer stole, he lied less, exhibited greater flexibility with adults, was less bossy with peers, and was having fewer problems at school. As he became more tractable in his outside life, however, he became much more volatile, impulsive, and aggressive during his sessions with me.

DEVELOPING AWARENESS OF HIS INTERNAL CONFLICT ABOUT SELF-CONTROL; A REENACTMENT OF THE PROCESS IN DEVELOPMENT BY WHICH SELF-CONTROL IS ACHIEVED

A new pattern developed in his analytic hours. Eddie alternately entertained me and provoked me. The latter became more physical. He snapped a handkerchief in my face and immediately apologized. I pointed out how he had gone too far and was now worried that I would retaliate. He started to do it again which I stopped by limit-setting and also interpreted the counterphobic motive for repeating the act. During the hours which followed, Eddie did things like batting the nerf ball (an indoor ball) in my face. The only way I could stop this was by challenging him with,

"Can you control yourself?" He would reply that he could, so I would respond, "Then do so." He claimed he did not want to stop but did. Such escalation of his provocativeness and impulsivity invariably occurred at times when his treatment was threatened, though he always discounted that. On this particular occasion his foster father had wanted to stop bringing him because Eddie was not appreciative. In the immediately ensuing sessions Eddie discharged much tension through physical activity, stopping only when challenged to do so.

He attempted to gain greater self-control by ritualizing his discharge of tension through such activities as shooting baskets. He also invoked good luck rituals, like touching me before each shot. These actions represented Eddie's efforts to master fears that his aggressive impulses had caused the threatened rupture of treatment and to assure himself that in the past his peskiness had not caused people to reject or abandon him.

Eventually he did things like hiding inside the window seat in my office. It was as if he felt at those moments only able to control himself by isolating himself from me. At the same time, by tucking himself into a corner of my office (as opposed to leaving), he was expressing his wish to stay with me.

Provocative play with the nerf ball escalated and my next tack was to suggest that these behaviors were out of his control.[3] That angered him and he became my jailer, thereby making me rather than himself the person who needed to be controlled. He then staged a fight between figurines of a dog and a man. I pointed out that he was depicting in elaborative play his internal struggle for self-control. Eddie listened and at the session's end wanted to take a couple of rubber bands from the office. His wish to keep something of mine, arising when we were addressing his wish to achieve self-control, suggested that retaining something of the parental figure, which is one result of identification, is important in achieving the capacity to control one's impulses.

---

[3]In retrospect I think a more accurate interpretation, in accord with the view of psychopathology presented in this book, would have been that he felt compelled to act uncontrolled. That was because he could not really believe and trust that I did not want to reject him as he had experienced everyone else in his early life having done. His out of control behavior was a compliance with what he had long ago concluded gratified adults' wishes to reject him.

At the next session he took apart and reassembled a scotch tape dispenser, asking me, "Aren't I smart?" (He sought my approval.) He put a piece of tape on me and ordered me to leave it there. (Feeling that he had secured my approval, he felt he could lay a claim on me.) Subsequently he inadvertently dropped an unopened package of graham crackers and opened it improperly. He blamed me for these mishaps. I was then able to point out how self-critical he could be, and that this might be a valuable clue toward understanding all of his previous activities. Namely, he had to repeatedly prove to himself that he wasn't afraid of making mistakes and that if he did make mistakes he could mend things again. He discounted my interpretation but started to make paper airplanes very carefully, claiming to be an expert at doing so. As he constructed planes expertly, which psychologically meant demonstrating his self-control, he told me menacingly to be quiet, that I was making him mad. Since I had been silent, Eddie was apparently attempting to reduce his own tension by controlling me. He wanted me to bring milk for him to drink with his graham crackers. We were witnessing a continuation of the prior session's theme; Eddie was further elaborating his attempts to master what was now slowly becoming experienced as internal conflict. The latter was being illustrated in the struggle he had dramatized between animal and man and disassembling and reassembling an object while seeking my approval. In his wish to demonstrate his self-control under my watchful, approving eye, to have me bear his tension (telling me to be quiet), to afford him nurturing interest (milk and graham crackers), and to have his mark on me (the tape), I believe that Eddie was illustrating and enacting features of the normal parent–child relationship which are involved in the acquisition of impulse control.

Initially I had interpreted Eddie's frequent efforts to enslave me as his attempts to develop self-control through controlling others (me). A more important meaning of that behavior was his wish to lay a claim on someone, to trust another enough to allow the intensity of his jealous, possessive feelings toward his parent. That wish reflected the young child's need to experience his parents as predictable and constant. Inconstancy on the part of parents may be experienced by the child as impulsivity in his environment. That quality in his environment supports impulsiveness in the child. Again, reviewing the sequence of this hour's material, after I had noted Eddie's efforts to master fears of his own destructiveness, he demonstrated how well he could make things (paper airplanes), implying that he was very self-controlled. And next, in his peevish reproach of me for not feeding him milk, we witnessed another expression of the importance of the constant parental influence in the development of impulse control, pride in mastery, and decent self-esteem regulation.

Eddie brought a sling shot to the next hour, "to keep the kids at school in order." He was still working on the same issue, but reverting to projecting his problem of lacking self-control onto others rather than himself. I believe that an element of sibling rivalry and his wish for the exclusive attention of the parent were also implicit in pronouncing himself different from the other kids. I focused on his wish to keep other people "in order," and he responded by changing and becoming a robber. He was soon firing pieces of crayon around the room. With this, as with much similar activity, I was only able to induce him to stop by challenging him: "Are you out of control? Can you control yourself? Then please do so." Frequently Eddie would continue the activity a little longer and then stop. He complained about not wanting to come anymore, but his social worker reported that all such complaints to her and his foster parents had ceased.

LAYING A CLAIM ON THE ANALYST: THE IMPORTANCE OF WANTING TO FEEL LOVED, CLAIMED, AND SPONSORED

Eddie brought some feathers and insisted on putting them in my hair, claiming at first that I looked like an Indian boy and then like a witch doctor. I said that I could not tell whether he was trying to make me look funny or giving me a gift. Eddie stumbled on this and changed the subject. He soon returned to it, insisting that I wear a headband of feathers which he had fashioned. He became angry, kicked at things, and threatened to make a mess when I declined. He wanted to see how I looked wearing the headband. I put it on and asked how I looked. Eddie replied, "Dumb," and then, "No, you look good." The headband had been a gift to me and we could now understand that Eddie had become upset because I had rejected his gift. In this as in other episodes Eddie's wish to retain my interest with his gifts was overshadowed by his intimidating attempts to control me. So, my initial impression had been that these were expressions of aggression rather than love. It was as if he felt that what he had to offer would not suffice to maintain my interest (and thus my presence). Accordingly, he accentuated the aggressive dimensions of his wish in the form of controlling me to insure my presence. In terms of my thesis about adolescent development, these were expressions of the child's overriding wish to please his parent in an effort to secure his sense of safety. Eddie's experience had obviously been that his efforts to do so had been in vain. As a result, in an effort to master the anxiety generated by the impulsive, capricious, domineering, and unpredictable qualities of his parenting environment, he had developed defensive identifications which embodied these very characteristics. These latter defensive identifications were adopted to deal with what Eddie experienced as aggression or hostility from the environment. By contrast Eddie's identification with his mother's touching and stroking was adopted to accommodate his wishes to retain feelings of love and security from the environment.

ISSUES INVOLVED IN SELF-ESTEEM REGULATION

Soon thereafter Eddie demonstrated the manner in which such phenomena are related to self-esteem regulation. On this occasion I declined Eddie's offer to make coffee for me after he found some in a closet. He responded that I did not like him, and started to make paper airplanes at which we knew he excelled. He insisted that I cheer "hooray" when he flew those airplanes. I suggested that his insistence that I cheer might be related to my having refused his offer to make coffee. He replied that I didn't think that he could make coffee right. We agreed that his feelings had been hurt and offended. So, Eddie managed his hurt feelings when he thought that I doubted his competence by exhibiting his competence in making airplanes. He managed his feelings that I didn't like him by having me demonstrate admiration for his productions in cheering for them.

Then, after feeling reassured that I was not rejecting him following those interpretations, Eddie showed me his hurt arm. That is, he could reveal hurt to me, at least for that moment, without fearing being overwhelmed by vulnerability and with less concern that I would make him feel worse.

Eddie's foster parents were now reporting that while he had become very fresh since learning of his paternity, he had also become extremely possessive and jealous of his foster mother's attention. This was markedly different from his earlier attitude, when his interest was focused on what she should do or was obligated to do for or give to him. That distinction is between an interest in another person as opposed to interest in what the other person will provide for him. In psychoanalytic terminology a libidinal relationship was developing from a previously narcissistic one.

REVERSAL OF THE ISOLATION OF EDDIE'S AFFECTS (FEELINGS)

Soon thereafter Eddie began to exhibit toward me in more subtle form the possessiveness he was exhibiting toward his foster mother. This took the form of wishing to be my son and fury at "those kids" (my other child patients). Eddie was expressing anger to his social worker for the first time. This constituted further evidence that the isolation of his affects was reversing. As these inner changes were occurring improvement was evident in his daily life. For example, his grades at school had improved significantly. At the same time he was experiencing jealous possessiveness of his foster mother and myself, Eddie's counterphobic defense was also abating. For example, in the 136th session Eddie laughed uproariously and rolled on the floor after a balloon he was inflating suddenly burst. He claimed it was funny. I wondered if his laughter might be covering up feelings of disappointment or being startled. He acknowledged the latter, and then said, "Phew . . . that scared me." This was his first acknowledgment of fear.

As his counterphobic behaviors were being relinquished, phenomena emerged which suggested that counterphobia had helped him avoid awareness of a very harsh, primitive conscience. For example, later during that same hour, Eddie disparaged my wife as pimply-faced and pimply-nosed. (His social worker had told him that I was married.) He then took back what he had said and mimicked a TV ad in which a man slaps his own face. When I wondered if he felt that he should punish himself for what he had said about my wife, Eddie fell out of the chair. It was as if he were confirming my interpretation, while at the same time trying to prove that he was not uncomfortable with these self-punitive feelings by continuing to engage in self-punishing behaviors. Undoing was replacing counterphobic behaviors, though both were being utilized.

EDDIE'S DEVELOPING AWARENESS THAT HIS CONFLICTS WERE INTRAPSYCHIC RATHER THAN INTERPERSONAL

During this same point in treatment Eddie's omnipotence fantasies became more obvious. He attributed great power to me, both positive and negative. I could make things go well for him or otherwise. When he began treatment Eddie acted as if no one could have any influence on him. Now he was reflecting what Freud identified as the overriding importance of the parents to the child. This circumstance rendered understandable the fact that threats to the treatment, that is, to the developing relationship to the analyst, were still the most clear-cut precipitants for provocative behavior on Eddie's part. Yet, he still could not acknowledge this but rather acted upon the underlying anxiety or guilt generated by the anticipation of our not meeting. For example, after announcing that he could meet only three times a week for a couple of months, Eddie began to hit the shelf which was attached to the analytic couch with his ringed fist, laughing as he did so. He then dramatized holding back his striking fist with his other hand. He gave a running commentary on what he was doing, saying that it was a hard struggle. He then said that he would go to sleep and keep his striking hand intertwined with the other one. His hands writhed around in this struggle as he feigned sleep, until eventually he hit the couch shelf once more. I told Eddie that he now seemed aware of how much he struggled to keep his impulsiveness under control. I added that his primary worry about going out of control used to be fear that I would retaliate. But now, since he knew that I did not retaliate, he was becoming more aware that he himself felt badly about losing control (i.e., his conflict was intrapsychic not interpersonal). As if to disavow what I had just said, Eddie attempted to pry the shelf away from the couch, back and forth, little by little, with a slight smile, more intentionally destructive. I commenced a commentary on this pattern of testing, to see how far he could allow himself to go without losing control or to test more strongly whether I might still be provoked to retaliate. I added that the problem was that this type of testing usually progressed to a point where he was out of control or something broke or happened which he did not really want to occur.

EVENTS IN EDDIE'S CURRENT LIFE REPLICATE EARLIER TRAUMATIC EXPERIENCES AND ARE BROUGHT INTO THE TREATMENT IN HIS BEHAVIOR TOWARD ME

Eddie was able to provide further understanding of the intensity and persistence of his provocative behaviors toward me. They reflected his efforts to deal with the distress his sister caused him whenever they were together, by turning passive into active. For behaviors like waving balloons in my face, trying to wrestle with me, and tweaking my nose were the ways his older sister behaved toward him whenever she visited their mother as she was at this time. After acknowledging this Eddie became more destructive, stripping varnish from the arm of a chair with his fingernails and sharp objects. He refused to explore or control this activity, but suddenly blurted out that I should make him stop and asked if I let my kids go out of control. I noted the relationship between his behaviors and thoughts about my purported family.[4] I asked

---

[4]In retrospect probably a more important determinant of this behavior and test of me involved his own earlier family life. The inference to be drawn from the fact that Eddie and his siblings were unmanageable when together was that his parents had not helped any of them develop adequate self-control. Eddie, the youngest, was not protected by his parents from tormenting and sadistic domination by his siblings. His own tendency to be uncontrolled almost certainly arose at least in part as a defensive identification with his siblings to reduce the frightening impact of those experiences from which his parents did not protect him. Eddie was now turning passive into active regarding these

how I could or should make him stop. He didn't know. So I allowed that the only way seemed to be to stop the hour prematurely and I preferred to understand his behavior rather than do that. He looked out the door before leaving that session, saw a woman therapist in the corridor, and related to me his fantasy that she was going to come in and punish him. So again, underneath his seeming insouciance regarding his destructive behavior, he feared being punished.[5]

CONTINUING REVERSAL OF THE ISOLATION OF EDDIE'S AFFECTS

Eddie was now expressing sadness in addition to acknowledging fright. For example, he allowed feeling sad when he was not able to reassemble something he had taken apart. This acknowledgment presented the opportunity to contrast and commend efforts to understand how he felt rather than dealing with tension by discharging it through activity; that is, talk versus play. On another occasion, after I failed to obey his command that I say "1-2-3" while he was drumming, Eddie looked morose, but claimed he was mad at me and turned away. He then banged so vigorously that he broke the pens he was using as drum sticks. I wondered from his expression if sadness and fright were interposed between my failure to be controlled by him and his resulting anger. His sadness seemed to be associated with an idea that if I did not comply with his requests I did not like him, or else that I couldn't be counted on by him. (I was not a reliable sponsor.) He offered no verbal response but moved away and started to take the telephone apart, ostensibly because he liked to dismantle things. As I reached over to stop him he blurted out, "Don't you touch me or I'll slap your hand." This had just slipped out, because he added that I would never find out what

---

issues in his analysis in an effort to reduce the impact of those traumatic experiences. His blurted-out instructions that I should make him stop being destructive suggested his wish that his parents had helped him and his siblings curtail their impulsiveness.

[5]What was not clear to me then is the degree to which such behaviors are compliances with rather than defiance of what the youth has concluded are the wishes of parent figures, if not as I mentioned, intense efforts to cure himself of the problem by turning passive into active in this behavior toward the therapist.

it was about. I suggested that it repeated some experience that he had had or had witnessed and he was doing to me what had been done or said to him in an effort to master the distress he had experienced from the original episode (i.e., turning passive into active). I added that the unhappy thing about this was that in all areas of his life he seemed obliged to repeat, from touching things to taking things apart, in order to assure himself that he would not be slapped and to reassure himself that other people would not lose interest in him. Eddie responded that he knew I would say that and wondered what obliged meant. I told him it meant that he was not in control of himself. He turned away, telling me not to say anything. He then went a little bit out of control, tossing things in the office. I could then demonstrate his pattern. He was trying to control me, by reversing what had been done to him, and then, if that failed, to go a little bit out of control.[6] Leaving that session Eddie jumped up happily to touch the overhead light. I suggested that it was more fun to do happy things than to consider unhappy experiences which had so influenced his life.

SECOND YEAR OF ANALYSIS

Eddie had now been in treatment for about a year (150 sessions). He was losing his exquisite ability to detect any changes in the office. I thought his reduced hypervigilance reflected lessening fearfulness of his environment, developing confidence that other people would not let him down, and an increasing inner sense of security and true self-confidence. He was better able to tolerate losing games. He made a cake for his foster mother's birthday and bought her a card with his own money; these were highly unusual gestures for him. Thus, he was beginning to exhibit a capacity for mutuality in relationships rather than simply having

---

[6]At the time I understood the latter to be a demonstration to himself that he was in control, that is, he controlled his going out of control. I now consider a more important determinant to be a compliance on his part, giving me what he thought I wanted in a perverse effort to please me and therefore secure the relationship with me. Recall that I had said that he couldn't control himself. Eddie did not like that interpretation whenever I made it.

to take and grab what he could for himself. He was now spontaneously revealing little bits about his outside life (e.g., feeling scared when he fell off his bike), but at the same time he was controlling me more in the office. He also would spend whole sessions reading or sometimes sleeping, huddled over the warm hot air register during early morning sessions in the winter. Before doing so he would always have me guess what was in his jacket pocket. I felt this pattern reflected increasing trust that I would not hurt him (in feeling comfortable enough to sleep) but lingering uncertainty about whether my interest in him would be sustained (in controlling me and having me guess what he had).

Eddie registered surprise one day when I reminded him that we would not meet for the next two sessions. He waved his arms happily but then disrupted the game we were playing. I pointed out how his happy reaction was followed by impulsiveness. Since he was becoming more impulsive at that moment there might be more to his response than simply happiness. Eddie prepared to leave the session five minutes early, going out to the porch to see if his foster parents were there. This plan to leave early was a turning passive into active mechanism.[7] He returned to the office, lay on the couch, and pantomimed breaking it. He put his head under the pillow and started to call "Help! Help!" He acted as if he were suffocating and wanted me to take the pillow off. Then he flung the pillow at me with great force and wanted me to toss it back to him. I told him that in spite of himself, that is, expressing happiness about not meeting, his reaction of wanting to break the couch and then wanting me to prevent him

---

[7]Eddie's consistent upsets around interruptions in treatment quite compellingly conveyed his extraordinary sensitivity to separations, even though he was unable to consciously acknowledge this and tended to voice indifference to such interruptions. In this sequence his anxiety about separating was reactivated by my reminder that we wouldn't meet for two sessions. Eddie responded, in an effort to master that anxiety, by perpetrating actively on me the equivalent of what he had experienced passively from me; he left early. His motive was to reduce his anxiety and in the context of the treatment to see whether I would react as he did to such experiences. If the therapist demonstrates his or her ability to deal with experiences that had traumatized the patient with greater equanimity than had the patient, then over time in analysis or therapy the patient can identify with the therapist's equanimity and in so doing, reverse the effects of the earlier life trauma which in Eddie had been the development of this behavioral pattern of impulsivity in the face of threatened separations.

from suffocating might be his way of telling us about times in the past when he desperately needed people to be there consistently and that these interruptions in our meetings seemed to bring back those feelings. Eddie quieted and soon was whining again for help and holding the pillow more tightly over his face. He turned away from me and then threw it at me again with great force. When I did not throw it back on command Eddie threatened to go out of control and kick the shelf off the couch to which it was attached. I suggested that he was angry because we were not going to be meeting. I also noted that he may have been telling us something important about his previous style of always appearing smiling and happy when that might not have been primarily what he was feeling.

THE INTENSITY OF THE CHILD'S WISH TO FEEL CLAIMED/WANTED BY HIS PARENT AND SECURE

At this point Eddie did not want anyone to know that he was a foster child. He demanded that his foster mother tell people that she was his grandmother, which she refused to do. He reminded her that she used to hold, hug, and rock him when he first lived there. She replied that he was a teenager now.

My original formulation of Eddie's impulsiveness had been that he gratified his impulses rather than the wishes of his important object relationships; that was because parents and their surrogates had not been sufficiently gratifying to motivate Eddie to forsake immediate gratification of his impulses in favor of pleasing them (parents). That formulation is more in line with classical psychoanalytic thinking which emphasizes the drives as the basic motivating forces in human experience and development. I now understand the situation differently. Eddie's failure to control his impulsiveness was based not simply on nongratifying parents but on ideas he had developed from experiences with inconstant parents. On the basis of his experiences he concluded that he could not expect what he sensed he needed from adults, namely a secure, constant relationship in which he felt valued by their appropriate protectiveness and sponsorship of him. In the absence of that, he struggled with the idea that he was somehow responsible for not having what he needed from parents. He massively warded off the idea of his culpability and responsibility by acting the opposite; namely, entitled and indifferent to adults rather than guilty and very needy of expressions of nurturance and security (as his lap-sitting requests suggest). In addition, as I noted earlier, his impulsiveness included significant elements of defensive identification derived from his earlier experiences with parents and older sibs; however, many of my interventions were based on my earlier formulation.

At moments of frustration Eddie now literally teeter-tottered between directing fury toward himself and toward me. Once he literally went back and forth saying, "Bloch is nice . . . Bloch is not nice" and between wanting to "protect Bloch" and to "get" Bloch. After hitting me near the eye with his slingshot he feigned firing it toward himself (i.e., undoing). He then told me about an animal whose bark is worse than its bite and put his slingshot inside *my* coat. I pointed out how he was using me as auxiliary ego to help him maintain self-control. He was also bespeaking the expectation of younger children that adults will help them control their impulsivity.

He went on to demonstrate that he had "deadly aim" in shooting gallery play (i.e., how dangerous he was). On occasion he fired rubber bands at me. I pointed out that now that he thought I liked him Eddie seemed to be showing me how impulsive and aggressive he could be; he responded, "Maybe." This persistence of his impulsivity toward me is better explained by my later, more complicated formulation, for it continued even after he seemed to experience me as constant, nonrejecting, and gratifying. Eddie's acknowledgment that "maybe" he was compelled to show me how unacceptable he was would more likely be motivated by underlying ideas that he was responsible for bad things which happened to him, and by lack of certainty that adults wanted better for him or that he deserved better treatment.

During the week prior to our second summer vacation Eddie was vilifying my other child patients. In elaborative play he treated me medically for malnutrition. He then became a restaurateur serving me meats from different lands. The first was "people stew" from a cannibalistic country. Under the impetus of an anticipated separation we could perceive in this metaphor his anxiety about being deprived of basic, oral supplies and his fear that separation was associated with destruction of others. One survives a separation at the expense of another (people stew). As if to illustrate the latter, Eddie became provocatively destructive in the office, scratching furniture while acknowledging anger toward me, but adding that we were not going to understand it. He made a fort and ensconced himself inside it. He dismissed any relationship between these behaviors and our imminent separation, avowing only pleasure about the vacation. I allowed his pleasure but reviewed the things he had done as the vacation approached: He had taken my role. He had taken home some play money from the office. He had hidden in the window seat and wanted me to search for him, and he had been provoking me to anger. Eddie responded by becoming hyperactive, so I wondered if hyperactivity was his way of avoiding the impending separation.[8] His response was to deny the event (i.e., the interruption of sessions) by playing a game right up to the end of the last hour before the vacation.

Upon resuming after that one-month vacation Eddie performed magic tricks, making objects disappear and reappear. This suggested that the issue and meaning of separation were still prominent in his sensibility. In sessions which followed he alternated between provoking and entertaining me. One day, during a moment of shared friendliness when we were both chuckling about a clever pun he had made using both of our names, Eddie impulsively marked my nose with a paint stick. As I walked toward the sink he forbade me to wash it off and climbed on my back as I continued in that direction. He feigned falling off my back, claiming I had pushed him. In sliding off he fell against the sink and cracked it. When he tried to fix it he broke it further. As I tried to interpret what had happened, Eddie drowned me out with a kazoo. While he was not out of control, as frequently happened, his behavior nevertheless eventuated in something breaking. It was as if he could not tolerate the shared feeling of closeness, yet wanted to control me and

---

[8]It would have been more accurate to tell him that the anticipated separation engendered anxiety in Eddie which, as is frequently the case, was communicated outwardly in hyperactivity.

not have me reject (walk away from) him. When he could not do so after putting his mark on me, he became anxious and then apparently angry and wanted both to control and hold onto me. Eddie said nothing but handed me a spent rifle shell. He then threatened to detonate an unfired shell. I observed that he seemed to be demonstrating concern about his destructive feelings or potential for being actually destructive.

This theme of wanting to lay his claim on me but fearing the destructiveness of doing so continued in sharper relief. It seemed that he had to test out via destructive provocativeness that he could not destroy me in his effort to master this anxiety. When confronted about provocative behavior, he now frequently responded that, "I *have* to do it." Thus, he was acknowledging the driven, compulsive aspect of this behavior. He began to scratch furniture with a sharp piece of steel. I interpreted the double aspect of such behaviors, provocation and leaving his mark. I suggested that such behaviors might have to do with concern about who would care for him. He was obliging me to treat him like a younger child to make him stop. In doing so, he might be reenacting worries from his past. He said he would not stop and didn't. I finally grabbed his wrist. He claimed that I had hurt him and he tried to hurt my hand. I noted his double-edged wish that I struggle with him (aggression) and that he have physical contact with me (nurturance). He claimed only to be mad (angry) because I had hurt him and he scratched the chair more after putting scotch tape on me. He became very frustrated because he could not hurt me physically. At that point I was furious.

During the next session (204th hour) Eddie took a knife from his pocket and began stabbing the shelf attached to the analytic couch, smiling at me as he did so. He then went to the patient's chair and began to shave the wooden arm of the chair with his knife. No manner of interpretation nor limit-setting was successful in getting him to stop doing so; finally, I took his wrist. He looked alarmed and relieved; I took the knife and locked it in the file cabinet. He asked why I took it, and also why I had let him do that much damage. Then he wanted me to approve of and admire his drawings. I pointed out how his behaviors alternated. I asked about his reaction to my having taken his knife from him. He had been scared and thought that I was going to stab him. Then he took that back, saying he hadn't felt that way. He wanted to leave twenty minutes early to get to a scout meeting and make up the time the following day. I reminded him that we were not meeting the next day and that he had made this same slip several times. He said that he was in "conflict" and then took that back, saying that he wanted to leave and I would not let him. I replied that since he knew my position, that it was his decision, he was in fact in conflict about it, and the conflict was inside himself and not between him and me. He took some things home from the office that day and called me Spencer for the first time. Again, such activities suggested that he wanted to maintain a connection with me at the same time he was agitating to leave early, that is, to reject me. I understood the latter to be a way of deceiving himself about the former.

A period of wanting to leave sessions early ensued. I told Eddie that I wanted us to have our full time together, but that the decision was his. Eddie's response was to literally obsess behaviorally: He would leave the office, then return, then leave, then return, then leave, linger at the door, and then return. At this time, Eddie allowed missing his foster mother when his foster parents were away for two days. I was able to demonstrate how Eddie's taking control of when our hours ended represented his reaction to his foster parents' having left him. I thought that such experiences tapped into deep feelings of powerlessness and helplessness to control the comings and goings of people who had been important to him early in his life. Eddie responded, "Good point—now can I leave?" His behavior confirmed that he tried to act powerful when he was scared and felt powerless (vulnerable). Again, we were seeing how pervasively Eddie resorted to reversal mechanisms, turning things into their opposite and counterphobia.

COMPLICATIONS FROM OUTSIDE THE ANALYSIS

For several months Eddie had been reporting that his mother was going to have her psychiatrist find out why he was being seen four times a week. That psychiatrist had gone so far as to call

Eddie's social worker demanding to know why; however, he had failed to take her suggestion that he ask me. Because there was at least a hint of complicity on his part with the efforts of Eddie's mother to undermine Eddie's analysis, I introduced myself to her psychiatrist at a professional meeting after one and a half years of treatment. I expressed my willingness to discuss Eddie's situation with him and requested his assistance in supporting Eddie's treatment. The other psychiatrist denied disagreement with the form of Eddie's treatment, though he questioned me superciliously about the indications for analysis in Eddie. He expressed his conviction that Eddie's mother and two siblings and Eddie also were all manic depressive. This contact proved to have no salutary influence on that psychiatrist's conduct.

EDDIE'S CONTINUING EFFORTS TO INTEGRATE SELF-CONTROL

Eddie was now frequently beginning hours by reversing our roles, ushering me into the office. The immediate precipitants for his impulsivity and provocativeness now seemed to be his frustration with other children he thought were my patients. His older brother was visiting their mother and Eddie was very jealous; so, that issue in his current life outside treatment intensified this issue in the transference. He threw clay around the office at the end of sessions and frequently tried to wrestle with me. He insisted that I feed him at the same time he wished to fight with me. Once he turned over some chairs and then wondered if I still wanted to see him. He was, therefore, addressing the issue of whether his behavior would drive me away (i.e., cause me to reject him). When I realized and told him that he often became impulsive at the end of sessions, after not having been so during the hour, Eddie responded, "Oh shut up, stupid." I noted that he was not out of control but rather impulsive at times of anticipated separations. He took out his knife just before leaving one day and touched the chair with it. I warned him with, "Remember what I said." He put the knife away but took out a piece of sandpaper and started to scratch the furniture. I had to take this away from him and urge him out the door. I was beginning to feel furious again.

I also realized that these most blatant provocations invariably occurred on Fridays. When I pointed this out, Eddie appeared startled, smiled disbelievingly, said it was a coincidence and that I made these things up. When I talked about these regressive wishes and needs for me and his tendency to push me away, he interrupted with, "You think I like coming here?" I replied that I thought he was of two minds about it; and when he became aware of wanting to be here, he became worried because that made him feel almost under my power. This was because I could leave or disappoint him. I pointed out that his reaction to this was to do the opposite, namely to control me or to act like he didn't want to be with me. I added that he also became impulsive at such times, and felt at risk for being sent away if he angered me. But, if he then could control me, he felt reassured that I was not angry or at least wouldn't leave. Eddie screamed at me to shut up. I said that guys don't mind listening to things that don't bother them. He tried to deceive himself into believing the conflict was interpersonal rather than internal, and that controlling others rather than self-control represented strength.

In the following hour (session 221), Eddie demonstrated one paradigmatic way in which children interact with parents to achieve self-control: Eddie had me sit next to him as he started to make a paper airplane. He folded the paper. Suddenly he blurted out, "It's wrong," and impulsively crumpled it into a ball. He threw it to me, ordering me to catch it, which I did. He held out his hand and told me to throw it back to him. I complied, but the wad deflected off his hand. He ordered me to do it again and I did, though inadvertently threw it further from his grasp. He missed it but retrieved it. He then told me to throw it right to him or he'd get impulsive. He made an effort to catch it that time and did so. He smiled, said "There," with satisfaction and relaxation of his tension and dropped it in the waste paper basket.

Upon experiencing frustration in making his airplane, I believe Eddie became overwhelmed with helplessness and then enraged which prompted him to destroy what he had made. In then throwing it to me, he turned his frustration from himself onto me. He then controlled me and I absorbed and bore his criticism for not doing (throwing) it right; that is, I bore with equanimity what Eddie had been unable to tolerate in himself, namely not doing something correctly. His attention then became directed from simply discharging his impulse to mastering the impulse through developing skill in the form of accurate control (sublimation). This occurred by a process of identifying with my reaction when he unleashed impulsiveness in smaller doses toward me in our game of catch. Eddie was eventually able to dispose of the crumpled paper properly, under his own willful control. Such a process must recur repeatedly between parents and their young children to help them integrate self-control.

Eddie entertained me with western songs. Frequently he rendered the lyics, "Release me so I can love again. Why should I keep loving you, since you're untrue?" On another occasion, as he prepared to leave, he pantomimed being tortured. I reflected that leaving was torture. He enacted his sleep walking and feigned being tortured in his sleep.

On another occasion at that time when I had just had a haircut which changed my appearance very little, Eddie asked, "Who are you?" His voice contained real emotion, as if there were some indefinable uncertainty or anxiety about my identity. He went on to reflect with a tone of disgusted disapproval that I had gotten a haircut. Eddie's reaction raised the question noted earlier about a subtle impairment of his object constancy based on the inconstancy of parenting figures during his first seven years of life.

A SECOND MEETING WITH EDDIE'S MOTHER

I met again with Eddie's mother. She still questioned why Eddie was seeing me four times a week, presenting herself as Eddie's advocate in the matter. Their social worker reported that Eddie's mother became irrationally enraged very readily and at such times the social worker felt like hitting her. The social worker's reaction to Eddie's mother was similar to what I experienced with Eddie. It suggested that this aspect of Eddie's behavior contained at least an element of identification with his mother.

Eddie's mother provided some history: He had been breast-fed for six or seven months and had been "serene" during infancy. He used a transitional object briefly, though she couldn't recall what it was. He became very active and precocious and was smarter and more capable than his brother. The family had been an affectionate one. Eddie's putative father would be away for three months at a time, though he was taking shorter trips toward the end of his life. When her husband was home he undertook much of the child care.

Eddie's biological father also met with me to discuss the frequency of Eddie's appointments. He recalled that Eddie was always in motion, "frisky," a "daredevil," and his mother's "pet" during his early childhood.

ADDITIONAL EXTERNAL CONTRIBUTANTS TO EDDIE'S HEIGHTENED AGGRESSIVENESS TOWARD ME

Eddie's ambivalence became more intense. He wondered why he had to meet so often since he was doing better. He became more physically aggressive, trying to wrestle with me to "overpower" me. No interpretation nor limit-setting would induce him to stop. As I simply fended him off, he complained that I had hurt his back and now he was really going to get me. I insisted that he stop but he did not. On this occasion I held him down on the floor with one hand for the remainder of the hour. As I let him up, he kicked and grazed my face. I told him to stop and let him go. He made a few more passes at me but did not grab me. He then professed ignorance about what had happened. It seemed to me that he was unable to stop until he felt he had hurt me. I was unable to find any day residue for this behavior, and only learned much later what was undoubtedly contributing to it from outside the office. I will mention that additional determinant for this behavior shortly.

In hours which followed, Eddie attempted to perfect his skill, by throwing toy Indians into a canister, rather than simply discharging his aggressive energy in cutting or biting them apart. My job in this game was to place the canister in certain positions. One day Eddie became very upset when the canister was not exactly where he had told me to put it. He seemed scared that I had not been completely, predictably reliable.

He spent more sessions reading. I wondered if he was now pulling away, after he had begun to feel friendlier, which had been manifested while we worked together perfecting his skill at tossing Indians into the canister. Eddie responded by trying to hold me immobilized while tormenting me by poking at my face. I pointed out his wishes both to hang onto me and to torment me. On another occasion he hit me very hard with the pillow and tried to smother me, all with a broad smile on his face. I had to resort to holding him down, asking if he was out of control. He responded no and I agreed. Finally the session neared its end. As I let him up I asked what was going on with him. He replied, "Lots of stuff," but would not elaborate. He began attacking again, by jumping over the arm of my chair into my lap, at which point I pushed him off. He kept repeating this activity. I finally told him that this was not helping us and we would have to stop a few minutes early. I opened the door but he closed it and remained inside, continuing to jump over the arm of the chair into my lap. After establishing that his mother and her boyfriend were picking him up, I said I'd accompany him to their car. He said he would go by himself. He pulled himself together, struck me very hard with the pillow, and left. At the beginning of the next session he feigned jumping on me, claiming he had really scared me. He had no ideas about what had happened the day before. He claimed not to have felt angry toward me until I hurt his legs.

Shortly after the Christmas vacation which occurred around that time, Eddie wanted to wrestle again. I was adamant about not doing so. Nevertheless, he slipped wrestling holds onto me and the chair in which I was sitting tipped over with Eddie landing on top of me in such a way that I was completely immobilized. I chose not to struggle. He regaled in his strength, indicating he could hit or do what he wished to me. He wanted me to apologize if I ever hurt him. He held me there until well after the session's end. I surmised, therefore, that one reason for this wish to overpower me was to remain with me.

During all these episodes of wrestling, nose tweaking, and so on, I experienced Eddie as strongly provoking me to hit or punish him. Then I learned from his social worker that Eddie had been witnessing a great deal of physical fighting on visits to his mother's apartment. His older brother and his mother's boyfriend were contending to the point of violence. In retrospect then, this was the currently traumatic experience from outside the analyis which had been contributing to the escalation of his aggression toward me during the prior couple of months. He was reenacting with me what he had witnessed, but in reverse, turning passive into active to master his anxiety by seeing if I could experience what he had with greater equanimity. If so, then he could identify with my better ability to deal with it.

Eddie began to yell angrily for me to let him demonstrate wrestling holds, but later would play peek-a-boo games. He attempted to engage me in real interactions. For example, he wanted me to give him change for a dollar and aspirin for his headaches. At this time Eddie forsook his foster mother's offer to have a birthday party for him in favor of having his mother give him a party; however, he had to make his own cake when he went to her apartment to celebrate his birthday. Such behavior on the part of his mother, abrogating parental duties despite protestations of her devotion to Eddie, may have contributed to his efforts to induce me to engage in real interactions like medicating his headache.

UNRAVELING THE MECHANISM OF EDDIE'S COUNTERPHOBIA

In hours shortly thereafter we unraveled the mechanism of Eddie's counterphobic style. I have pointed out that Eddie was basically worried that I would get angry at him; but he coped with this by acting as if he were trying to provoke me to become angry toward him, that is, counterphobia. He seemed to be trying to prove to himself that nothing bad would happen. There seemed to be another ingredient involved which related to a feature of Eddie's perceptual memory.

After a two-week spring vacation, Eddie commented that he had not seen me for a long time and he almost had not wanted to come. At the next session he implored me to let him go through the folder of the artwork he had done since beginning treatment. He examined his previous artwork carefully. I wondered why he wanted to do this now and he replied because they might be moving; then he added that that was a joke. I wondered if perhaps he was reviewing all the things he had drawn here to reacquaint himself with his treatment and with me; that is, he wanted to ascertain that things were the same here. He replied, "You're smart." From this and other examples described earlier, it was almost as if Eddie, despite being intelligent and acutely perceptive, had some subtle breach in his object constancy both as described by Anna Freud, the ability to retain visual memory of someone in their absence, and in his libidinal object constancy as described by Mahler, an ability to experience the security-providing qualities of the mother in her absence. If the prosaic example of his mother refusing to make Eddie's birthday cake after offering to celebrate him typified her behaviors when she was raising him, then we might surmise that Eddie's developing capacity to recognize and trust the familiar without feeling anxious had been impaired by the combination of her compromised security-engendering qualities and premature separations from both parents.

Physical attacks, under the guise of wrestling, intensified again. His ostensible motive was to control me. He accused me of wanting to hurt him when I held him at bay. I suggested that he might feel that way because he experienced his own demands upon me as too great, and that I would feel overwhelmed and want to retaliate. I extended the interpretation to relate his need to control me to not having been able to control people earlier in his life. He might feel frightened if he trusted me. He said he did not trust me, adding, "You might be a thief!" I asked what a thief does. He retorted, "Steals." So, if he trusted me, then he would have to worry that I would take advantage of him. He wondered if I thought he hated me. I responded that I didn't know, but thought his feelings were mixed. He wanted me to explain that and I did. He then started to take the telephone apart and I ordered him to stop. He threatened to cut my necktie with scissors. I had to push the scissors away, and he became furious, claiming that I had hurt him. I said I was sorry, that it had not been my intent. He then took out the Chinese checker set and began compulsively to color the holes on the playing board. He was literally unable to stop himself until he had colored all of them. Purportedly this was because someone else might finish the job. When I told him the board would be here tomorrow, he replied that maybe he wouldn't be; either of us could have an accident or get hit. In his manner of coloring the game board I believe we were witnessing the development of compulsive mechanisms to bind anxiety and tension which ordinarily would have been discharged directly on me.

Eddie became even more unmanageable—squirting me with a trick ring, inadvertently damaging my necktie with water, breaking pencils defiantly, throwing things around, surreptitiously wiping paint on the seat cushion. Yet, he became worried whenever I became stern or angry. Then he would try to insure my attention, as by having me name tunes he played on his kazoo. It seemed that if he could maintain my attention in that manner, namely by controlling me in such a way that I was exhibiting interest in what he was doing, then he felt reassured that I was not angry at him and would not retaliate. He wondered if I'd kick him out if he didn't want to learn about the basis of his behaviors. I said I would not.

A likely contributant to the escalation of these destructive, challenging behaviors became apparent when his mother requested another meeting. She planned to appeal for custody of Eddie. Her psychiatrist supported this and wanted to meet with Eddie and her. While she had ostensibly come for my opinion, she afforded no opportunity for discussion. Rather, she filled the time with insistences about the rectitude of her decision and repeated that she would not be deterred. She thought I favored his remaining with the foster parents. I suggested that she might want to consider not whether she should have custody of Eddie but when would be the optimum timing for such transfer of custody. She paid no attention.

When I next saw Eddie I suggested that he must be in a terrible dilemma, concerned about hurting either his foster parents' or his mother's feelings. He would not talk about it. I also wondered if his provocativeness from the week before could be related to this; that is, he was dealing with fears of separation by trying to make it happen with me, the mechanism known as turning passive into active. He asked about my water-stained necktie and wondered about having to replace the pencils he had broken. Rather than answering directly I observed that in the latter activity he might have been communicating that he felt broken up about this matter. At that point Eddie broke a stirring rod. He tossed pencils around. I asked him to please not do so. He did it less. He refused to discuss this because "you're a dummy." I noticed an old pattern of putting on a happy face in situations of distress, but observed to him that he had come further than that now and knew his feelings. With that he started to sing the song, "Put On a Happy Face," but with his own lyrics. They were about, "If you want to talk to Dr. Proctor and Blocker, put on a happy face, etc." He went on and on in a crescendo-ing, shrieking manner. At the end I told him that it sounded like an anguished cry, not a happy song, and maybe it was like laughing on the outside and crying on the inside—broken up inside like the pencil he had broken. It was time to stop but Eddie would not leave. He was trying to put wrestling holds on me. He asked if he would have to see me if he lived with his mother. He thought he would not. I indicated my hope that we would be able to complete our work together. I identified his evident conflict, not wanting to be here but literally trying to cling to me with arm locks. He said that because I wouldn't let him put a wrestling hold on me, I had to pay the consequences. He took a new pencil, broke it in two and walked out with a smile.

In hours which followed, whenever I raised his dilemma and probable confusion with respect to his custody, Eddie became provocative and he picked up pieces of furniture and balanced them. I said this was what he was presumably experiencing in his outside life, namely, just trying to balance things between his mother and foster mother and keep himself on an even keel. I reflected my wish to help him in any way I could. He said that I could not and became even more provocative—hitting my nose, hitting my face with his shoes, shadow boxing at me, pushing my nose. I became angry and told him to stop. He said, "You can't make me." I responded that if he could not stop we would have to stop the hour and continue tomorrow. He told me he could not leave and continued this behavior. He kept putting his feet on the freshly painted walls, trying to throw the couch pillow at me with great force and pushing it in my face. Eventually I took him by the arms, sat him in the analyst's chair, and told him to stay there. He was taken aback and said I couldn't make him, which I agreed, and started to talk to him: I wondered why he tried to get people mad at him and to reject him. He said that it was only toward me that he acted this way. I recalled evidence to the contrary, that he had alienated many people who didn't realize what he and I knew, namely, that those behaviors were his way of keeping out of sight his feelings of confusion, his fears, and his loneliness. I told him I was sure that he could cause me to terminate his treatment prematurely but I hoped that he would not. I did not see his situation as hopeless, nor did I think he would end up with the kind of illness that other members of his family had suffered. I wanted to work with him and help him get over his difficulties. While we understood that his wrestling and bumptious behaviors reflected his inner discomfort and at the same time ways of avoiding thinking about his feelings, such behaviors were not helpful, and I would do whatever was necessary to maintain control. I also told him that if he could understand just one question—why he was driven to try to get people angry at him and drive them away—then he might well be able to finish his treatment, which is what he claimed to want. He asked again what was that question, and had been silent with moist eyes, looking down without moving for the duration of my five-minute, earnest and emphatic talk to him. I told him that I would see him tomorrow. He got up silently and left.

IN CHAOTIC CASES EXPECT CHAOTIC EXTERNAL CONDITIONS

Eddie's mother would not be dissuaded from her efforts to gain custody. Their social worker was certain that the court referee would award her custody, unless Eddie did not want to go with her, or unless I made a strong statement, which the social worker did not ask for.

Shortly thereafter the psychiatrist of Eddie's mother had his secretary call and ask something of me which could then have been construed as my agreeing that he see Eddie in consultation. I had him speak to me directly. He was confident of being able to determine, on the basis of a single interview with Eddie and his mother together, the most appropriate disposition for the child. He saw nothing inappropriate in his request, and in fact, asked if I were feeling a bit insecure when I questioned his approach. I discussed such a meeting with Eddie. He wanted to meet his mother's psychiatrist and became preoccupied with whether I liked that psychiatrist. Eddie and his mother met jointly with him for a half-hour shortly thereafter. Eddie's foster mother and his social worker reported that Eddie's mother was undermining Eddie's treatment and that her psychiatrist seemed to be abetting her attitudes and actions.

THE INABILITY OF IMPULSE-RIDDEN ADOLESCENTS TO SPONTANEOUSLY IDENTIFY THEIR FEELINGS

Eddie continued with the curious pattern of intense provocation alternating with insistence upon staying past the end of sessions, and having me approve of and be interested in his projects. Once when I tried to stop his wrestling he told me I couldn't make him and said softly, "You're not my father." I was able to identify a pattern: Even after a tranquil session, Eddie became hyperactive and destructive at the end of hours, as if to induce me to kick him out. Often I was furious at such times. In fact, literally ushering him out physically before the end of the hour was the only way I could sometimes stop his wrestling. This pattern in the office replicated the way he felt and handled the situation in his life outside treatment. He was, therefore, apprising us of a powerful relationship in his mind between separation and destruction. This issue was now thrown into sharper relief by the impending custody hearing. On this occasion I had to push him out as he continued to break toy soldiers and then was hitting at me.

At the next session I introduced this association between separation and destruction to suggest that he might be in conflict over with whom he would live. He disclaimed any reaction to having been separated from his mother (at age 5), but laughed as I responded, "Oh yes, any mother is as good as any other." He had adopted just that stance, never getting close to anyone after he left his home, and acting as he did now, as if nothing bothered him and that he was confidently self-sufficient. I said that he knew that was a way to avoid his underlying fears. He responded that he was not going to talk to me about these things. I pointed out how it was conveyed in his behavior toward the end of sessions. I wondered how he felt about leaving his foster parents. He asked how he should feel. I could not tell if he had no feelings about it, did not know how he felt, or was simply withholding his feelings from me. He wanted me to tell him what feelings people have. He was lying prone on the couch, and his expression was so glum that I concluded that he was serious. He insisted that I name different feelings, and he allowed the ones he felt toward his foster mother—anger sometimes, sadness, positive feelings, and he wondered why he should feel jealous. He disclaimed any conflict, however, for even though he liked both, he preferred to be with his mother. He wondered what he had to work on here to finish. This led to a discussion of his school performance and his interpersonal relationships as the latter were reflected in his transference to me. Regarding school, he said he only cared about getting by and regarding relationships with others, I didn't count, I was "nothing."

EVIDENCE THAT THIS WAS A TREATMENT IN PROGRESS

The following hour we tripped over each other entering the office and Eddie apologized. Later he offered a package of candy which he had brought for me, "Because I like to share" (referring to himself). He wanted to play hockey with the candy wafers, and was soon pulverizing them against the wall, making a mess. Again, all interpretive efforts, this time identifying the issue of control and smearing and wondering at what age children did that, were to no avail. He grabbed my ankle from the floor and started to wrestle me down. He refused to stop and I had to pull away from him. He claimed I had hurt his sore thumb and started to attack me with a vengeance. He continued until I literally opened the door and dragged him outside and tossed his coat out to him. He struggled until the moment he was outside (and therefore in view of anybody who should happen by on the street), and then stopped immediately and acted normally. I said I would see him the next day. He said good-bye and left with a smile. On this occasion, unlike several previous ones, I had not been roused to anger.

He arrived a half-hour late for the next session and was reluctant to discuss what had happened the previous day. He insisted upon playing the same hockey game with candy wafers. At the end he observed that I was angering him but he hadn't done anything to me in response to that feeling. I wondered why and he responded that it was because I hadn't made him mad. That suggested that the intensity of his reactions may have paralleled his perception of the level to which I had been aroused to anger. When he sensed that I had become angry he became more aggressive. Such a response would be compatible with a defensive identification basis for his aggressive behaviors.

He brought me a piece of fudge the next day, and by previous agreement we alternately talked and played the hockey game. Eddie allowed wishing to have a much older brother or a young father, someone about 30 years of age. He professed no understanding of his behavior at the end of our sessions—his hyperactivity, destructiveness, provocativeness, and physical aggressiveness toward me. In the heat of the table hockey game he gouged my hand, causing it to bleed. He seemed genuinely concerned, apologized, and said that he had not meant to do that. He immediately looked over his own hands to find evidence that I had done the same thing to him. His apology, followed by efforts to prove I had done the same to him, suggested that guilt was associated with fears of retaliation, which he was attempting to deal with by claiming he had already received equivalent punishment.

During this whole period of analysis when Eddie was so intensely aggressive and unable to be reasoned with, it was little episodes like these—acting truly sorry for having gouged me, apologizing when we tripped over each other, bringing me pieces of candy, and ceasing his aggressive and regressive behaviors as soon as he left the office—that reassured me that the intensity of his hostility was a reflection of transference and that this was a therapeutic experience for him and not simply an orgy of sadism or of ego regression. This had been our last session before a one-week spring vacation. As it drew to a close, Eddie began to feign sleep and dreaming of torture with agonizing sounds and movements. I noted that this behavior followed talking about his paternity and leaving his foster home, so perhaps he was trying to tell me that to think and feel about these things was torture. If so, I could see why he would want to just shut out his thoughts and feelings and simply act.[9] As he left, he wondered where I was going when I left the office. That question was consistent with his overriding concerns about separation, continuity of experience, and his efforts to overcome the problems created for him by separation.

EVIDENCES OF IMPROVEMENT IN EDDIE'S LIFE

At school Eddie's graded performance was mediocre because he was not turning in his work, but his reading had improved to the first-year college level on achievement tests during the course of this year. He had progressed from fifth grade level to eighth grade level in math. His relationships with teachers and peers had improved greatly; he no longer clowned or misbehaved.

EDDIE TURNS TO SUBLIMATION

Eddie brought a chess set to our first postvacation session and we played during every session for a month. Eddie was very engrossed in these games, playing aggressively, happy when he won, frustrated when losing. He also brought us snacks. In sharp contrast to his prevacation behavior, he was attempting to sublimate his aggressive impulses. He was battling me in a board game rather than physically fighting. He announced that he had made a soccer team and that this might conflict with some of our meetings. That attitude represented a dramatic departure from his likely response in the past when he would not have considered continuing treatment if there was a conflict with soccer. He now frequently skipped soccer practices to attend our meetings. Also, he began for the first time to ask my permission to do things (e.g., "Can I be excused to go to the restroom?").

---

[9]That interpretation is more consistent with the approach recommended in the discussion of therapy in chapter 9. Specifically, I underscored to Eddie the sense rather than the non-sense of his behaviors or, in this case, his dramatization.

As we continued to play chess, Eddie began to again express admiration to the point of overvaluing me. I knew a lot; I thought twenty moves ahead (not accurate) whereas he himself thought only one move ahead; I gave him the games he won; I should wish him good luck before a soccer match because once when I had he was the high scorer. There were evidences of a wish to be "chummy." For example, he devised a signal to announce his arrival each time. He exhibited greater trustworthiness. He apologized whenever he was late. He more frequently expressed wishes for my approval of such things as his high achievement in reading. He was feeling closer to me, wanting to feel a sponsoring attitude on my part toward his progress. Feeling more secure he exhibited attitudes which would be considered in psychoanalytic terms indicative of oedipal concerns (fear of hurting me in friendly competition) and negative oedipal or latency interests (his admiration of me).

CHANGE OF CUSTODY

Following another week's planned absence, Eddie and his foster mother arrived late to the waiting room. His foster mother, a large, obese woman, was moist eyed as she told me that a lot had happened that day. There had been a court hearing and Eddie was going to live with his mother. She immediately went on to talk about the other children she was now baby-sitting and how much money she made from that, and that her previous foster daughter now wanted to return to live with her. I invited them both into the office. Eddie looked at her blankly off and on as she fell into the patient chair and continued. Eddie's mother had a lawyer with her in court and she herself, his foster mother, had said nothing. The judge had taken Eddie aside and asked where he wanted to go and he said with his mother. She added that Eddie wanted to go with her because his mother let him do anything that he wanted to and gave him what he wanted. It had been said in court that Eddie had been helped a lot by treatment and that treatment was to continue. I told her that Eddie had had good foster mothering. She replied that they had said that, too. Tears brimmed in her eyes. Eddie had set up the chess set.

His foster mother continued, saying that Eddie thought she was mad at him, but she wasn't. It was just the mean things that he did sometimes. I told her that Eddie might object to my saying this, but I believed that he handled his discomfort and sadness by trying to keep people apart and to create anger, which was easier to bear than sadness. She nodded. He looked at me blankly. She didn't know what she would do, but added quickly that she still had her license to provide foster care. She had quit her job after twenty-two years, had recently had her sixty-second birthday, but she would be working again soon, not just social security. She had these three kids to baby-sit now and her foster daughter was coming back to her. She reached a stopping point and heaved a sigh. We were smiling at each other. "I guess that's it," she said, "and why we were twenty minutes late." I responded that she had gotten here and that's what was important. I thanked her for coming in to let me know what had happened. She hove-up from her chair, saying that Eddie's mother and her boyfriend would pick him up, and that he could go with them anytime. She left. Her own pain over the separation, indicating the intensity of the emotional investment she had made in Eddie, was clear, as was her compensatory effort to deal with it by replacing Eddie. She would have other things to take Eddie's place in her life. Eddie pushed the chess board toward me. I tried to explore the day's events, but he would only say that he was happy to be going with his mother. In the hours which followed he lost many chess games. He had laryngitis and reminded me that this was the first cold he had had since last fall. This was remarkable, since in the past he had frequent colds. He discounted any possibility that the recent stresses in his home life had predisposed him to catching a cold at this time.

The summer vacation was rapidly approaching. Eddie wondered if I'd be meeting periodically with his mother as I had with his foster parents. He didn't care. When he became frustrated during games he called out names like "bumble-ass." Until recently any vulgarity had been eschewed. I thought this most likely indicated that he was feeling a little freer internally rather than greater permissiveness from his mother for such language.

Eddie graduated from ninth grade. He described the commencement briefly. Then we played chess and he beat me handily. I pointed out the difference compared to his recent frequent losses. He acknowledged that he "came to life today." I wondered if everything that had been going on recently, including the court proceeding, had made it difficult for him to keep his mind on the game. He shrugged and I raised the matter of leaving his foster parents. He became fidgety. He calculated that he had lived with them from the second through the ninth grades, more than half his life. He began to gouge the arm of the chair. When I called attention to this, he responded that he was leaving his mark here. I wondered if he had left his mark on his foster parents and he responded yes with a laugh. He described the stickers and scratches in his room. It was time to stop but he insisted upon remaining. This mirrored what we had just been talking about, namely, his response to leaving his foster parents. By the next time I saw him, he had moved into his mother's apartment. Whenever I would ask about missing his foster parents, Eddie would shrug and wonder, "So what?" It was all in the past, but he would become mildly hyperactive at those moments.

Evidences began to emerge that Eddie was identifying with men in his life—the manager of the apartment complex where he now lived, his mother's boyfriend (i.e., his biological father), a new friend. These might have constituted the first vestiges of the adolescent process of emancipation. He began arriving late. He described more events from his outside life, particularly new experiences, and his manner was more conversational. He began to play chess differently. Previously he had been primarily interested in controlling the game in order to win. He would take back moves or make me change my moves. Now he played by the rules, accepting his poor moves, and playing cautiously. He always anticipated that I would make some spectacular move which would disarm him. In terms of psychoanalytic developmental psychology this reflected a shift from preoedipal to oedipal conflicts. He was now more concerned about castration than about control. In terms of the thesis of this book, more basic was his sense of stability in the therapeutic relationship and that I wanted him to succeed. Then, during one game when Eddie was far behind, he made up his mind to fight back and to win, which he did. He was happy. At that point he wanted to play a different game. We had been playing chess almost every session for three months. Now we played a different game for many sessions. He asked how long we had played chess. I asked how he recalled interacting with me before we began playing chess. He pawed the air with a smile, acknowledging the fighting. I observed that it was as if he had changed from handling his fighting feelings by actually fighting, to doing so in chess. He had never thought about it that way, and after a moment of restless reflection, he returned to the game. When he lost that game he said, "God darn it." His frustration was expressed solely in words.

THE END OF TREATMENT

Eddie began to miss appointments without calling and at the next session would report with embarrassment what had happened. Frequently he had been with his mother.

I met with his mother and their social worker. His mother wanted to know whether Eddie had said anything about living with her. She also wanted the frequency of his appointments reduced. I explained why I thought they should not be curtailed, at least not to less than three times weekly. His mother claimed to understand and accept my reasoning. She expressed curiosity about Eddie's failure to contact his foster mother, and claimed to have encouraged him to do so. I underscored this as an area in which further work was warranted; it reflected Eddie's need to put his feelings out of mind for fear of being overwhelmed by them. When she brought up Eddie's difficulty in accepting her rules at times, I underscored his need to further consolidate impulse control and improve his frustration tolerance. When she reported his expressions of anxiety about "making it" in high school, I emphasized that his ability to experience and acknowledge his anxiety represented important progress. I also talked about the preventive aspects of further work now, noting the intensity of his attachment to her and relating this to emancipation issues of adolescence. She responded that she had never been possessive. I assured her that that was not what I had implied. Rather, I had been stressing the intensity of Eddie's devotion to her. It was decided that she and I would meet monthly.

Eddie was becoming quite compulsive. For example, he counted play money in ways he had never done before. He put pieces of games away in separate bins with unnecessary care, and he generally acted in an overly orderly manner. After losing a number of games he accused me of cheating. I wondered why I would do that; he claimed it was because I had lost so many games to him. He disregarded my attempt to demonstrate his projection, attributing his own motive to me. Then he began to say, as he lost games, that he had messed it up for himself, suggesting that his resort to projection to lessen his own excessive, internal self-criticism by blaming me was abating. During these hours Eddie demonstrated a fixed intensity in his efforts to win and to improve himself when he lost. I wondered to myself if this pattern, particularly persisting at games until he would beat me handily, reflected oedipal concerns now that he was with his mother. Specifically, he wanted to see if I could survive his beating me in competition. From time to time he would voice his wish not to have to come here anymore—someday; but he would not explore what needed to be accomplished before terminating.

As our three-week summer vacation approached, Eddie continued to miss sessions occasionally and it was easy to identify the psychological significance in these failures to apprise me of his absences. I stressed how these behaviors were communicating something about his feelings while at the same time substituting for his feelings. He responded that anything was possible, adding that we could be dead tomorrow. I used this to suggest that this whole pattern of behavior may have developed in order to avoid his feelings about very significant events—the sudden, unexpected death of his father and the later removal of his mother from their home. He held his head, telling me that I always said weird things like that which didn't make sense. At our last session before vacation Eddie denied any reaction to the anticipated separation and wondered how he should react. He acted as if we were not going to have an interruption by concentrating on a game. We agreed to meet three weeks hence.

Eddie failed that appointment and the next one, during which I telephoned. His mother said he was asleep and busy getting started in school. She also was very busy at school, doing field work in public health. She assured me that Eddie would call before the next appointment. He neither called nor showed and I called again during the fourth consecutive missed session.

This time his mother launched into a tirade about Eddie not needing four weekly appointments. She was going to call their social worker and her lawyer to get it changed. She knew he didn't need psychoanalysis and could see a therapist once every week or two. She disputed my contention that the matter could be negotiated, saying that she had tried. She dismissed my assertion that it was important for Eddie and me to work this out, and she put no stock in my explanation of why it was not in his best interest to stop suddenly. She had been incensed at my assertion during our last meeting that Eddie needed help in his adolescence to be able to become more independent from her. He had always been very independent. This was the most telling evidence of her motivation, namely, possessive jealousy. She added that if the treatment is not going well, then a patient has the right to choose his own doctor. I allowed that, but reflected puzzlement about how that would apply here. For everybody who knew of the situation felt that Eddie's improvement had been remarkable. She agreed but indicated that if the situation changed, like living in a different home and not needing treatment as much, he should be able to change doctors. Two and a half years of analysis was enough and she was now in the mental health field and knew that people had rights. I contacted their social worker who was unable to get Eddie back to treatment since his mother's public defender was as adamant as the mother. We decided to attempt to work out a termination. I received a message from his mother that Eddie would be in twice the next week, twice the week after that, and once the third week hence.

Eddie ambled into the next appointment and sat in the analyst's chair. He was bigger and looked more clearly adolescent. He sat smiling, looking around, and wondered why I wasn't talking. At his request I reviewed my conversations with his mother and spelled out his options: to continue his treatment to completion; to terminate within a specific period of time; or, I supposed, to stop was a third option. He asked if I meant just stopping rather than tapering. I said yes, for to do otherwise would amount to hanging on rather than letting go, and I thought we would need to meet regularly in order to deal with the issues of termination. Eddie equivocated. He knew that his mother wanted him to stop with the tapered meetings over three weeks.

He was reluctant to say that he wanted to stop, but we were unable to understand his reticence. Rather, he became curious about my other analysands, and also wondered what he still needed to work on, so that he could fix it right away he added with a laugh. I attempted to describe those areas, and he seemed to understand. I also described his considerable gains, upon which he amplified. He told me that his mother claimed that I had yelled at her over the phone. He didn't know what to make of that, because while he didn't know why she would lie, she could have. And I had never yelled at him, though I had talked "sternly" to him at times when he was out of control. He wondered if I would be disappointed if he didn't finish his treatment. I told him that he had hit upon a crucial issue in termination and that we should talk more about it. (This was the adolescent issue of emancipatory guilt.) He wondered if he was taller than me, and evinced a mixed reaction (glad and not glad) after deciding that he wasn't yet.

At our next meeting he was weighing what he wanted to do. His mother wanted him to stop and if anything else were done, then she was going to her lawyer. He disavowed concern about incurring her disfavor if he should decide to complete a termination. We talked about a number of other matters. His mother had explained to Eddie that her own illness and that of his sister and brother were the result of a blood deficiency for which they had to take pills. Since Eddie had a different father he was not affected. I wondered if he now believed that his mother's boyfriend was his father. Eddie didn't know, but he couldn't bring back his putative father in any event. His eyes became slightly moist. He was going to find out when he was older, and would have access to records when his father was working away, and so on. I tried to explore again his question of whether I would be disappointed if he stopped. He wondered if I would feel that I had not succeeded, but wouldn't elaborate on this. By the end of that hour he still had not reached a decision. When I said that the tapering would be of no value to him, he responded with an anxious "gulp," "You mean just stop?" We decided to meet again and make that decision.

That next meeting was our 360th session. Eddie sat again in the analyst's chair, looked around, and wondered if I had anything to say. He wanted to stop and wondered if this would be our last meeting. I asked his reaction to this being our last meeting and he hesitatingly replied that he was happy. I tried to explore his hesitation as a reflection of discomfort about feeling or acknowledging happiness to be leaving, but we were not able to take this further. I observed other things he was doing, many of an obsessional nature, which kept his attention away from his reaction to stopping. He denied feeling uncomfortable. We were silent and he allowed not liking silence, and would think of things to say if I wasn't going to talk. He recounted his outside activities, including his relationship with his sister who had a violent temper. He felt awful when she hit their mother. He felt very angry because he could not do anything about it and would leave the scene. He talked, again in response to questions, about his frustration with his mother's boyfriend who angrily ordered him around. He described his mother as even-tempered but not easy-going, and recounted experiences when she angered him. He talked openly and exhibited appropriate feelings. I returned a number of his games which he had not remembered leaving in the office. He compulsively counted the pieces and said he'd play them with the manager of their apartment complex. With five minutes left, he wanted to see his folder of artwork and insisted upon staying later to do so. He wondered what some of it was, and expressed embarrassment about some of it. Each time I mentioned that it was time to stop, he responded, "Just a minute." He finally gathered up his things and I shook his hand and wished him well, as he walked with a smile out into the early autumn evening, and I closed the door behind him.

EDDIE'S LATER LIFE

Eddie's social worker reported that within several months Eddie reestablished social contact with his foster parents. He functioned well in all areas in high school, during which he held a part-time job and made an all-star soccer team. Upon graduating from high school he became employed, subsequently married, and his former social worker thought that he also attended college. There was no further delinquent or later criminal behavior.

BRIEF SUMMARY

Eddie was an impulse-ridden, delinquent-oriented, friendless 12-year-old who was referred for analysis because of failure in school and stealing from his long-time foster parents, fighting, lying, and alienating peers at school. His putative father had been killed when Eddie was 18 months old. His mother had been hospitalized intermittently for manic depressive illness from the time he was 5 years old, at which time he and his siblings were placed in foster care. His older brother and sister, both of whom exhibited severe impulsive behavior, were being treated for manic depressive pychosis and schizophrenia respectively. Eddie had several foster home placements between ages 5 and 7 years when a permanent placement was found with foster parents who could tolerate him.

Eddie initially acted impervious to any outside influence. He rationalized and justified all his behaviors by blaming others. Although usually presenting himself with a smile, Eddie did experience anger which he always understood to be caused by others; that is, "you made me angry." Other emotions were isolated from his conscious awareness. Eddie had adapted to the world around him by impulsive behavior which substituted for awareness of inner feelings and conflicts, by behaviors based on turning passively experienced traumatic experiences into ones of an equivalent nature that he actively perpetrated onto others, and by recourse to counterphobia, a variation of the latter mechanism in which people exhibit behaviors opposite from what they basically fear. Eddie attempted to maintain these defensive and adaptive mechanisms in therapy by literally controlling my behaviors.

The bulk of the therapeutic work devolved around dealing with Eddie's enactments with the analyst of traumatic experiences from his current and past life. Eddie presented these in reverse; he perpetrated upon me the types of experience he had witnessed or experienced passively. His motive was to reduce his tension and then to be able to identify with the therapist's ability to deal with these experiences with greater equanimity than he himself had experienced when faced with them. These behaviors revealed the degree to which Eddie was searching for a constant, dependable, positive relationship in which he felt sponsored. As he began to experience that, his provocative destructiveness intensified in an effort to prove to himself that the therapist neither wanted to punish him nor would abandon him. This aggressiveness was augmented by Eddie's efforts to deal with current traumata in his life; namely, aggression he witnessed between his older brother and his mother's boyfriend, and his older sister's aggressive behavior toward him and their mother. In becoming so aggressive toward me he was also revealing the depth of his underlying conviction that he had been responsible for the bad things which had happened in his life, specifically separations, abandonments, and destruction of his parents. This issue was not analyzed.

Eddie also engaged with me in behaviors that replicated the ways by which we think parents normally help their young children to comfortably integrate self-control. Through these interactions Eddie became convinced that he would not destroy or drive me away. Thus, having reduced his concern about his destructiveness, he could now be helped to identify, to face, and to experience emotions of fear, anxiety, and sadness, which his impulsiveness had enabled him to keep repressed. He could then accept responsibility for his misdeeds, shortcomings, and mistakes without feeling in danger of being overwhelmed by overweening, intense guilt. The companion outcome was acquiring self-control over his impulsivity through identification with the analyst, and by substituting some compulsivity for his impulsivity. Even as Eddie improved significantly and we might have expected memories to replace reenacting, the therapeutic work was still accomplished almost entirely through examining Eddie's behavior toward the analyst.

Factors outside the office which had threatened to disrupt the analysis from its outset ultimately forced a premature termination, but not before Eddie had achieved remarkable improvement which was sustained into adulthood, enabling him to complete his development.

DISCUSSION

Eddie's treatment demonstrates that impulse-ridden youth can be successfully treated by intensive therapy. It seems reasonable to make this point at a time when such cases are becoming more numerous and this type of treatment has fallen out of favor. Unfortunately, there may be no substitutes for the intensive involvement and time required to accomplish certain cures. So, at least some of our dwindling resources may be as well spent in teaching people how to treat such patients and paying them to do so as in looking for more superficial or social or medicinal treatments.

A specific approach has been espoused for cases in which one can expect the treatment to be undermined by dysfunctional families, by well-intentioned but overzealous public agencies (in this case the public defenders' office) and by competitive colleagues (the mother's psychiatrist). Specifically, it is possible and even advised to direct one's therapeutic efforts exclusively toward strengthening the patient's ego to deal with 'the slings and arrows of outrageous fortune' and not attempting to work with the dysfunctional family as well. Clearly the efforts of Eddie's perspicacious welfare department social worker who initiated Eddie's treatment and continually intervened on the side of keeping it going were crucial and cannot be minimized. However, the clinical work was done almost exclusively with the patient.

The interaction between patient and therapist (as opposed to exploring the relationship between memories of one's past and one's current behaviors), may remain the relatively exclusive focus in the therapy of such individuals, whose modus operandi has been to substitute action for recollection, thought, and feeling. Since Eddie was verbalizing more around the time of his premature termination, it is possible that remembering would have continued to replace repeating (acting). However, by then Eddie was no longer impulsive or aggressive. So again, remembering may not form a significant part of the treatment of such individuals, but they will get better.

Unlike Eddie, most of the other cases were individuals whose difficulties had arisen in adolescence when they faced the crucial developmental imperative to emancipate psychologically. These individuals had concluded, accurately or inaccurately, from their experiences with parents that moving toward greater psychological independence threatened the stability of the relationship and sponsorship they still felt in need of from their parents. Thus, they experienced emancipatory guilt that often took the form of fears that becoming more autonomous would be hurtful to their parents or themselves.

By contrast Eddie began his chronological adolescent years with a different relationship to parenting figures. His overt attitude was that caretaking adults were simply need-fulfilling objects toward whom he experienced no emotional attachment nor interest. He acted and apparently felt beholden to no one; at the same time he exhibited no impetus to emancipate. You will recall that Eddie played like a much younger child than a $12^1/2$- to 14-year-old during the first year and a half of his treatment. This in itself bespoke his underlying expectation that people should treat him as they would a much younger child.

His avowed singular interest was to reunite with his mother. However, she herself had historically proven inconstant by virtue of illness and hospitalizations. Moreover, the unruliness and lack of self-control exhibited by her other children from early in their lives, albeit complicated later by mental illnesses, is presumptive evidence that she had not been a stabilizing influence. This factor, together with her penchant for becoming irrationally enraged, suggests another basis for Eddie to have adopted a defensive identification with her early in his life which took the form of impulsivity.

Defensive identification, based on turning passive into active, was a mechanism Eddie shared with the other adolescent patients. It was one important determinant of his aggressiveness toward me, and perhaps most clearly correlated with his response to the violence he witnessed at his mother's apartment between his brother and his mother's boyfriend and in his sister's attacks on their mother and himself. He identified with their aggression, a defensive identification, and turned it onto me to see how I would respond when faced with what he had witnessed and experienced. He was never able to talk about this. The work was done exclusively by reenacting something that he claimed was between him and me, rather than recognizing that it was the displacement or externalization of a traumatic experience from his current life outside treatment.

Even though he warded-off conscious awareness of them, Eddie had to reduce his fears of his own destructiveness and the intense self-punitiveness aroused by the latter experiences. Only then was he able to feel sufficiently internally secure and externally sponsored to move toward adolescent emancipation. He disclaimed a need for this latter sense of security. Yet, the thrust of his treatment was to establish and guarantee the presence of such a relationship with the analyst while he overtly rejected that idea and attacked me, purportedly so I would discharge him. One important source of his aggression during treatment was an effort to see if I would reject him. Deep down he thought that he deserved this because he had caused the destructive things that had happened in his life. The guilt associated with this idea had not been analyzed by the time his treatment was stopped. It was so frightening to him that the work on this issue too was almost entirely carried out in his interaction with me.

Whether or not Eddie intended to provoke me to fury, I reacted with fury on several occasions in response to his enactments of behaviors based on defensive identifications. It is my sense that such patients have to evoke in the therapist the intensity of emotion they themselves had experienced or witnessed in order for the therapeutic experience to be authentic. In a seeming paradox, Eddie needed to evoke that level of intensity in the therapist, but he denied or minimized this response. You will recall that Eddie experienced me as having been less angry (i.e., "stern") than I had felt at times (i.e., "furious"). The implication is that he did not want me to become angry with him or to reject him while at the same time needing me to experience a higher level of intensity of emotion. I had to truly "get it," that is, experience what he struggled with, in order for him to authentically feel that it was possible for him to change.

Another aspect of the therapeutic process, at least for this impulse-ridden youth, involved enacting the type of interactions in which much younger children normally engage with their parents to acquire self control. This is accomplished through identifying with the parents' ability to tolerate frustration, blame, and being controlled. Compulsive mechanisms to deal with impulsivity also emerged.

An additional, important feature of the therapeutic process is helping the patient become acquainted with the range of his emotions. Eddie's affects were in part isolated and also in a curious way not quite spontaneously comprehensible to him. You will recall that he needed me to identify the feelings one might have when separating from long-time foster parents; as I did so, Eddie was able to recognize and acknowledge those which he felt.

As a last word of clarification, I was developing the ideas about adolescence presented in this book at the time when I treated Eddie. For that reason, some of my interpretations were more in line with a traditional psychoanalytic understanding and others with the viewpoint emphasized in this book. I noted these differently oriented interpretations in the narrative to reduce any difficulty they may have created in following the treatment and to further distinguish my approach from that of the longer-standing theory.

Epilogue

A view of adolescent development has been presented based on two premises. One is that adolescents' psychological development is propelled by an inherent, maturational factor, termed "strivings to complete development." The other is that adaptation of the adolescent's maturing ego to his or her environment plays a more crucial role in psychological development than has been posited by other clinical theories. Adolescents carry over from earlier childhood the idea that pleasing their parents is necessary to maintain their own sense of security and to assure their developmental progress. Then, as they act upon their maturational urges to emancipate to an adult level of autonomy, they experience a normal internal conflict. This conflict takes the form of concern that what is required to retain a positive relationship with parents is not compatible with their strivings to move ahead as they themselves see fit. In the face of this potential conflict, parental sponsorship of their adolescents' strivings to progress reduces the likelihood that problems will result from this developmental conflict.

Current academic researchers have been more impressed by the diversity than by the similarities of adolescents' experiences (Feldman and Elliott, 1990). The diversity to which they refer is both between groups of adolescents (e.g., socioeconomic, ethnic, minority, etc.), and also within the same individual adolescent. The latter differences within the same individual depend upon the specific conditions under which the adolescent is being studied.[1] Thus, there has been a move away from the search for unified developmental processes in favor of examining responses

---

[1] You will recall, as an example, that adolescents' modes of thinking are no longer considered to develop and be sustained in a predictable (Kohlberg and

that may be specific to a given situation. As a result of this trend in research, Feldman and Elliott (1990) conclude that the field of adolescent study currently lacks theories to guide its questions and "rules for understanding exactly how youth are influenced by specific situations and settings and, in turn, influence them" (p. 487).

Humans share similar needs and have species-limited means of accommodating them. Thus, it should be possible to articulate a theory which encompasses these disparate research findings and relates them to clinical observation. A theory which remains close to experience has a better chance of being overarching; that is, a model that represents a low level of abstraction can be more confidently applied to research data than a theory which represents a high level of abstraction. Traditional psychoanalysis, for example, the only comprehensive theory of adolescence presented to date, represents a higher level of abstraction than my thesis. To wit, it is easier to agree upon evidence of parental sponsorship than of unconscious sexual drive from behavioral observations.

The clinically derived thesis I have presented offers a model for reconciling the academic research with features of long-standing psychodynamic theory that have proven serviceable. How does my thesis accomplish this? First, the importance of adolescents' adaptation to their environment, that is, to the attitudes and behaviors of their parents and to a lesser degree of their peers, has been emphasized. Much of the recent academic research has an adaptational, and therefore interpersonal, base. Thus, the adaptational perspective represents a common framework for translating the research findings into the terms of my clinical overview.

At the same time, in my model the adolescent's intrapsychic experience is the ultimate source of his or her responses and behaviors. This aspect of my thesis represents the potential common ground with psychodynamic theory. Traditional psychoanalytic theory underscores the need to escape from an internally

---

Gilligan, 1971), sex-specific (Gilligan 1982, 1986) manner. Rather, the way in which adolescents reason depends upon their familiarity with the specific situation under consideration, and, for example, whether it is real or hypothetical (Keating, 1990; Torney-Purta, 1990).

generated, basically hostile relationship with parents. I have, by contrast, emphasized that adolescents wish to retain a supportive relationship with their parents while emancipating. This shift in emphasis renders my view more congruent with academic research, since much of it focuses on the importance of environmental factors. Also, the research literature contains broad support for the companion second element of my thesis, parental sponsorship which serves to maintain a positive relationship between adolescent and parents.

The other basic element of my model is that progression in adolescents is propelled by strivings to complete development. The relative importance to adolescent psychological development of an ego maturational factor might be questioned by both traditional psychoanalytic theory which emphasizes libidinal maturation and by research which stresses environmental influences on adolescent development. Nonetheless, the existence of a maturational component in adolescent psychological development would not be discounted by either of the other approaches.

I have illustrated the applicability of this model to the behavior of well-functioning adolescents, to those exhibiting the psychopathology of everyday life, to those suffering mild and severe psychological illnesses, and to those exhibiting delinquent behavior. Identifying the same conflict amongst adolescents in such different states of health and psychological trouble supports my point. Namely, this thesis offers a way of drawing into a psychodynamic theory the data from current research on infancy (e.g., Stern, 1985; Emde, 1991; Lichtenberg, 1982, 1989) and academic research on adolescents (e.g., Offer and Offer, 1975; Feldman and Elliott, 1990; Hauser, Powers, and Noam, 1991), as well as empirical (e.g., Weiss, Sampson, and the Mt. Zion Psychotherapy Research Group, 1986) and clinical (e.g., Langs, 1985) research on the therapeutic process in adults. Basically my thesis addresses one of the two fundamental questions in developmental clinical psychiatry and psychology; that is the manner in which the interpersonal influences the intrapsychic; it is an issue on the border of individual psychology and group psychology, sociology, and cultural anthropology.

I have devoted much less attention to the other basic issue in developmental psychiatry, namely the question of what is psychic structure. This issue is at the interface of psychology and neurophysiology; and, in all likelihood, the subject of medication for adolescents ultimately relates to this question. Because of the current interest in treating adolescents medicinally, this issue should not go undiscussed, even in a book which has emphasized psychotherapeutic treatment. This area is currently popular for several reasons. Medications which had previously been reserved for adults are now being prescribed for adolescents; and the dual pressures to meet increasing demands for services and to reduce costs of treatment make the medicinal approach appealing. Despite considerable advances in understanding some biochemical actions of psychiatric medications, the clinical question of when to prescribe medicine for adolescents still remains more trial-and-error based than determined by data-derived indications.

In inaugurating a new journal devoted to psychopharmacological approaches to children and adolescents, Popper (1990) has framed the dilemma. He notes that empirical trials of psychiatric medications for treating adolescents (and children), which rely on the technical competence and judgment of physicians, are currently being conducted on such a widespread basis that this empirical approach has replaced the traditional medical dictum to diagnose before treating as the standard for prescribing. Yet, the medical literature contains only the most sketchy documentation of the safety and effectiveness of even some of the most commonly used treatments. Popper also points out that in this field clear diagnostic criteria are available but not always applicable, and in some situations the diagnostic criteria are highly debatable. He observes that this widespread empiricism exposes many children to medical risks, but also brings medical help to many children whose treatability is only speculative today. Popper concludes that:

> In view of the scientific unknowns in applying these psychopharmacological treatments to children, the traditional cautionary approach would lead to waiting for more data. Yet a further delay in the application of these treatments would mean that another generation of children and adolescents may be "protected" from the fruits of the biological revolution in psychiatry and the behavioral revolution in pediatrics. . . . Genuine standards are not available, but there are some reasonable approaches [p. 3].

When prescribing is done on an empirical basis without clear indications, then therapists feel hard pressed not to recommend medicine when faced with symptomatic adolescents. This is particularly so in light of the other considerations noted in addition to the current popularity of medicating, namely, treatment time and costs, and the appropriate therapeutic wish to relieve suffering expeditiously.

The critical question from my perspective is not whether to medicate but when to treat with medicine. I presented an acutely psychotic patient who responded dramatically to medicine. Acute psychosis probably represents the diagnosis for which there is the most clear-cut indication for medicating adolescents. In comparing that patient with another acutely psychotic adolescent who was treated successfully psychotherapeutically, I emphasized that factors in addition to the symptom diagnosis should be considered in deciding upon the treatment modality. Important amongst these factors is whether you think the patient can work psychotherapeutically; often this cannot be determined without a trial of therapy. I also presented other patients who were successfully treated psychotherapeutically but for whom medication would probably be prescribed in today's therapeutic climate. In presenting those cases of depression and anxiety, obsessionalism, substance abuse, and impulse pathology which responded to psychotherapy and psychoanalysis, I hope to encourage the following approach to adolescent patients: Whenever there is any doubt about the need for or value of medication (and today there most often will be), one's adolescent patients are best served by first working psychotherapeutically from the vantage of the psychodynamic perspective I have presented in this book. Add medication to the therapeutic regimen only after you have persuaded yourself that intensive therapy is not proving salutary or that the patient cannot work psychotherapeutically. That is, retain medication as a later or last resort rather than considering it an initial treatment of choice.

Preliminary indications from formal research on drugs and on psychotherapy for depressed adolescents support this position. Controlled studies, albeit with modest numbers of patients, have not shown medication to be effective in treating depressed adolescents (Kutcher, Boulos, Ward, Marton, Simeon, Ferguson,

Szalai, Katic, Roberts, Dubois, and Reed, 1994; see also Campbell and Spencer, 1988). On the other hand, initial studies of psycho-therapeutic interventions, comprising very small samples but which are being conducted with the same research methodology that is used for drug studies, indicate that interpersonal therapy is effective treatment for depressed adolescents (Mufson, Mo-reau, Weissman, Wickramaratne, Martin, and Samoilov, 1994). Moreover, even if not a sea change, a shift in the prevailing winds may be occurring in the direction of renewed interest in the efficacy of psychotherapy in conditions for which psychiatry has been more exclusively searching for medicinal solutions in re-cent years (see, for example, Markowitz, 1994).

A current proponent of medication usage shares my reluc-tance to prescribe for adolescents; he attributes his reservations to a cultural mistrust of psychiatric medication rather than to objective clinical judgment (Kramer, 1993, pp. 100–103). There are several reasons why I advocate the Hippocratic approach of trying to avoid the possibility of harm or at least risking only when all else has failed. In addition to issues mentioned in chap-ter 8 (p. 234), my rationale includes the fact that devastating long-term and late-onset side effects are often not discovered un-til years after some medications have achieved wide acceptance. My recourse to medication in most cases only when all else has failed also reflects a persuasion regarding the manner in which we can best serve present and future generations of adolescents and the adults they go on to become. The questions that I ask myself are: Can adolescents face new worlds most bravely by strengthening themselves internally on the basis of their own grit and insight, prompted by their therapists' confidence in their ability to do so? And, do we subtly subscribe and thus contribute to obliging adolescents to face the brave new world Huxley (1932) envisioned in which drugs regulate experience?

In our lifetime we have witnessed significant sectors of soci-ety plunge headlong into drug use to no avail and with untold emotional havoc and financial costs. Clearly the judicious pre-scription of psychotropic medication is not abusive use of pre-scription drugs; nor is it the same as abandonment to street and designer drug use. But the trend and direction are the same. That is, there is great danger that the message conveyed to the suggestible adolescent recipient of medication from the adult prescriber is that one looks to pills for solutions to developmental problems. Given the importance I have placed on achieving internal psychological independence as the entree to mature interdependency, I am sure that the approach I am advocating comes as no surprise.

References

Adatto, C. (1958), Ego reintegration observed in analysis of late adolescents. *Internat. J. Psycho-Anal.*, 39:172–177.

———— (1966), On the metamorphosis from adolescence into adulthood. *J. Amer. Psychoanal. Assn.*, 14:485–509.

———— (1980), Late adolescence to early adulthood. In: *The Course of Life: Psychoanalytic Contributions Toward Understanding Personality Development*, Vol. 2, ed. S. Greenspan & G. Pollock. Washington, DC: NIMH, pp. 463–476.

Adelson, J. (1971), The political imagination of the young adolescent. In: *12 to 16: Early Adolescence*, ed. J. Kagan & R. Coles. New York: W. W. Norton, 1972, pp. 106–143.

Adler, A. (1938), *Social Interest: A Challenge to Mankind.* New York: Putnam, 1939.

Aichhorn, A. (1925), *Wayward Youth.* Cleveland: World Publishing, 1963.

American Psychiatric Association (1987), *Diagnostic and Statistical Manual of Mental Disorders*, 3rd ed. rev. (DSM-III-R). Washington, DC: American Psychiatric Press.

Ames, R. (1957), Physical maturing among boys as related to adult social behavior. *Calif. J. Ed. Res.*, 8:69–75.

Anderson, S. (1939), *Memoirs.* New York: Readers Digest.

Anthony, E. (1970), The reactions of parents to adolescents and to their behavior. In: *Parenthood: Its Psychology and Psychopathology*, ed. E. Anthony & T. Benedek. Boston: Little, Brown, pp. 307–324.

Ariès, P. (1960), *Centuries of Childhood*, tr. R. Baldick. New York: Alfred J. Knopf, 1962.

Arnstein, R. (1989), Overview of normal transition to young adulthood. In: *Adolescent Psychiatry*, Vol. 16, ed. S. Feinstein, A. Esman, J. Looney, G. Orvin, J. Schimel, A. Schwartzberg, A. Sorosky, & M. Sugar. Chicago: University of Chicago Press.

Bakan, D. (1971), Adolescence in America: From idea to social fact. In: *12 to 16: Early Adolescence*, ed. J. Kagan & R. Coles. New York: W. W. Norton, 1972, pp. 73–89.

Bell, A. (1961), The role of parents. In: *Adolescents: Psychoanalytic Approach to Problems and Therapy*, ed. S. Lorand & H. Schneer. New York: Harper & Row, pp. 273–281.

Beres, D. (1958), Vicissitudes of superego functions and superego precursors in childhood. *The Psychoanalytic Study of the Child*, 13:324–351. New York: International Universities Press.

Bernfeld, S. (1923), Uber eine typische form der männlichen pubertät. (A typical form of male puberty.) *Imago*, 9:169–188.

——— (1935), On simple male adolescence, tr. R. Ekstein. *Seminars in Psychiatry*, 1:113–126, 1969.

Bibring, E. (1937), Symposium on the therapeutic results in psychoanalysis. *Internat. J. Psycho-Anal.*, 18:170–189.

Blaine, G., Jr., & Farnsworth, D. (1980), Personality development in the young adult. In: *The Course of Life: Psychoanalytic Contributions Toward Understanding Personality Development*, Vol. 2, ed. S. Greenspan & G. Pollock. Washington, DC: NIMH.

Bloch, H. A., & Niederhoffer, A. (1958), *The Gang: A Study of Adolescent Behavior*. New York: Philosophical Library.

Bloch, H. S. (1970), The psychological adjustment of normal people during a year's tour in Vietnam. *Psychiatric Quart.*, 44:613–626.

——— (1981), The role of strivings to complete development in the therapeutic process of child analysis. *Internat. Rev. Psychoanal.*, 8:203–218.

——— (1989), The common core of paranoia and depression. *Psychoanal. Inq.*, 9:427–449.

Block, J., with the collaboration of Haan, N. (1971), *Lives Through Time*. Berkeley, CA: Bancroft Books.

Bloom-Feshbach, J., & Bloom-Feshbach, S. (1987), *The Psychology of Separation and Loss*, ed. J. Bloom-Feshbach, S. Bloom-Feshbach, & Associates. San Francisco: Jossey-Bass.

Blos, P. (1957), Preoedipal factors in the etiology of female delinquency. *The Psychoanalytic Study of the Child*, 12:229–249. New York: International Universities Press.

——— (1958), Preadolescent drive organization. *J. Amer. Psychoanal. Assn.*, 6:47–56.

——— (1962), *On Adolescence*. New York: Free Press of Glencoe.

——— (1967), The second individuation process of adolescence. *The Psychoanalytic Study of the Child*, 22:162–186. New York: International Universities Press.

—— (1976), Postscript. In: *The Adolescent Passage*. New York: International Universities Press, 1979, pp. 246–253.

—— (1977), When and how does adolescence end? Structural criteria for adult closure. In: *Adolescent Psychiatry*, Vol. 5, ed. S. Feinstein & P. Giovacchini. New York: Jason Aronson, pp. 5–17.

—— (1985), Influence of the early father on the development of the male adolescent. The 1st Annual Ralph Greenson Lecture, presented at the Adolescent Day Treatment Center, Children's Hospital, San Francisco, CA, April 27.

Blum, G. (1949), A study of the psychoanalytic theory of psychosexual development. *Genet. Psychol.* Monograph, 39:3–99.

Bornstein, B. (1951), On latency. *The Psychoanalytic Study of the Child*, 6:279–285. New York: International Universities Press.

Bowlby, J. (1969), *Attachment and Loss*, Vol. 1. New York: Basic Books.

—— (1973), *Attachment and Loss*, Vol. 2. New York: Basic Books.

—— (1980), *Attachment and Loss*, Vol. 3. New York: Basic Books.

Braungart, R. (1980), Youth movements. In: *Handbook of Adolescent Psychology*, ed. J. Adelson. New York: John Wiley, pp. 560–597.

Breuer, J., & Freud, S. (1893–1895), Studies on Hysteria. *Standard Edition*, 2. London: Hogarth Press, 1955.

Brockman, D. (1984), Introduction. In: *Late Adolescence: Psychoanalytic Studies*. New York: International Universities Press.

Brooks-Gunn, J., & Reiter, E. (1990), The role of pubertal processes. In: *At the Threshold: The Developing Adolescent*, ed. S. Feldman & G. Elliott. Cambridge, MA: Harvard University Press, pp. 16–53.

Bruch, H. (1977), Anorexia nervosa. In: *Adolescent Psychiatry*, Vol. 5, ed. S. Feinstein & P. Giovacchini. New York: Jason Aronson, pp. 293–303.

Brunswick, R. M. (1940), The preoedipal phase of the libido development. *Psychoanal. Quart.*, 9:293–319.

Bühler, C. (1935), *From Birth to Maturity*. London: Routledge & Kegan Paul.

Calogeras, R., & Schupper, F. (1972), Origins and early formulations of the Oedipus complex. *J. Amer. Psychoanal. Assn.*, 20:751–775.

Campbell, M., & Spencer, E. (1988), Psychopharmacology in child and adolescent psychiatry: A review of the past five years. *J. Amer. Acad. Child & Adol. Psychiatry*, 27:269–279.

Conrad, J. (1927), *The Shadow Line*. New York: Doubleday.

Cooper, C., Grotevant, H., & Condon, S. (1983), Individuality and connectedness both foster adolescent identity formation and role-taking skills. In: *Adolescent Development in the Family: New Directions for Child Development*, ed. H. Grotevant & C. Cooper. San Francisco: Jossey Bass, pp. 43–59.

Coppolillo, H. (1984), Integration, organization and regulation in late adolescence. In: *Late Adolescence: Psychoanalytic Studies*, ed. D. Brockman. New York: International Universities Press, pp. 123–151.

Coren, H., & Saldinger, J. (1967), Visual hallucinosis in children. *The Psychoanalytic Study of the Child*, 22:331–356. New York: International Universities Press.

Cramer, B. (1987), Objective and subjective aspects of parent-infant relations: An attempt at correlation between infant studies and clinical work. In: *Handbook of Infant Development*, 2nd ed., ed. J. Osofsky. New York: John Wiley, pp. 1037–1057.

Davis, N. (1975), The reasons of misrule. In: *Society and Culture in Early Modern France*. Stanford, CA: Stanford University Press.

Deutsch, H. (1944), *The Psychology of Women*, Vol. 1. New York: Grune & Stratton.

Devereux, G. (1953), Why Oedipus killed Laius. *Internat. J. Psycho-Anal.*, 32:132–141.

Eccles, J., Midgley, C., Wigfield, A., Buchanan, C., Reuman, D., Flanagan, C., & MacIver, D. (1993), Development during adolescence: The impact of stage-environment fit on young adolescents' experiences in schools and in families. *Amer. Psychologist*, 48:90–101.

Ehrhardt, A., Meyer-Bahlburg, H., Bell, J., Cohen, S., Healey, J., Stiel, R., Feldman, J., Morishima, A., & New, M. (1984), Idiopathic precocious puberty in girls: Psychiatric follow-up in adolescence. *J. Amer. Acad. Child Psychiatry*, 23:23–33.

Eichorn, D., Clausen, J., Haan, N., Honzik, M., & Mussen, P. (1981), *Present and Past in Middle Life*. New York: Academic Press.

Eissler, K. (1958), Notes on problems of technique in the psychoanalytic treatment of adolescents: With some remarks on perversions. *The Psychoanalytic Study of the Child*, 13:223–254. New York: International Universities Press.

Elder, G. (1980), Adolescence in historical perspective. In: *Handbook of Adolescent Psychology*, ed. J. Adelson. New York: John Wiley, pp. 3–46.

Ellis, H. (1939), *My Life*. Houghton Mifflin.

Emde, R. (1985), From adolescence to midlife: Remodeling the structure of adult development. *J. Amer. Psychoanal. Assn.*, 33:59–112.

—— (1988a), Development terminable and interminable. I. Innate and motivational factors from infancy. *Internat. J. Psycho-Anal.*, 69:23–42.

—— (1988b), Development terminable and interminable: II. Recent psychoanalytic theory and therapeutic considerations. *Internat. J. Psycho-Anal.*, 69:283–296.

—— (1991), Positive emotions for psychoanalytic theory: Surprises from infancy research and new directions. *J. Amer. Psychoanal. Assn.*, 39(Suppl.):5–44.

Enright, R., Levy, Jr., V., Harris, D., & Lapsley, D. (1987), Do economic conditions influence how theorists view adolescents? *J. Youth & Adol.*, 16:541–559.

Erikson, E. (1950), *Childhood and Society.* New York: W. W. Norton.

—— (1956), The problem of ego identity. In: *Identity and the Life Cycle. Psychological Issues*, Monogr. 1. New York: International Universities Press, 1959.

Esman, A. (1979), Adolescence and the "new sexuality." In: *On Sexuality: Psychoanalytic Observations*, ed. T. Karasu & C. Socarides. New York: International Universities Press, pp. 19–28.

—— (1980), Mid-adolescence—Foundations for later psychopathology. In: *The Course of Life: Psychoanalytic Contributions Toward Understanding Personality Development*, Vol. 2, ed. S. Greenspan & G. Pollock. Washington, DC: NIMH, pp. 419–430.

—— (1983), The "stimulus barrier": A review and reconsideration. *The Psychoanalytic Study of the Child*, 38:193–207. New Haven, CT: Yale University Press.

Fairbairn, W. R. (1952), *Psychoanalytic Studies of the Personality.* London: Tavistock/Routledge & Kegan Paul.

—— (1963), Synopsis of an object relations theory of the personality. *Internat. J. Psycho-Anal.*, 44:224–225.

Fechner, G. (1873), *Einege Ideen zur Schopfungs—und Enwicklungs—geschichte der Organismen.* Leipzig.

Feldman, S., & Elliott, G. (1990), Progress and promise of research on adolescence. In: *At the Threshold: The Developing Adolescent*, ed. S. Feldman & G. Elliott. Cambridge, MA: Harvard University Press, pp. 479–505.

Fisher, S. (1970), *Body Experience in Fantasy and Behavior.* New York: Appleton-Century-Crofts.

—— (1973), *The Female Orgasm.* New York: Basic Books.

—— Greenberg, R. (1977), *The Scientific Credibility of Freud's Theories and Therapy.* New York: Basic Books.

Fonagy, P., & Target, M. (1994), The efficacy of psychoanalysis for children with disruptive disorders. *J. Amer. Acad. Child & Adol. Psychiatry*, 33:45–55.

Fountain, G. (1961), Adolescent into adult: An inquiry. *J. Amer. Psychoanal. Assn.*, 9:417–433.

Fraiberg, S. (1955), Some considerations in the introduction to therapy at puberty. *The Psychoanalytic Study of the Child*, 10:264–286. New York: International Universities Press.

Frankel, S. (1994), Not knowing. The analytic relationship as guide and solution. Typescript.

—— Sherick, I. (1979), Observations of the emerging sexual identity of three and four year old children: With emphasis on female sexual identity. *Internat. Rev. Psychoanal.*, 6:299–309.

Freedman, D. (1983), Of instincts and instinctual drives: Some developmental considerations. *Psychoanal. Inq.*, 2:153–167.

Freud, A. (1936), The Ego and the Mechanisms of Defense, *Writings*, Vol. 2. New York: International Universities Press, 1966.

—— (1958), Adolescence. *The Psychoanalytic Study of the Child*, 13:255–278. New York: International Universities Press.

—— (1965), Normality and Pathology in Childhood. *Writings*, Vol. 6. New York: International Universities Press.

—— (1966), Adolescence as a developmental disturbance. *Writings*, Vol. 7. New York: International Universities Press, pp. 39–47.

—— (1968), Difficulties in the path of psychoanalysis: A confrontation of past and present viewpoints. In: *Problems in Psychoanalytic Training, Diagnosis, and the Technique of Therapy. Writings*, Vol. 7. New York: International Universities Press, 1969, pp. 124–156.

Freud, S. (1895), A reply to criticisms of my paper on anxiety neurosis. *Standard Edition*, 3:121–139. London: Hogarth Press, 1962.

—— (1896), The aetiology of hysteria. *Standard Edition*, 3:189–221. London: Hogarth Press, 1962.

—— (1897), Extracts from the Fliess papers (1950 [1892–1899]). *Standard Edition*, 1:259–260; 263–266. London: Hogarth Press, 1966.

—— (1900), The Interpretation of Dreams. *Standard Edition*, 4 & 5. London: Hogarth Press, 1953.

—— (1905a), Fragment of an analysis of a case of hysteria. *Standard Edition*, 7:3–122. London: Hogarth Press, 1953.

—— (1905b), Three essays on the theory of sexuality. *Standard Edition*, 7:125–245. London: Hogarth Press, 1953.

—— (1906), My views on the part played by sexuality in the aetiology of the neuroses. *Standard Edition*, 7:270–279. London: Hogarth Press, 1953.

—— (1908), On the sexual theories of children. *Standard Edition*, 9:205–226. London: Hogarth Press, 1959.

—— (1909), Analysis of a phobia in a five-year-old boy. *Standard Edition*, 10:3–149. London: Hogarth Press, 1955.

—— (1910), Leonardo da Vinci and a memory of his childhood. *Standard Edition*, 11:59–137. London: Hogarth Press, 1957.

—— (1911), Formulations on the two principles of mental functioning. *Standard Edition*, 12:213–226. London: Hogarth Press, 1958.

—————— (1912), On the universal tendency to debasement in the sphere of love (contributions to the psychology of love II). *Standard Edition*, 11:177–190. London: Hogarth Press, 1957.

—————— (1913), Totem and taboo. *Standard Edition*, 13:ix–162. London: Hogarth Press, 1955.

—————— (1915), Instincts and their vicissitudes. *Standard Edition*, 14:109–140. London: Hogarth Press, 1957.

—————— (1920), Beyond the pleasure principle. *Standard Edition*, 18:3–64. London: Hogarth Press, 1955.

—————— (1923), The ego and the id. *Standard Edition*, 19:3–66. London: Hogarth Press, 1961.

—————— (1924), The dissolution of the Oedipus complex. *Standard Edition*, 19:173–179. London: Hogarth Press, 1961.

—————— (1925a), An autobiographical study. *Standard Edition*, 20:3–74. London: Hogarth Press, 1959.

—————— (1925b), Some psychical consequences of the anatomical distinction between the sexes. *Standard Edition*, 19:243–258. London: Hogarth Press, 1961.

—————— (1926), Inhibitions, symptoms and anxiety. *Standard Edition*, 20:77–175. London: Hogarth Press, 1959.

—————— (1928), Dostoevsky and parricide. *Standard Edition*, 21:175–196. London: Hogarth Press, 1961.

—————— (1930), Civilization and its discontents. *Standard Edition*, 21:59–145. London: Hogarth Press, 1961.

—————— (1931), Female sexuality. *Standard Edition*, 21:223–243. London: Hogarth Press, 1961.

—————— (1933), New Introductory Lectures. *Standard Edition*, 22:3–182. London: Hogarth Press, 1964.

—————— (1940), An outline of psychoanalysis. *Standard Edition*, 23:141–207. London: Hogarth Press, 1964.

Furstenberg, F. (1990), Coming of age in a changing family system. In: *At the Threshold: The Developing Adolescent*, ed. S. Feldman & G. Elliott. Cambridge, MA: Harvard University Press.

Gagnon, J. (1971), The creation of the sexual in early adolescence. In: *12 to 16: Early Adolescence*, ed. J. Kagan & R. Coles. New York: W. W. Norton, 1972, pp. 231–257.

Galdston, R. (1974), Mind over matter: Observations of 50 patients hospitalized with anorexia nervosa. *J. Amer. Acad. Child Psychiat.*, 13:246–263.

Galenson, E., & Roiphe, H. (1976), Some suggested revisions concerning early female development. *J. Amer. Psychoanal. Assn.*, 24(Suppl. 5):246–263.

Garver, P. (1982), Washington talk. *New York Times.* December 17:A26.

Geleerd, E. (1957), Some aspects of psychoanalytic technique with adolescents. *The Psychoanalytic Study of the Child,* 12:263–283. New York: International Universities Press.

Ghannam, J. (1985), The origins and development of the castration theme in Freud's writings. Typescript. San Francisco.

Gilligan, C. (1982), *A Different Voice.* Cambridge, MA: Harvard University Press.

———— (1986), Exit-voice dilemmas in adolescent development. In: *Development, Democracy and the Art of Trespassing: Essays in Honor of Albert O. Hirschman,* ed. A. Foxley, M. McPherson, & G. O'Donnell. Notre Dame, IN: University of Notre Dame Press.

Gitelson, M. (1948), Character synthesis: The psychotherapeutic problem of adolescence. *Amer. J. Orthopsychiatry,* 18:422–436.

Goethe, J. (1774), *The Sorrows of Young Werther,* tr. C. Hutter. New York: New American Library/Signet Classics, 1962.

Grotevant, H., & Cooper, C. (1985), Patterns of interaction in family relationships and the development of identity exploration in adolescence. *Child Develop.,* 56:415–428.

———— ———— (1986), Individuation in family relationships: A perspective on individual differences in the development of identity and role-taking skill in adolescence. *Hum. Develop.,* 29:82–100.

Group for the Advancement of Psychiatry (GAP) (1968), *Normal Adolescence: Its Dynamics and Impact. Report No. 68.* New York: Group for the Advancement of Psychiatry.

Hall, G. S. (1904), *Adolescence: Its Psychology and Its Relations to Physiology, Anthropology, Sociology, Sex, Crime, Religion and Education.* New York: D. Appleton.

Hampson, J., Hampson, J., & Money, J. (1955), The syndrome of gonadal agenesis (ovarian agenesis) and male chromosomal pattern in girls and women: Psychologic studies. *Johns Hopkins Hosp. Bull.,* 97:207–226.

———— Money, J. (1955), Idiopathic sexual precocity in the female. *Psychosomat. Med.,* 17:16–35.

Harlow, H., & Harlow, M. (1962), The effect of rearing conditions on behavior. *Bull. Menninger Clinic,* 16:213–224.

Harter, S. (1990), Self and identity development. In: *At the Threshold: The Developing Adolescent,* ed. S. Feldman & G. Elliott. Cambridge, MA: Harvard University Press, pp. 352–387.

Hartmann, H. (1939), *Ego Psychology and the Problem of Adaptation.* New York: International Universities Press, 1958.

———— (1964), *Essays on Ego Psychology: Selected Problems in Psychoanalytic Theory.* New York: International Universities Press.

Hauser, S., & Bowlds, M. (1990), Stress, coping, and adaptation. In: *At the Threshold: The Developing Adolescent,* ed. S. Feldman & G. Elliott. Cambridge, MA: Harvard University Press, pp. 388–413.

———— with Powers, S., & Noam, G. (1991), *Adolescents and Their Families: Paths of Ego Development.* New York: Free Press/Macmillan.

Hendrick, I. (1942), Instinct and ego during infancy. *Psychoanal. Quart.,* 11:33–58.

———— (1943), Work and the pleasure principle. *Psychoanal. Quart.,* 12:311–329.

Higgins, L. (1994), Mentoring moves mountains. *Stanford Med.,* 11/3:4–8.

Holder, A. (1982), Preoedipal contributions to the formation of the superego. *The Psychoanalytic Study of the Child,* 37:245–272. New Haven, CT: Yale University Press.

Huxley, A. (1932), *Brave New World.* New York: Harper & Row, 1946.

Isay, R. (1980), Late adolescence: The second separation stage of adolescence. In: *The Course of Life: Psychoanalytic Contributions Toward Understanding Personality Development,* Vol. 2, ed. S. Greenspan & G. Pollock. Washington, DC: NIMH, pp. 511–522.

Itard, J. (1802), *The Wild Boy of Aveyron,* tr. G. & M. Humphrey. New York: Appleton-Century-Crofts, 1931.

Jacobson, E. (1964), *The Self and the Object World.* New York: International Universities Press.

Jones, E. (1922), Some problems of adolescence. In: *Papers on Psychoanalysis,* 5th ed. London: Bailliére, Tindall & Cox, 1948, pp. 389–406.

Jones, M. (1965), Psychological correlates of somatic development. *Child Develop.,* 36:899–911.

Josselson, R. (1987), *Finding Herself: Pathways to Identity Development in Women.* San Francisco: Jossey-Bass.

———— (1989), Identity formation in adolescence: Implications for young adulthood. In: *Adolescent Psychiatry,* Vol. 16, ed. S. Feinstein, A. Esman, J. Looney, G. Orvin, J. Schimel, A. Schwartzberg, A. Sorosky, & M. Sugar. Chicago: University of Chicago Press, pp. 142–154.

Jung, C. (1917), Psychology of the unconscious. In: *Collected Papers on Analytic Psychology.* New York: Moffat, Yard.

Kagan, J. (1971), A conception of early adolescence. In: *12 to 16: Early Adolescence,* ed. J. Kagan & R. Coles. New York: W. W. Norton, 1972, pp. 90–105.

———— Moss, H. (1962), *Birth to Maturity: A Study in Psychological Development,* 2nd ed. New Haven, CT: Yale University Press, 1983.

Kaplan, E. (1980), Adolescents, age fifteen to eighteen: A psychoanalytic developmental view. In: *The Course of Life: Psychoanalytic Contributions Toward Understanding Personality Development*, Vol. 2, ed. S. Greenspan & G. Pollock. Washington, DC: NIMH, pp. 373–396.

——— (1989), Career change in early adulthood: Developmental considerations. In: *Adolescent Psychiatry*, Vol. 16. ed. S. Feinstein, A. Esman, J. Looney, G. Orvin, J. Schimel, A. Schwartzberg, A. Sorosky, & M. Sugar. Chicago: University of Chicago Press, pp. 259–277.

Katan, A. (1937), The role of "displacement" in agoraphobia. *Internat. J. Psycho-Anal.*, 32:41–50, 1951.

Katchadourian, H. (1990), Sexuality. In: *At the Threshold: The Developing Adolescent*, ed. S. Feldman & G. Elliott. Cambridge, MA: Harvard University Press, pp. 330–351.

Keating, D. (1980), Thinking processes in adolescence. In: *Handbook of Adolescent Psychology*, ed. J. Adelson. New York: John Wiley, pp. 211–246.

——— (1990), Adolescent thinking. In: *At the Threshold: The Developing Adolescent*, ed. S. Feldman & G. Elliott. Cambridge, MA: Harvard University Press, pp. 54–90.

Kernberg, O. (1966), Structural derivatives of object relationships. *Internat. J. Psycho-Anal.*, 47:236–253.

——— (1976), *Object Relations Theory and Clinical Psychoanalysis*. New York: Jason Aronson.

Kestenberg, J. (1961), Menarche. In: *Adolescents: Psychoanalytic Approach to Problems and Therapy*, ed. S. Lorand & H. Schneer. New York: Harper & Row, pp. 19–50.

Kiell, N. (1964), *The Universal Experience of Adolescence*. New York: International Universities Press.

Kleeman, J. (1976), Freud's view of early female sexuality in the light of direct child observation. *J. Amer. Psychoanal. Assn.*, 24(Suppl.): 3–27.

Klein, M. (1934), A contribution to the psychogenesis of manic-depressive states. In: *Contributions to Psycho-Analysis, 1921–1945*. London: Hogarth Press, 1948, pp. 282–310.

———(1975), *Envy and Gratitude and Other Works, 1946–1963*. New York: Delacorte Press/Seymour Lawrence.

Kohlberg, L., & Gilligan, C. (1971), The adolescent as a philosopher: The discovery of the self in a post-coventional world. In: *12 to 16: Early Adolescence*, ed. J. Kagan & R. Coles. New York: W. W. Norton, 1972, pp. 144–179.

Kohut, H. (1982), Introspection, empathy, and the semi-circle of mental health. *Internat. J. Psycho-Anal.*, 63:395–407.

Kramer, P. (1993), *Listening to Prozac: A Psychiatrist Explores Antidepressant Drugs and the Remaking of the Self.* New York: Viking.

Krasnow, C. (1989), Joseph Conrad's *The Shadow Line:* From late adolescence to early adulthood. In: *Adolescent Psychiatry,* Vol. 16, ed. S. Feinstein, A. Esman, J. Looney, G. Orvin, J. Schimel, A. Schwartzberg, A. Sorosky, & M. Sugar. Chicago: University of Chicago Press, pp. 202–215.

Krims, M. (1962), Psychiatric observations of children with precocious physical development. *J. Amer. Acad. Child Psychiatry,* 1:397–413.

Kutcher, S., Boulos, C., Ward, B., Marton, P, Simeon, J., Ferguson, H. B., Szalai, J., Katic, M., Roberts, N., Dubois, C., & Reed, K. (1994), Response to desipramine in adolescent depression: A fixed-dose, placebo-controlled trial. *J. Amer. Acad. Child & Adol. Psychiatry,* 33:686–694.

Langs, R. (1985), *Madness and Cure.* Emerson, NJ: Newconcept Press.

Lauer, R. (1973), *Perspectives on Social Change.* Boston: Allyn & Bacon.

Levin, A. (1948), The Oedipus myth in history and psychiatry. *Psychiatry,* 2:283–299.

Levin, R. (1966), An empirical test of the female castration complex. *J. Abnorm. Psychol.,* 71:181–188.

Levinson, D., Darrow, C., Klein, E., Levinson, M., & McKee, B. (1978), *The Seasons of a Man's Life.* New York: Alfred J. Knopf.

Lewis, S. (1969), *Experimental Induction of Castration Anxiety and Anxiety Over Loss of Love.* Unpublished doctoral dissertation. Yeshiva University, New York.

Lichtenberg, J. (1982), Continuities and transformations between infancy and adolescence. In: *Adolescent Psychiatry,* Vol. 10, ed. S. Feinstein, J. Looney, A. Schwartzburg, & A. Sorosky. Chicago: University of Chicago Press, pp. 182–198.

———— (1983), *Psychoanalysis and Infant Research.* Hillsdale, NJ: Analytic Press.

———— (1989), *Psychoanalysis and Motivation.* Hillsdale, NJ: Analytic Press.

———— Kindler, A. (1994), A motivational systems approach to the clinical experience. *J. Amer. Psychoanal. Assn.,* 42:405–420.

Lieberman, A. (1987), Separation in infancy and early childhood: Contributions of attachment theory and psychoanalysis. In: *The Psychology of Separation and Loss,* ed. J. Bloom-Feshbach, S. Bloom-Feshbach, & Associates. San Francisco: Jossey-Bass, pp. 109–135.

Looney, J., & Lewis, J. (1985), Competent adolescents from different socioeconomic and ethnic contexts. In: *Adolescent Psychiatry,* Vol. 11, ed. M. Sugar. Chicago: University of Chicago Press, pp. 64–74.

Lowery, R. (1965), *Male-Female Differences in Attitude Toward Death*. Unpublished doctoral dissertation. Brandeis University, Waltham, MA.

Mack, J. (1986), Adolescent suicide: An architectural model. In: *Suicide and Depression among Adolescents and Young Adults*, ed. G. Klerman. Washington, DC: American Psychiatric Press, pp. 53–76.

———— Hickler, H. (1981), *Vivienne: The Life and Suicide of an Adolescent Girl*. Boston: Little, Brown.

Mahler, M., Pine, F., & Bergman, A. (1975), *The Psychological Birth of the Human Infant*. New York: Basic Books.

Manosevitz, M., & Lanyon, R. (1965), Fear survey schedule: A normative study. *Psycholog. Reports*, 17:699–703.

Marasse, H., & Hart, M. (1975), The oedipal period. In: *Personality Development and Deviation*, ed. G. Wiedeman. New York: International Universities Press, pp. 110–122.

Marcia, J. (1980), Identity in adolescence. In: *Handbook of Adolescent Psychology*, ed. J. Adelson. New York: John Wiley, pp. 159–186.

Marin Independent Journal (1991), Lifestyles sect. San Rafael, CA. April 19:D14.

Markowitz, J. (1994), Psychotherapy of dysthymia. *Amer. J. Psychiatry*, 151:1114–1121.

Masterson, J. (1967), *The Psychiatric Dilemma of Adolescence*. Boston: Little, Brown.

———— (1969), A point of view on diagnosis and treatment of adolescents. *Seminars in Psychiatry*, 1:57–65.

Meltzoff, A., & Borton, W. (1979), Intermodal matching by neonates. *Nature*, 282:403–404.

Menand, L. (1994), Listening to bourbon. *New Yorker Magazine*, April 19, p. 108.

Meyer-Bahlburg, H., Ehrhardt, A., Bell, J., Cohen, S., Healey, J., Feldman, J., Morishima, A., Baker, S., & New, M. (1985), Idiopathic precocious puberty in girls: Psychosexual development. *J. Youth & Adol.*, 14:339–353.

Modell, A. (1965), On having the right to a life: An aspect of the superego's development. *Internat. J. Psycho-Anal.*, 46:323–331.

———— (1971), The origin of certain forms of pre-oedipal guilt and the implications for a psychoanalytic theory of affects. *Internat. J. Psycho-Anal.*, 52:337–346.

Modell, J., & Goodman, M. (1990), Historical perspectives. In: *At the Threshold: The Developing Adolescent*, ed. S. Feldman & G. Elliott. Cambridge, MA: Harvard University Press, pp. 93–122.

Mogul, S. (1969), Clinical assessment of adolescent development. *Seminars in Psychiatry*, 1:24–31.

—— (1980), Asceticism in adolescence and anorexia nervosa. *The Psychoanalytic Study of the Child*, 35:155–175. New Haven, CT: Yale University Press.

Moller, H. (1968), Youth as a force in the modern world. *Compar. Studies in Soc. & Hist.*, 10:237–260.

Money, J., & Hampson, J. (1955), Idiopathic sexual precocity in the male. *Psychosom. Med.*, 17:1–15.

—— Walker, P. (1971), Psychosexual development, maternalism, nonpromiscuity, and body image in 15 females with precocious puberty. *Arch. Sex. Behav.*, 1:45–60.

Muensterberger, W. (1961), The adolescent in society. In: *Adolescents: Psychoanalytic Approach to Problems and Therapy*, ed. S. Lorand & H. Schneer. New York: Harper & Row, pp. 346–368.

Mufson, L., Moreau, D., Weissman, M., Wickramaratne, P., Martin, J., & Samoilov, A. (1994), Modification of interpersonal psychotherapy with depressed adolescents (IPT-A): Phase I and II studies. *J. Amer. Acad. Child & Adolesc. Psychiat.*, 33:695–705.

Murphy, S. (1994), Quoted in "Is your child a star?" by Karen S. Peterson. Gannett News Service. *Marin Independent J.*, February 17: D1.

Niederland, W. (1981), The survivor syndrome: Further observations and dimensions. *J. Amer. Psychoanal. Assn.*, 29:413–425.

Noshpitz, J. (1991), Disturbances in early adolescent development. In: *The Course of Life: Psychoanalytic Contributions Toward Understanding Personality Development*, Vol. 4, ed. S. Greenspan & G. Pollock. Madison, CT: International Universities Press, pp. 119–180.

Offer, D. (1969), *The Psychological World of the Teenager: A Study of Normal Adolescent Boys*. New York: Basic Books.

—— Offer, J. (1975), *From Teenage to Young Manhood: A Psychological Study*. New York: Basic Books.

—— Schonert-Reichl, K. (1992), Debunking the myths of adolescence: Findings from recent research. *J. Amer. Acad. Child & Adol. Psychiat.*, 31:1003–1014.

Ogden, T. (1983), The concept of internal object relations. *Internat. J. Psycho-Anal.*, 64:227–241.

Oldham, D. (1978), Adolescent turmoil: A myth revisited. In: *Adolescent Psychiatry*, Vol. 6, ed. S. Feinstein & P. Giovacchini. Chicago: University of Chicago Press, pp. 267–279.

Osofsky, J., Ed. (1987), *Handbook of Infant Development*, 2nd ed. New York: John Wiley.

Panel (1980), Conceptualizing the nature of the therapeutic action of child analysis. L. Sabot, reporter. *J. Amer. Psychoanal. Assn.*, 28:161–179.

———— (1987), Psychoanalysis of the young adult: Theory and technique. J. Chused, reporter. *J. Amer. Psychoanal. Assn.*, 35:175–187.

Parens, H. (1986), Review of *Adolescence and Developmental Breakdown: A Psychoanalytic View*, by M. & M. E. Laufer. *Internat. J. Psycho-Anal.*, 67:522–525.

———— Pollock, L., Stern, J., & Kramer, S. (1976), On the girl's entry into the Oedipus complex. *J. Amer. Psychoanal. Assn.*, 24(Suppl.): 79–107.

Perun, P., & Erkut, S. (1986), Well-being in adolescence: Past and present. In: *Suicide and Depression among Adolescents and Young Adults*, ed. G. Klerman. Washington, DC: American Psychiatric Press, pp. 255–276.

Peskin, H. (1972), Multiple prediction of adult psychological health from preadolescent and adolescent behaviors. *J. Consult. & Clin. Psychology*, 38:155–160.

———— (1973), Influence of the developmental schedule of puberty on learning and ego functioning. *J. Youth & Adol.*, 2:273–290.

Plato, *The Dialogues of Plato*. New York: Bantam Books, 1986.

Popper, C. (1990), Introduction: Therapeutic empiricism and therapeutic basics. *J. Child & Adol. Psychopharmacol.*, 1:3–5.

Provence, S., & Lipton, R. (1962), *Infants in Institutions*. New York: International Universities Press.

Roper Starch, Worldwide (1994), *Teens Talk About Sex: Adolescent Sexuality in the 90's. A Survey of High School Students*. New York: SIECUS Publications.

Rosenbaum, M-B. (1979), The changing body image of the adolescent girl. In: *Female Adolescent Development*, ed. M. Sugar. New York: Brunner/Mazel, pp. 234–252.

Saint Augustine (397–398), *Confessions*, tr. R. Pine-Coffin. New York: Penguin Books, 1961.

Salinger, J. (1945), *The Catcher in the Rye*. New York: New American Library/Signet Books, 1953.

Sandler, J., & Rosenblatt, B. (1962), The concept of the representational world. *The Psychoanalytic Study of the Child*, 17:128–145. New York: International Universities Press.

Sarnoff, C. (1976), *On Latency*. New York: Jason Aronson.

Sarnoff, I., & Corwin, S. (1959), Castration anxiety and the fear of death. *J. Personal.*, 27:374–385.

Scheffler, R. (1971), *From Five to Six: A Longitudinal Study of Psychodynamic Change*. Unpublished doctoral dissertation. Harvard University, Cambridge, MA.

Schill, T. (1966), Sex differences in identification of the castrating agent on the Blacky test. *J. Clin. Psychol.*, 22:324–325.

Schweitzer, A. (1949), *Memoirs of Childhood and Youth*. New York: Macmillan.

Seidman, S., & Rieder, R. (1994), A review of sexual behavior in the United States. *Amer. J. Psychiatry*, 151:330–341.

Selvini, M. (1974), *Self-Starvation: From the Intrapsychic to the Transpersonal Approach to Anorexia Nervosa*. London: Chaucer.

Settlage, C. (1974a), Danger signals in the separation–individuation process: The observations and formulations of Margaret S. Mahler. In: *The Infant at Risk*, ed. B. Bergsma, R. Gross, C. Settlage, & A. Solnit. New York: Intercontinental Books, pp. 63–75.

—— (1974b), The technique of defense analysis in the psychoanalysis of an early adolescent. In: *The Analyst and the Adolescent at Work*, ed. M. Harley. Chicago: Quadrangle, pp. 3–39.

Shapiro, T., & Perry, R. (1976), Latency revisited: The age 7 plus or minus 1. *The Psychoanalytic Study of the Child*, 31:79–105. New Haven, CT: Yale University Press.

Sklansky, M., & Rabichow, H. (1980), *Effective Counseling of Adolescents*. Chicago: Association Press/Follett.

Solyom, A., Austad, C., Sherick, I., & Bacon, G. (1980), Precocious sexual development in girls: The emotional impact on the child and her parents. *J. Pediatric Psychol.*, 5:385–393.

Sonis, W., Comite, F., Pescovitz, O., Hench, K., Rahn, C., Cutler, G., Loriaux, D., & Klein, R. (1986), Biobehavioral aspects of precocious puberty. *J. Amer. Acad. Child Psychiatry*, 25:674–679.

Spiegel, L. (1951), Review of contributions to a psychoanalytic theory of adolescence. *The Psychoanalytic Study of the Child*, 6:375–393. New York: International Universities Press.

Staples, H., & Smarr, E. (1980), Bridge to adulthood: Years from eighteen to twenty-three. In: *The Course of Life: Psychoanalytic Contributions Toward Understanding Personality Development*, Vol. 2, ed. S. Greenspan & G. Pollock. Washington, DC: NIMH, pp. 477–496.

Steinberg, L. (1990), Autonomy, conflict, and harmony in the family relationship. In: *At the Threshold: The Developing Adolescent*, ed. S. Feldman & G. Elliott. Cambridge, MA: Harvard University Press, pp. 255–276.

Stern, D. (1985), *The Interpersonal World of the Infant*. New York: Basic Books.

Stewart, W. (1976), *The Formation of the Early Adult Life Structure in Women*. Unpublished doctoral dissertation in clinical psychology. Teachers College, Columbia University, New York.

Stoller, R. (1976), Primary femininity. *J. Amer. Psychoanal. Assn.*, 24(Suppl.):59–78.

Strachey, J. (1955), Editor's introduction. In: Studies on Hysteria, by J. Breuer & S. Freud. *Standard Edition*, 2. London: Hogarth Press, 1955.

——— (1961), Editor's introduction. In: S. Freud (1930), Civilization and its discontents. *Standard Edition*, 21. London: Hogarth Press, 1961.

Sutherland, J. (1980), The British object relations theorists: Balint, Winnicott, Fairbairn, Guntrip. *J. Amer. Psychoanal. Assn.*, 28:829–860.

Tanner, J. (1971), Sequence, tempo, and individual variation in growth and development of boys and girls aged twelve to sixteen. In: *12 to 16: Early Adolescence*, ed. J. Kagan & R. Coles. New York: W. W. Norton, 1972, pp. 1–24.

——— (1975), Growth and endocrinology of the adolescent. In: *Endocrine and Genetic Diseases of Childhood and Adolescence*, 2nd ed., ed. L. Gardner. Philadelphia: W. B. Saunders, pp. 14–64.

Target, M., & Fonagy, P. (1994), Efficacy of psychoanalysis for children with emotional disorders. *J. Amer. Acad. Child & Adol. Psychiatry*, 33:361–371.

Thomas, R., with Folkart, L., & Model, E. (1963), The search for a sexual identity in a case of constitutional sexual precocity. *The Psychoanalytic Study of the Child*, 18:636–662. New York: International Universities Press.

Torney-Purta, J. (1990), Youth in relation to social institutions. In: *At the Threshold: The Developing Adolescent*, ed. S. Feldman & G. Elliott. Cambridge, MA: Harvard University Press, pp. 457–477.

Vaillant, G. (1977), *Adaptation to Life*. Boston: Little, Brown.

——— (1987), A developmental view of old and new perspectives of personality disorders. *J. Personality Disorders*, 1:146–156. New York: Guilford Press.

Volkmar, F. (1994), Review of *At the Threshold: The Developing Adolescent*, ed. S. Feldman & G. Elliott. *Amer. J. Psychiatry*, 151:445–446.

Waller, J., Kaufman, M., & Deutsch, F. (1940), Anorexia nervosa: A psychosomatic entity. *Psychosom. Med.*, 2:3–16.

Weiss, J., Sampson, H., & the Mount Zion Psychotherapy Research Group (1986), *The Psychoanalytic Process: Theory, Clinical Observation and Empirical Research*. New York: Guilford Press.

Weissman, S., Cohen, R., Boxer, A., & Cohler, B. (1989), Parenthood experience and the adolescent's transition to young adulthood: Self psychological perspectives. In: *Adolescent Psychiatry*, Vol. 16, ed. S. Feinstein, A. Esman, J. Looney, G. Orvin, J. Schimel, A. Schwartzberg, A. Sorosky, & M. Sugar. Chicago: University of Chicago Press, pp. 155–174.

Werkman, S. (1966), Identity and the creative surge in adolescence. In: *Science and Psychoanalysis*, Vol. 9, ed. J. Masserman. New York: Grune & Stratton, pp. 48–57.

West, A. (1994), When the disease doesn't read the textbook: Focus and timing in the career of Julianne Imperato-McGinley. *Cornell University Medical College Alumni Magazine*, November: 2–6.

Wilson, D. (1994), The not-so-opposite sexes (based on an interview with psychology professor Elizabeth J. Aries). *Amherst*, 46:20–22.

Winnicott, D. W. (1958), *Through Paediatrics to Psychoanalysis*. New York: Basic Books, 1975.

————— (1965), *The Maturational Processes and the Facilitating Environment*. New York: International Universities Press.

Wolf, E., Gedo, J., & Terman, D. (1972), On the adolescent process as a transformation of the self. *J. Youth & Adol.*, 1:257–273.

Wolff, P. (1966), The Causes, Controls, and Organization of Behaviors in the Neonate. *Psychological Issues*, Monograph 17. New York: International Universities Press.

Name Index

Subject Index

403